The Foot and Ankle

AANA Advanced Arthroscopic Surgical Techniques

AANA Advanced Arthroscopic Surgical Techniques
Series

Series Editors, Richard K. N. Ryu, MD and Jeffrey S. Abrams, MD

The Foot and Ankle

AANA Advanced Arthroscopic Surgical Techniques

EDITED BY

JAMES W. STONE, MD
Midwest Orthopedic Specialty Hospital
Franklin, Wisconsin

JOHN G. KENNEDY, MD, MCH, FRCS
Hospital for Special Surgery
New York, New York

MARK GLAZEBROOK, MD
Queen Elizabeth II Health Sciences Center
Halifax, Nova Scotia

CRC Press
Taylor & Francis Group
Boca Raton London New York

CRC Press is an imprint of the
Taylor & Francis Group, an **informa** business

First published 2016 by SLACK Incorporated

Published 2024 by CRC Press
2385 NW Executive Center Drive, Suite 320, Boca Raton FL 33431

and by CRC Press
4 Park Square, Milton Park, Abingdon, Oxon, OX14 4RN

CRC Press is an imprint of Taylor & Francis Group, LLC

Library of Congress Cataloging-in-Publication Data

AANA advanced arthroscopic surgical techniques. The foot and ankle / edited by James W. Stone, John G. Kennedy, Mark Glazebrook.

p. ; cm.
Advanced arthroscopic surgical techniques
Foot and ankle
Preceded by AANA advanced arthroscopy. The foot and ankle / [edited by] Annunziato Amendola, James W. Stone. Philadelphia : Saunders/Elsevier, c2010.
Includes bibliographical references and index.
ISBN 9781617119989 (alk. paper)
X. Stone, James W., editor. II. Kennedy, John G. (Orthopaedic surgeon), editor. III. Glazebrook, Mark, editor. IV. Arthroscopy Association of North America. V. AANA advanced arthroscopy. The foot and ankle. Preceded by (work): VI. Title: Advanced arthroscopic surgical techniques. VII. Title: Foot and ankle.
[DNLM: 1. Ankle Joint--surgery. 2. Foot--surgery. 3. Arthroscopy--methods. WE 880]
RD563
617.5'85059--dc23

2015036224

ISBN: 9781617119989 (hbk)
ISBN: 9781003524205 (ebk)

DOI: 10.1201/9781003524205

DEDICATION

To my wife, Joan, and children, Jonathan and Melissa, for allowing me the time to work on projects such as these, but most importantly, for your unconditional love and support.

James W. Stone, MD

This book is dedicated to my mother, Marquerite Kennedy, who has recently passed, and to my father, who is fighting on. Both members of the "greatest generation," they taught me the value of hard work and dedication and the importance of a spirit of team collaboration. They taught me to give up is not an option and to value friends who are there in times of need. To this end, they would be proud of our team's achievement in completing this excellent book.

John G. Kennedy, MD, MCh FRCS

I dedicate my work spent on this text book to my wife, Kathie, and our children, Haley, Jonah, and Zachary, whom I have robbed precious family time from to complete the project. I also dedicate this to my mom, Dianne Glazebrook, and deceased father, "Mick" Glazebrook, whom I am sure never thought the "Son of a Taxi driver" could edit a textbook while being an MD, Orthopedic surgeon, and PhD researcher.

Mark Glazebrook, MD

Contents

Acknowledgments

As our understanding of the problems of the foot and ankle improves and our ability to treat many of these conditions with minimally invasive arthroscopic surgery increases, it is appropriate to look back and acknowledge the contributions of the surgical pioneers who have made these advances possible. Dr. Richard Ferkel in the United States and Dr. Niek van Dijk in the Netherlands have been two giants in the field. Without their research, hard work, and innovation, very few of the procedures we describe in this book would be possible. We are privileged to have both of these physicians contribute chapters to this book.

To all of the contributors to this book, we acknowledge the time taken away from your families and your personal life in order to produce this excellent educational volume. We would like to acknowledge not just the contribution of the authors, but also that of their families, who willingly sacrifice this time with their fathers, mothers, sons, and daughters, so that this book could be produced to the highest possible standard. Our gratitude and appreciation are also extended to our patients who have placed their trust and faith in us to perform these pioneering procedures.

We take this opportunity to thank Drs. Richard Ryu and Jeffrey Abrams for placing their faith in us to complete this project and to the team at SLACK Incorporated, including especially Carrie Kotlar and Dani Malady, for their professional assistance and persistence in pushing this project to completion.

James W. Stone, MD
John G. Kennedy, MD, MCh, FRCS
Mark Glazebrook, MD

About the Editors

James W. Stone, MD received his BA degree from Williams College in Williamstown, MA and his MD degree from Harvard Medical School in Boston, MA. He completed his Orthopedic Surgery residency at Barnes Hospital, Washington University in St. Louis, MO, followed by a sports medicine fellowship at Massachusetts General Hospital in Boston. He is in private practice orthopedic surgery in Milwaukee, WI, specializing in orthopedic sports medicine with a special interest in ankle arthroscopy. He is an Assistant Clinical Professor of Orthopedic Surgery at the Medical College of Wisconsin in Milwaukee. He currently serves on the Board of Directors of the Arthroscopy Association of North America (AANA) and has served on numerous committees of that association. He regularly instructs at arthroscopy and sports medicine courses both in the United States and internationally on current techniques in ankle arthroscopy and has published extensively in peer-reviewed journals, book chapters, and as an editor of ankle arthroscopy texts.

John G. Kennedy, MD, MCh, FRCS is an ankle surgeon working primarily in sports injuries at Hospital for Special Surgery in New York City, NY.

Dr. Kennedy graduated from the Royal College of Surgeons in Dublin in 1989 and has since trained both in Ireland and in the United States. Having access to both European and American training has provided a unique opportunity to blend the best aspects of both systems. Pragmatic solutions combined with innovative surgery have therefore been the hallmark of Dr. Kennedy's practice. Arthroscopy of the joint and tendon are a backbone of Dr. Kennedy's practice, and the indications and practical therapies using the arthroscope are constantly evolving. To date, he has authored over 140 peer-reviewed publication, in addition to multiple book chapters and books on this area of expertise.

Dr. Kennedy is a Master Instructor at the Arthroscopy Association of North America (AANA) foot and ankle arthroscopy course, where he feels that he learns as much as he teaches from participants who attend from all over the world. This commitment to global teaching is further emphasized by the presence of several international orthopedic surgeons and researchers who train with Dr. Kennedy each year at his practice in New York City. This book from AANA on techniques in arthroscopy of the foot and ankle provides an excellent account for both basic and advanced arthroscopists to learn and further develop their skill set. It provides a comprehensive account of the most up-to-date concepts and procedures written by the foremost surgeons in the world.

Mark Glazebrook, MD is a full time Associate Professor of Orthopaedic Surgery at Dalhousie University in Nova Scotia, Canada with a cross appointment to the School of Biomedical Engineering. He completed his medical training in 1994 and completed specialty training in Orthopaedic Surgery in 1999 at Dalhousie. He then went on to complete a fellowship in Orthopedic Foot & Ankle and Sports Medicine at the University of Western Ontario. This was followed with a PhD in Achilles Tendon Disease at Dalhousie University while working part time in his clinical practice. Dr. Glazebrook devotes 80% of his working time to clinical practice focusing on Orthopedic Foot & Ankle Reconstruction and Sports Medicine. During research time, focus is on outcome studies on Evidence-Based Medicine, Ankle Arthritis, MTP Arthritis, Bone Graft Substitutes, and Achilles tendon rupture care.

Dr. Glazebrook has authored 51 peer reviewed paper publications, 12 textbook chapters, and 77 published abstracts. He has completed 167 invited guest speaker engagements, including international sites in Columbia, UK, Australia, Lebanon, Africa, and USA. Dr. Glazebrook was an American Foot &Ankle Society (AOFAS) Travelling Fellow in 2006 and an American

British Canadian (ABC) Travelling Fellow in 2009. He has 24 committee appointments (9 local, 15 national, and 8 international).

Dr. Glazebrook has been Chairman of the American Orthopedic Society Foot and Ankle Society (AOFAS) Annual Summer Precourse Meeting "Innovations in Orthopedic Foot and Ankle Surgery" in Washington, DC; Co-Chairman of the Arthroscopy Association of North America (AANA) Annual Fall Foot and Ankle Curriculum in Phoenix, AZ; and Master Instructor Faculty Member of the Combined AANA/AOFAS Annual Masters Foot and Ankle Course in Chicago, IL. He is also an invited faculty of American Academy of Orthopedic Surgeons (AAOS) 16 ICLs and 5 symposia as well as a North American Foot and Ankle Federation Representative to the International Federation of Foot & Ankle Societies (IFFAS).

Contributing Authors

Jorge I. Acevedo, MD (Chapter 10)
Co-director, Foot and Ankle Center
Southeast Orthopedic Specialist
Jacksonville, Florida

Francesco Allegra, MD (Chapter 7)
University Orthopedic Department
Università La Sapienza
Polo Pontino, ICOT Latina
Italy

Annunziato Amendola, MD (Chapter 14)
Professor and Vice Chair
Chief, Division of Sports Medicine
Department of Orthopedic Surgery
Duke University
Durham, North Carolina

William Bugbee, MD (Chapter 8)
Attending Physician
Joint Reconstruction
Director of Cartilage Transplantation Program
Division of Orthopaedic Surgery
Scripps Clinic
La Jolla, California

James D. F. Calder, MD, FRCS(Tr & Orth), FFSEM(UK) (Chapter 19)
Consultant Orthopaedic Surgeon
Fortius Clinic
London, England

Woojin Choi, MD, PhD (Chapter 3)
Clinical Associate Professor
Foot & Ankle Service/Diabetic Foot Clinic
Department of Orthopaedic Surgery
Yonsei University College of Medicine
Seoul, Korea

Mark E. Easley, MD (Chapter 13)
Associate Professor
Co-director, Foot and Ankle Fellowship Program
Department of Orthopaedic Surgery
Duke University Medical Center
Durham, North Carolina

Richard D. Ferkel, MD (Chapter 4)
Sports Medicine Fellowship Director
Southern California Orthopedic Institute
Van Nuys, California
Assistant Clinical Professor of Orthopedic Surgery
UCLA Center for the Health Sciences
Los Angeles, California

Ethan J. Fraser, MD, MBBS (Chapters 6, 20, 21, 22)
Research Fellow
Office of Dr JG Kennedy
Foot and Ankle Service
Hospital for Special Surgery
New York, New York

Richard Freeman, MBBS, FRCS(Tr & Ortho) (Chapter 19)
Fortius Clinic
London, England

Arianna L. Gianakos, BS (Chapter 6)
Research Fellow
Office of Dr JG Kennedy
Foot and Ankle Service
Hospital for Special Surgery
New York, New York

Alberto Gobbi, MD (Chapter 5)
Orthopaedic Arthroscopic Surgery International (OASI) Bioresearch Foundation, Gobbi Onlus
Milan, Italy

Christopher E. Gross, MD (Chapter 13)
Medical University of South Carolina
Department of Orthopaedics
Charleston, South Carolina

Stephane Guillo, MD (Chapter 11)
Orthopaedic Surgeon
Assistant Professor
Sport's clinic of Bordeaux Mérignac
Aquitaine, France

Beat Hintermann, MD (Chapter 12)
Associate Professor
University of Basel
Chairman
Clinic of Orthopaedic Surgery and Traumatology
Kantonsspital Baselland
Liestal, Switzerland

Georgios Karnatzikos, MD (Chapter 5)
Orthopaedic Arthroscopic Surgery International (OASI) Bioresearch Foundation, Gobbi Onlus
Milan, Italy

Dnyanesh Lad, MD (Chapter 5)
Orthopaedic Arthroscopic Surgery International (OASI) Bioresearch Foundation, Gobbi Onlus
Milan, Italy

Peter Mangone, MD (Chapter 10)
Co-director, Foot and Ankle Center
Blue Ridge Bone and Joint Clinic
Volunteer Clinical Attending
MAHEC Family Practice Residency Program
Volunteer Clinical Attending
MAHEC Family Practice Sports Medicine Fellowship
Asheville, North Carolina

Alberto Marangon, MD (Chapter 22)
Clinic San Francesco
Verona, Italy

Adam F. Meisel, MD (Chapter 4)
MidAmerica Orthopaedics
Palos Hills, Illinois

Gokhan Meric, MD (Chapter 8)
SCORE Research Institute
La Jolla, San Diego, California

Xavier Martin Oliva, PhD (Chapter 16)
Foot and Ankle Unit
Remei Hospital
Professor, Anatomy Department
Barcelona University
Barcelona, Spain

Jason A. Patterson, MD (Chapter 14)
OrthoArizona, Mezona Division
Gilbert, Arizona

Phinit Phisitkul, MD (Chapter 18)
Clinical Associate Professor
Department of Orthopaedics and Rehabilitation
University of Iowa Hospital and Clinics
Iowa City, Iowa

Steven M. Raikin, MD (Chapter 9)
Director, Foot and Ankle Service
Rothman Institute
Professor of Orthopaedic Surgery
Jefferson Medical College
Director, Foot and Ankle Fellowship Program
Thomas Jefferson University Hospital
Philadelphia, Pennsylvania

Andrew W. Ross, BA (Chapter 21)
Research Fellow
Office of Dr JG Kennedy
Foot and Ankle Service
Hospital for Special Surgery
New York, New York

Chamnanni Rungprai, MD (Chapter 18)
Orthopaedic Foot and Ankle Fellow
Department of Orthopaedics and Rehabilitation
University of Iowa Hospital and Clinics
Iowa City, Iowa
Orthopaedic Foot and Ankle Surgeon
Department of Orthopaedics
Phramongkutklao Hospital and College of Medicine
Bangkok, Thailand

Masato Takao, MD, PhD (Chapters 9, 11)
Professor
Department of Orthopaedic Surgery
Department of Sport & Medical Science
Teikyo Institute of Sports Science & Medicine
Chief in Foot & Ankle Unit
Teikyo University School of Medicine
Tokyo, Japan

C. Niek van Dijk, MD, PhD (Chapters 1, 17)
Orthopaedic Research Centre Amsterdam
Department of Orthopaedic Surgery
Academic Medical Center
University of Amsterdam
Amsterdam, the Netherlands

Jin Woo Lee, MD, PhD (Chapter 3)
Professor
Director of Foot & Ankle Clinic
Department of Orthopaedic Surgery
Yonsei University College of Medicine
Seoul, Korea

Youichi Yasui, MD (Chapters 6, 20, 22)
Foot and Ankle Service
Hospital for Special Surgery
New York, New York
Department of Orthopedics
Teikyo University Hospital
Tokyo, Japan

Alastair Younger, MB, ChB, ChM, MSc, FRCSC (Chapters 23, 24)
Professor
Department of Orthopaedics
University of British Columbia
Vancouver, British Columbia, Canada

Ruben Zwiers, MSc, PhD-candidate (Chapters 1, 17)
Orthopaedic Research Centre Amsterdam
Department of Orthopaedic Surgery
Academic Medical Center
University of Amsterdam
Amsterdam, the Netherlands

Foreword

Since its introduction, the field of arthroscopic surgery has changed dramatically. This is especially true in the foot and ankle. Today, the arthroscope is used extensively for numerous foot and ankle conditions. This monograph, entitled *The Foot and Ankle: AANA Advanced Arthroscopic Surgical Techniques*, reflects the innovative ways the field has evolved. Since its previous edition in 2010, many newer techniques have been introduced.

The book's editors, Drs. Stone, Kennedy, and Glazebrook, have done a wonderful job in selecting the world's experts to explain these new advanced methods of treatment. Each chapter is beautifully organized similarly from Introduction, Indications, Pertinent Physical Findings, Imaging, Equipment, Positioning and Portals, Step-by-Step Description of the Procedure, Postoperative Protocol, Potential Complications, and Top Technical Pearls.

Each section of the book deals with the problems most commonly seen by the foot and ankle arthroscopist. There are 9 chapters detailing different methods to address osteochondral lesions of the talus and tibia, giving readers numerous options to treat their patients with the latest innovations. Moreover, the second section on ankle stabilizations shows the latest methods to stabilize the medial and lateral sides of the ankle via the arthroscope or through arthroscopically assisted stabilization. Arthroscopic ankle ligament stabilization is expanding rapidly and is beautifully described here.

Subtalar and great toe arthroscopy have also become more popular, done supine or prone, and are described clearly here. Prone arthroscopy is one of the most significant newer techniques for the foot and ankle and its use with tendoscopy. Achilles disorders and posterior impingement teach the reader the fine points of each indication. In addition, the chapters on arthroscopic treatment of foot and ankle fractures show its utility and tricks to fix these injuries.

Overall, this text presents critical new information in each chapter that will teach the reader how to perform state-of-the-art arthroscopic techniques that are needed to treat today's patients. In 2016, we must continue to "push the envelope" and expand the indications for arthroscopic treatment of all foot and ankle problems. Thirty years ago, we only dreamed of the techniques described in this book, but today they are a reality and excellently detailed in each chapter. Every foot and ankle arthroscopist should study this book and its wonderful videos carefully and learn all of the pearls to give our patients the absolute best surgical care.

Each book in the AANA series in an important cornerstone in building our arthroscopic foundation, and this book solidifies the foot and ankle portion of this field.

Richard D. Ferkel, MD
Sports Medicine Fellowship Director
Southern California Orthopedic Institute
Van Nuys, California
Assistant Clinical Professor of Orthopedic Surgery
UCLA Center for the Health Sciences
Los Angeles, California

Introduction

The *AANA Advanced Arthroscopic Surgical Techniques Series* represents the very best that AANA has to offer the practicing orthopedic surgeon. With premier arthroscopic surgeons taking the lead, each book in the series presents the latest diagnostic, therapeutic, and reconstructive techniques available in arthroscopic surgery today.

Each technique-based chapter is consistently organized with a user-friendly interface allowing for a quick reference or for prolonged study. Bulleted lists of easily accessed, high-yield information, including preoperative planning, patient selection, equipment checklists, step-by-step descriptions of procedures, and essential technical pearls, in addition to indications, contraindications, postoperative protocols, and potential complications, make this an invaluable resource for surgeons who want to improve not only their skill level, but also their mastery of the fundamentals that define arthroscopic surgery. Well-edited videos, accompanied by narration, further serve to support the materials systematically outlined in each chapter for each volume.

Education and innovation continue to be the top priority for AANA and its leadership. As such, all proceeds from this Series will be donated to the AANA Education Foundation, which, among other endeavors, helps support resident education at the Orthopedic Learning Center, The Traveling Fellowship, the Society of Military Orthopedic Surgeons (SOMOS)–AANA collaboration, resident scholarships to the Annual Meeting, as well as numerous research grants and awards. With the purchase of this textbook series, AANA will also provide free electronic access to the text and videos from the same book in their initial series, *AANA Advanced Arthroscopy* (2010).

We believe that this 5-volume series is a "must have" resource for those who rely on their arthroscopic skills and knowledge to improve patient outcomes. Concise, current, and cogent help describe the impact that these textbooks will have on your practice and in your clinical successes. AANA is delighted to have again taken on this critical leadership position in surgeon education, and is proud of the quality and immediacy of these 5 outstanding volumes.

Richard K. N. Ryu, MD
Jeffrey S. Abrams, MD
Series Co-Editors

1

Posterior Ankle Impingement
Two-Portal Hindfoot Endoscopy

Ruben Zwiers, MSc, PhD-candidate and C. Niek van Dijk, MD, PhD

Introduction

In general, patients with posterior ankle impingement problems are treated conservatively first. Conservative interventions include rest, nonsteroidal anti-inflammatory drugs, physical therapy modalities, or intra-articular cortisone injections. When conservative treatment fails, endoscopic surgery is indicated in these patients. Good functional and clinical outcomes have been described after endoscopic excision of an os trigonum, hypertrophic posterior talar process, posterior tibial or talar osteophytes, and soft tissue overgrowth.[1-6] In cases where athletic patients require a prompt return to athletic play, surgery is often recommended initially or very early in the treatment process without a significant time period spent attempting conservative therapy. If complaints of posterior ankle impingement cause a substantial decrease in functioning and imaging reveals a bony cause, surgical resection is indicated.[7]

Indications

- Bony soft tissue impingement including os trigonum or symptomatic hypertrophic posterior talar process, posterior tibial osteophytes, and posterior talar osteophytes
- Posterior soft tissue impingement
- Chronic flexor hallucis longus (FHL) tenosynovitis

Pertinent Physical Findings

- Tenderness to palpation on the posterior aspect of the talus with bony or soft tissue impingement ankle and subtalar joint

Stone JW, Kennedy JG, Glazebrook M, eds. *The Foot and Ankle: AANA Advanced Arthroscopic Surgical Techniques* (pp 1-6).

- Tenderness to palpation over the FHL with increased discomfort and possible crepitus with flexion and extension of the great toe in cases of FHL tenosynovitis
- Posterior impingement sign: Patients suffering from posterior ankle impingement usually present with posterior ankle pain on (hyper-)plantarflexion of the ankle. The diagnosis can be made by means of physical examination using a hyperplantarflexion test. The hyperplantarflexion test is determined to be positive when the patient experiences recognizable pain on sudden passive hyperplantarflexion of the ankle. A negative test rules out posterior ankle impingement syndrome. After a positive test is elicited, a diagnostic infiltration with a local anesthetic can be given in order to confirm the diagnosis.

Pertinent Imaging

- Plain radiographs: After a clinical diagnosis is made, imaging should be utilized to determine the absence or presence of bony pathology. To differentiate between a hypertrophied posterolateral talar process and os trigonum, the posterior impingement view—a lateral radiograph with the foot in 25 degrees of external rotation in relation to the standard lateral radiograph—is recommended.[8] This provides a more comprehensive view of the posterior talus.
- Computed tomography: In cases where standard radiographs are not definitive or further information is required, additional imaging techniques can be obtained. Especially following trauma, a computed tomography scan can help to ascertain the extent of injury and exact location of calcifications or bony fragments.
- Magnetic resonance imaging (MRI): MRI is useful for evaluating soft tissue pathology. MRI may demonstrate capsular or ligament thickening. FHL pathology can also be evaluated. In addition, MRI shows the presence of bone marrow edema, a fracture line, or fluid in the synchondrosis.

Equipment

For irrigation, a saline bag with gravity flow is used. A 4.0-mm, 30-degree arthroscope is routinely used for posterior ankle arthroscopy. A good alternative is a 2.7-mm arthroscope of 11 cm in length in combination with a 4.6-mm, high-volume arthroscope sheath. Apart from the standard excisional and motorized instruments for the treatment of osteophytes and ossicle, a 4-mm osteotome and small periosteal elevator can be useful.[9]

Positioning and Portals

The procedure is carried out as outpatient surgery under general or spinal anesthesia. The patient is placed in the prone position. The involved leg is marked with an arrow to avoid performing surgery on the wrong side. A tourniquet is inflated around the thigh for hemostasis. A small support is placed under the lower leg, making it possible to move the ankle freely (Figure 1-1).[10]

Step-by-Step Description of the Procedure

Important anatomical landmarks for this procedure are the lateral malleolus, the Achilles tendon, and the sole of the foot. With the ankle in the neutral position, a line is drawn from the tip

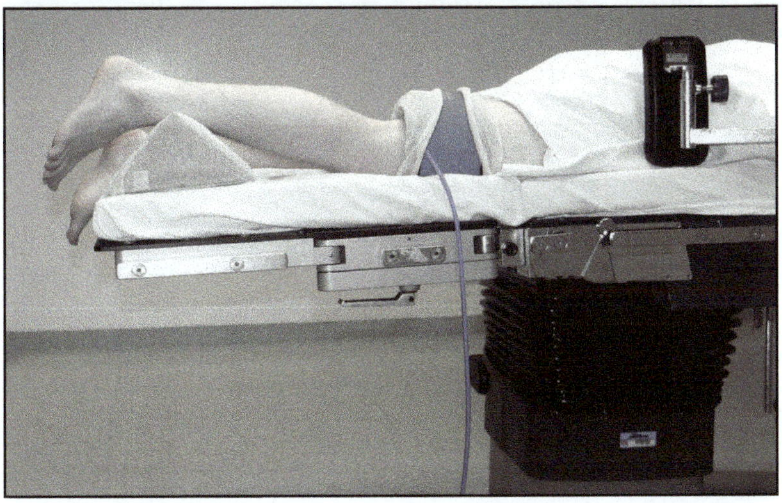

Figure 1-1. The patient is placed in the prone position for posterior hindfoot endoscopy.

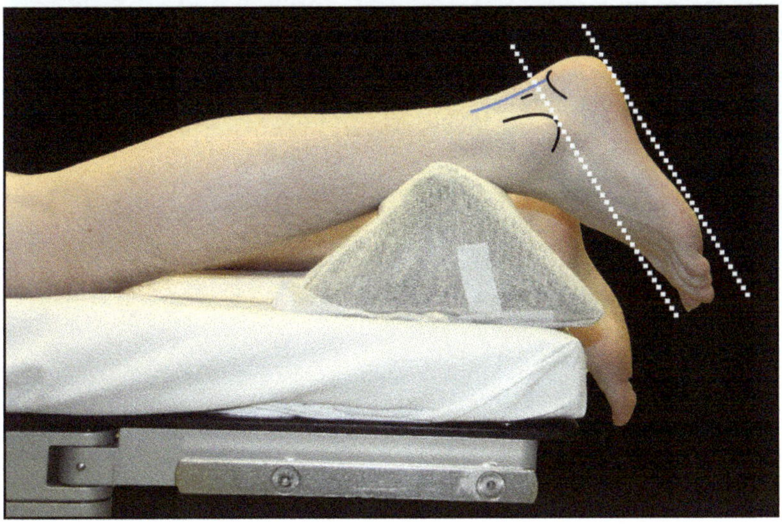

Figure 1-2. With the ankle in the neutral position, a line is drawn from the tip of the lateral malleolus to the Achilles tendon, parallel to the sole of the foot. The posterolateral portal is positioned just above this line and anterior to the border of the Achilles tendon.

of the lateral malleolus to the Achilles tendon, parallel to the sole of the foot. The posterolateral portal is positioned above this line and anterior to the border of the Achilles tendon (Figure 1-2). A stab incision is made and followed by blunt dissection of the subcutaneous layers using a mosquito clamp. Then, a 4.6-mm arthroscope shaft with a blunt trocar is introduced in the direction of the first interdigital web space. At this point, the arthroscope is exchanged for the trocar. It is likely that the surgeon will have poor visualization initially due to the fatty tissue overlying the joint capsule prior to resection.

At this point, the posteromedial portal is created at the same level just medial to the Achilles tendon. After a stab incision is made, the subcutaneous layer is bluntly dissected. A mosquito forceps is introduced and directed toward the arthroscope shaft in a 90-degree angle. The shaft of the laterally placed arthroscope is then used to guide the mosquito clamp anteriorly to the bone. The tip of the mosquito then comes to view and is used to spread the extra-articular soft tissue in front of the tip of the arthroscope. Once the mosquito clamp is visualized, a 5.5-mm resector is introduced in exchange for the clamp. To introduce the shaver, the scope is brought back to the starting position, and again the scope is used as a guide. When the tip of the shaver comes into view, the shaver is directed in a lateral and slightly plantar direction. With a few turns of

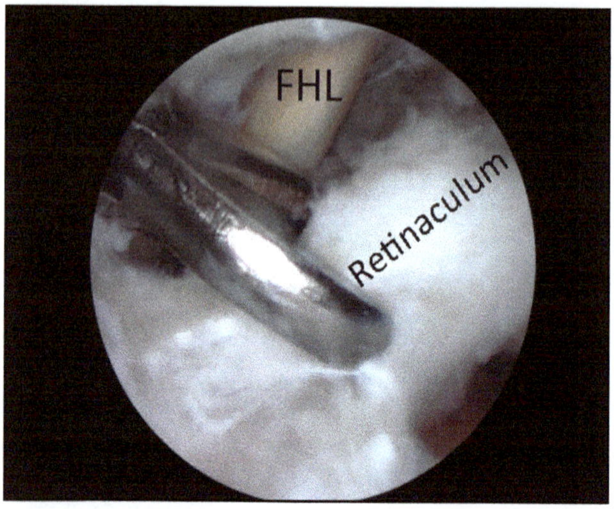

Figure 1-3. Endoscopic view of the FHL retinaculum. The retinaculum is cut using a punch.

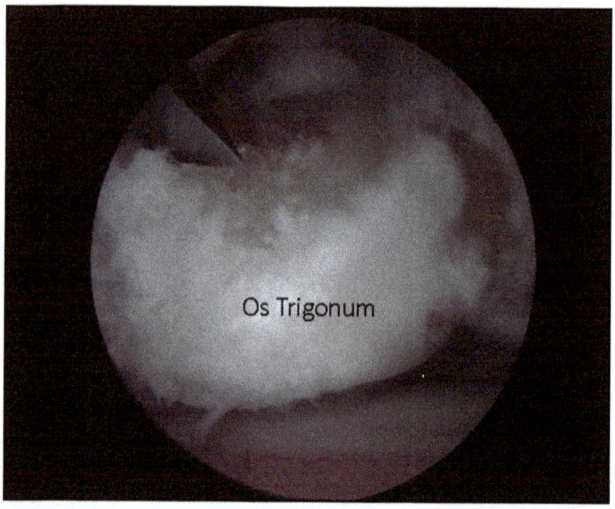

Figure 1-4. Endoscopic view of the os trigonum. The fragment is detached using an osteotome.

the shaver, the fatty tissue and thin joint capsule are removed. The posterior compartment of the subtalar joint can be visualized. The FHL tendon is an important landmark to prevent damage to the more medially located neurovascular bundle.

Os Trigonum

Removal of a symptomatic os trigonum or a nonunion of a fracture of the posterior talar process involves partial detachment of the ligaments attached to the os trigonum. Consecutively, the flexor retinaculum, posterior talocalcaneal ligament, and posterior talofibular ligament are cut by means of a punch (Figure 1-3).

The remnants of these 3 ligaments from the posterior talar prominence can be cleaned by means of a shaver. The os trigonum can be lifted from the subtalar joint using a small-sized bone elevator. The periosteal elevator can be used to identify the fibrotic zone between the os trigonum and talus from above. The os trigonum can be mobilized and removed by using a grasper (Figure 1-4). The talus is now inspected for any remnants of the os trigonum.

Hypertrophic Posterior Talar Process

In the case of a bony prominence/hypertrophic posterior talar process, removal can best be performed by means of a 4.0-mm osteotome. By using the osteotome, it is important not to start too far anteriorly to prevent damage to the subtalar joint. First, the superior part of the talar process is freed from soft tissue by using a shaver. The ligaments attached to the posterior talar prominence are detached. A 4.0-mm osteotome is now introduced through the posteromedial portal. The osteotome is positioned relatively posterior on the posterior prominence. The posteroinferior part of the posterior talar process is thus removed. The superior remnants of the posterior talar process can be removed by a shaver.

Soft Tissue

In the case of soft tissue impingement, a soft tissue distractor is applied. The posterior syndesmotic ligaments are inspected (tibial slip and intermalleolar ligaments). If hypertrophic, they are partially resected. Any soft tissue covering the posterior talar process is removed. The Rouvière ligament attaches to the posterior talar process.[11] It is partially resected in order to be able to inspect and enter the ankle joint. Especially in cases where this Rouvière ligament is thickened, it can be part of the pathology.

After finishing the procedure, stab incisions are closed with 3.0 Ethilon (Ethicon) to prevent sinus formation. A sterile compression dressing is applied.[12]

Postoperative Protocol

There is a general consensus in the literature to allow weightbearing as tolerated from the first postoperative day with a compression bandage. The dressing can be taken off after 3 days. Range of motion exercises are started on the day of surgery. Full weightbearing is expected by 4 to 5 days postoperatively.[10]

Potential Complications

The principle concern of the hindfoot endoscopy is due to the proximity of the medial neurovascular bundle to the posteromedial portal and the sural nerve to the posterolateral portal. The majority of neurovascular injuries occur as a result of inaccurate portal placement, improper use of joint distraction, inadequate monitoring of soft tissue fluid extravasation, or improper use of a tourniquet. However, Zengerink and van Dijk showed the complication rate to be 2.3%.[13]

Top Technical Pearls for the Procedure

1. Create the posterolateral portal just proximal and lateral to the imaginary intersection of the horizontal line, parallel to the foot sole, from the tip of the lateral malleolus to the Achilles tendon with the ankle in the neutral position.
2. The posteromedial portal is located at the same level as the posterolateral portal, just medial to the Achilles tendon.

(continued)

3. Use the arthroscopic shaft, inserted through the posterolateral portal and directed toward the interdigital web space in between the first and second toe, as a guide to travel anteriorly with the instruments inserted through the posteromedial portal.
4. Use an arthroscopic punch to detach the flexor retinaculum from the posterior talar process and to release the tendon sheath in case of tendinopathy of the FHL.
5. Use the FHL tendon as a landmark. Stay lateral to the FHL tendon.

References

1. Scholten PE, Sierevelt IN, van Dijk CN. Hindfoot endoscopy for posterior ankle impingement. *J Bone Joint Surg Am.* 2008;90(12):2665-2672.
2. Willits K, Sonneveld H, Amendola A, Giffin JR, Griffin S, Fowler PJ. Outcome of posterior ankle arthroscopy for hindfoot impingement. *Arthroscopy.* 2008;24(2):196-202.
3. Jourdel F, Tourne Y, Saragaglia D. [Posterior ankle impingement syndrome: a retrospective study in 21 cases treated surgically]. *Rev Chir Orthop Reparatrice Appar Mot.* 2005;91(3):239-247.
4. Noguchi H, Ishii Y, Takeda M, Hasegawa A, Monden S, Takagishi K. Arthroscopic excision of posterior ankle bony impingement for early return to the field: short-term results. *Foot Ankle Int.* 2010;31(5):398-403.
5. Calder JD, Sexton SA, Pearce CJ. Return to training and playing after posterior ankle arthroscopy for posterior impingement in elite professional soccer. *Am J Sports Med.* 2010;38(1):120-124.
6. Galla M, Lobenhoffer P. Technique and results of arthroscopic treatment of posterior ankle impingement. *Foot Ankle Surg.* 2011;17(2):79-84.
7. Smyth NA, Zwiers R, Wiegerinck JI, et al. Posterior hindfoot arthroscopy: a review. *Am J Sports Med.* 2014;42(1):225-234.
8. Wiegerinck JI, Vroemen JC, van Dongen TH, Sierevelt IN, Maas M, van Dijk CN. The posterior impingement view: an alternative conventional projection to detect bony posterior ankle impingement. *Arthroscopy.* 2014;30(10):1311-1316.
9. van Dijk CN. Instrumentation. In: *Ankle Arthroscopy: Techniques Developed by the Amsterdam Foot and Ankle School.* Berlin, Germany: Springer; 2014:67-80.
10. van Dijk CN. Posterior ankle impingement. In: *Ankle Arthroscopy: Techniques Developed by the Amsterdam Foot and Ankle School.* Berlin, Germany: Springer; 2014:231-259.
11. Golano P, Vega J, de Leeuw PA, et al. Anatomy of the ankle ligaments: a pictorial essay. *Knee Surg Sports Traumatol Arthrosc.* 2010;18(5):557-569.
12. van Dijk CN, Scholten PE, Krips R. A 2-portal endoscopic approach for diagnosis and treatment of posterior ankle pathology. *Arthroscopy.* 2000;16(8):871-876.
13. Zengerink M, van Dijk CN. Complications in ankle arthroscopy. *Knee Surg Sports Traumatol Arthrosc.* 2012;20(8):1420-1431.

Please visit www.routledge.com/9781617119989 to access additional material.

Section I

Osteochondral Lesions of the Talar Dome

2

Debridement With Stimulation of the Subchondral Bone

James W. Stone, MD

Introduction

Osteochondral lesions of the talar dome may occur anywhere on the talus, but they occur most commonly on the posteromedial or anterolateral surface. Most are secondary to trauma, which may be an acute injury or the result of cumulative injuries to the surface of the bone. Other factors that may contribute to their development include genetic, hormonal, hematologic, and drug-related influences. Anterolateral lesions are most frequently secondary to acute injuries, whereas posteromedial lesions are more commonly chronic in nature and more likely to be associated with subchondral cyst formation. The choice of surgical treatment may be influenced by several factors, including the size and location of the lesion, chronicity of the lesion, response to previous surgery, presence of a subchondral cyst, and quality of the subchondral bone attached to the chondral portion of the lesion. Surgery is indicated for symptomatic lesions. Traditional treatment includes debridement of the loose osteochondral fragments, which may cause mechanical symptoms in the ankle. The base of the lesion is treated with abrasion, drilling, or microfracture to stimulate the development of fibrocartilaginous repair tissue. Numerous studies have documented that first-time treatment of an osteochondral lesion of the talar dome using debridement with abrasion, drilling, or microfracture of the base yields good to excellent results in approximately 80% of patients.[1-10] Although some studies have suggested deterioration of results over time, others have suggested maintenance of results over time.[11,12]

Indications

- Symptomatic osteochondral lesions of the talar dome: Asymptomatic small lesions of the talar dome do not necessarily require surgery. Patients who present with osteochondral lesions causing persistent pain, instability, or mechanical symptoms are candidates for surgery.
- Talar dome location: Lateral lesions are generally acute whereas medial lesions are more commonly chronic. The lateral lesions may be associated with a sizeable bony fragment and, in

Stone JW, Kennedy JG, Glazebrook M, eds. *The Foot and Ankle: AANA Advanced Arthroscopic Surgical Techniques* (pp 9-17).

the acute situation, may be amenable to internal fixation either arthroscopically or open. This can be performed using absorbable pins or headless screws. The medial lesions are generally characterized by poor-quality articular cartilage and underlying bone, which is necrotic and will not support healing of the fragment even with internal fixation and bone grafting. These lesions are best treated with debridement of the loose fragments and treatment of the base of the lesion with marrow stimulation using abrasion, drilling, or microfracture.

- Lesion size: Studies have suggested that lesions with a threshold size of approximately 150 mm^2 (approximately 14-mm diameter) have a poor prognosis for the resolution of symptoms after simple debridement procedures. Consideration should be given for procedures that reconstruct bone and/or articular cartilage in these larger lesions.
- Associated cyst: The presence of an associated subchondral cyst has been correlated with poorer results after simple debridement with stimulation of the base. Consideration should be given to treatment with bone grafting of these lesions. In addition, procedures to reconstruct the articular cartilage may be considered.

Pertinent Physical Findings

- Tenderness: A patient's complaint of pain may be poorly localized and not even correspond to the side of the osteochondral lesion. However, if tenderness is present, it will generally correlate with the side of the lesion. For medial lesions that are generally located more posteriorly on the talar dome, ankle dorsiflexion with posterior joint palpation may elicit tenderness. In contrast, lateral lesions that are generally located more anteriorly on the talar dome may be associated with tenderness to palpation at the lateral joint line with the ankle in a position of plantarflexion.
- Swelling: Generalized ankle swelling may be present with a joint effusion associated with synovitis secondary to a loose fragment.
- Alignment: A careful assessment of hindfoot alignment must be performed to rule out the presence of abnormal varus or valgus inclination, which might place abnormal stress on the medial or lateral talar dome, respectively, and the presence of which may require consideration for tibial osteotomy or another realignment procedure to restore physiologic lower extremity alignment.
- Joint flexibility: The subtalar joint should be examined for normal range of motion to rule out tarsal coalition or significant degenerative change, which may limit motion, causing increased stress transfer to the ankle joint.
- Joint laxity: A careful examination of the lateral ligament structures should be performed with the anterior drawer performed with the ankle in slight plantarflexion and inversion stress at neutral. Comparison with the opposite ankle is important, along with an assessment for possible congenital ligament laxity. An associated surgical procedure to address chronic ligament laxity in the presence of a chronic medial talar dome lesion must be considered in these patients.

Pertinent Imaging

- Plain radiographs: Anteroposterior, mortise, and lateral radiographs should be obtained on every patient. Weightbearing views may assist in assessing joint alignment. In addition to basic information regarding an osteochondral lesion, plain radiographs may show coexisting abnormalities such as osteophytes, joint space narrowing, or abnormalities of other joints of

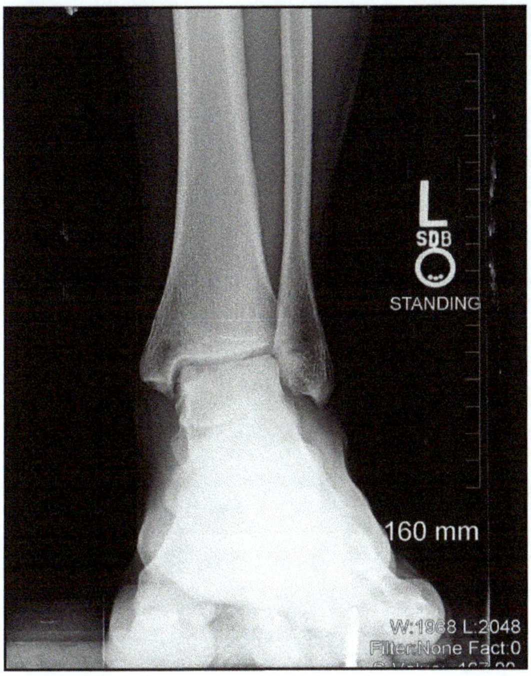

Figure 2-1. Preoperative anteroposterior radiograph demonstrates a medial talar dome osteochondral lesion with loose fragment.

the hindfoot and midfoot, which may affect the assessment and treatment of the osteochondral lesion of the talar dome (Figure 2-1).

- Magnetic resonance imaging (MRI): MRI is helpful in assessing the size and location of the lesion.[13-15] It may also show the presence of fluid beneath the lesion, which suggests a loose fragment. MRI is also useful in detecting the presence and size of an associated subchondral cyst. Large cysts have been associated with poorer prognosis after traditional surgical treatment with debridement and base stimulation, and their presence may lead the surgeon to select a more aggressive approach to surgical treatment. MRI may help to assess the quality of the articular cartilage and has been found to correlate with arthroscopic findings. A weakness of MRI is that the presence of bone marrow edema may exaggerate the size of the lesion (Figure 2-2).
- Computed tomography (CT): CT may be utilized to specifically address lesion size as it provides the most precise assessment of bone fragment size and quality while also providing accurate assessment of associated cysts (Figure 2-3).

Equipment

Although some authors suggest that the procedure can be performed with standard (4-mm diameter) arthroscopic instrumentation used for larger joints,[16] this author recommends small joint arthroscopes of an approximately 2.4- to 2.7-mm diameter. Modern small arthroscopes with wide angle views provide excellent visualization while minimizing iatrogenic articular cartilage injury. Both a standard 30-degree angle viewing arthroscope and a 70-degree arthroscope should be available, particularly for posteromedial lesions. Availability of a selection of straight and angled curettes is crucial for debridement of these lesions. Several vendors have developed small joint kits that include specialized curettes, instruments that accommodate the curvature of the talar dome to allow forward and backward debridement of the articular cartilage, small-diameter micro picks for microfracture, and drill guides for precise antegrade or retrograde drilling.

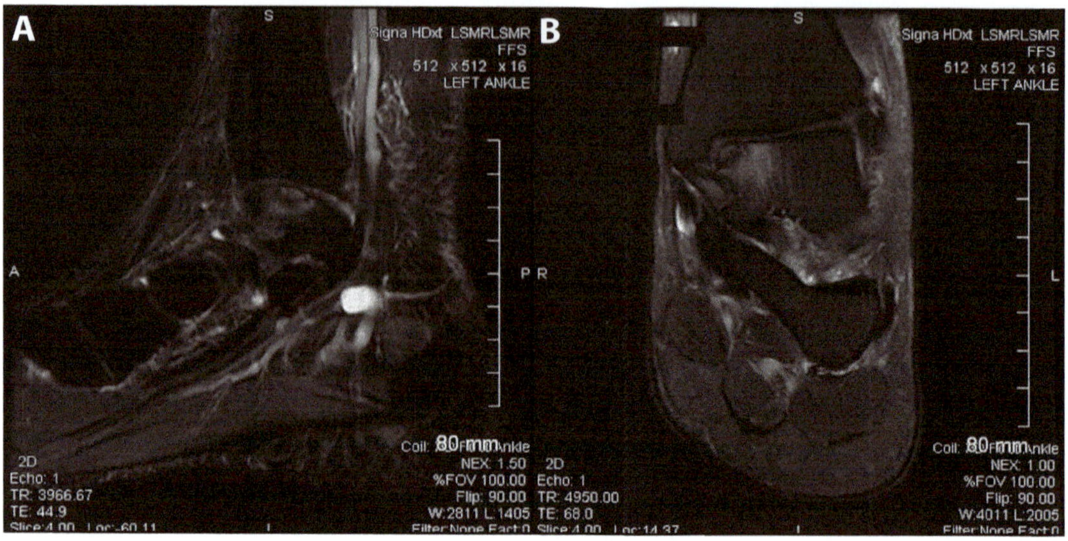

Figure 2-2. (A) Sagittal and (B) coronal T2 fat-suppressed MRI images delineate the lesion and the associated bone edema in the body of the talus.

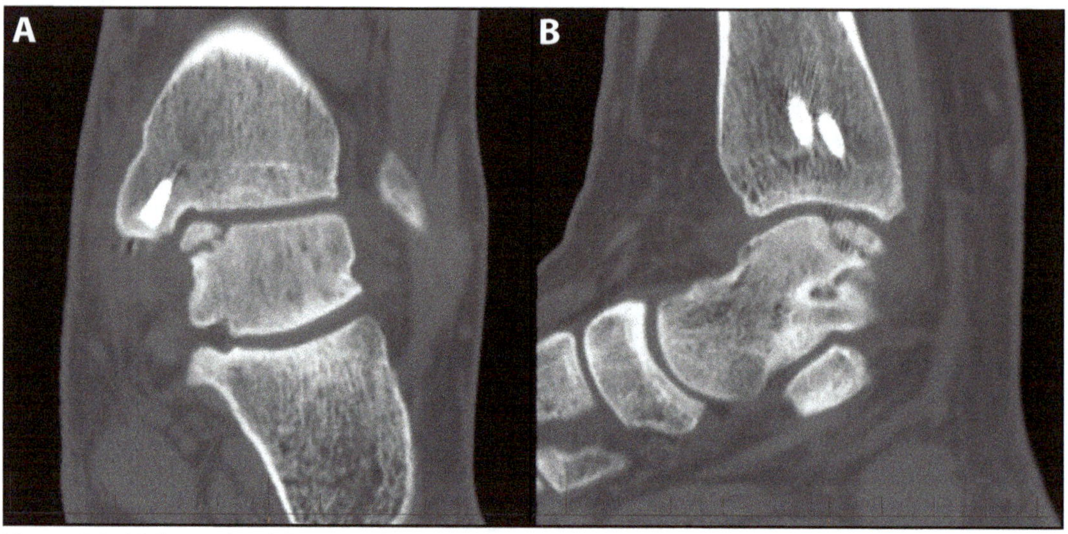

Figure 2-3. (A) Coronal and (B) sagittal CT scans delineate the bony fragment of the talar dome lesion. The CT gives the best visualization of the bone fragment and estimate of the size and location of the lesion.

Positioning and Portals

The patient is positioned supine on the operating table with the ipsilateral hip and knee flexed and supported by a well-padded leg holder. The leg holder should have a long thigh segment and a short leg segment so that the force applied for distraction is distributed over a wide area of the thigh rather than concentrating in the popliteal space. This may diminish the risk of deep vein thrombosis (DVT) secondary to venous stasis.

The foot, ankle, and leg are prepped and draped up to the leg holder. A commercially available sterile distraction strap is placed around the hindfoot and midfoot. It is connected to a sterile bar using a piece of sterile Velcro, which allows the surgeon to apply the desired degree of distraction force to the ankle. This setup provides a stable platform for surgery without the need for application of distraction by an assistant while allowing free intraoperative motion of the ankle joint in dorsiflexion and plantarflexion.

Step-by-Step Description of the Procedure

An 18-gauge needle is used to determine the optimal location for the anteromedial portal, which is placed at the medial border of the tibialis anterior tendon and inferior to the tibial plafond at the position that best allows needle passage across the joint. The portals are created using the "nick and spread" technique; only the skin is penetrated by the #11 blade, and then the subcutaneous tissues are bluntly dissected to the level of the joint capsule. The capsule is then penetrated using a blunt trocar to avoid iatrogenic articular cartilage injury. The arthroscope is introduced through this portal and the joint may be visualized dry.

The author recommends placing the posterolateral portal at this point. The location is at the lateral border of the Achilles tendon approximately 1 to 2 cm distal to the anterior portal. The 18-gauge needle is utilized to determine the location that allows easy passage into the joint beneath the posterior syndesmotic ligament as visualized using the arthroscope in the anteromedial portal. This portal is used for dedicated inflow using an arthroscopic fluid pump set on low pressure (approximately 25 mm Hg) and low flow. The leg is monitored throughout the case to be certain that excessive swelling of the soft tissues does not occur.

An anterolateral portal is created in a similar fashion just lateral to the peroneus tertius and common extensor tendons under direct arthroscopic visualization using transillumination from the arthroscope to avoid injury to neurovascular structures, also using a hypodermic needle to determine optimal portal placement.

An organized diagnostic arthroscopy is performed with the arthroscope in the anteromedial portal. The arthroscope may also be placed in the anterolateral and posterolateral portals if required to visualize the entire joint. A probe is placed in the anterolateral portal to palpate the surface of the talus. In general, when performing the surgical procedure, the arthroscope will be placed on the side opposite the lesion and the instruments will be introduced through the portal on the same side as the lesion. The 70-degree arthroscope may be substituted for the 30-degree scope to better visualize posteromedial lesions. In some cases, improved visualization of posteromedial lesions can be achieved by placing the arthroscope into the posterolateral portal and instrumenting from 1 of the 2 anterior portals. Becoming facile using all 3 portals allows the arthroscopic surgeon to successfully approach most osteochondral lesions of the talar dome.

The probe is used to palpate the surface of the talus to identify the margins of the lesion (Figure 2-4). The free fragment is elevated with the probe to assess the quality of the articular cartilage attached to the lesion, the quality of the underlying subchondral bone, and the quality of the bone at the base of the lesion. The most common finding is poor-quality subchondral bone on a chronic medial lesion with necrotic, flaking bone at the base of the lesion. In this situation, fragment excision is appropriate. Reduction and fixation of a lesion is only appropriate to consider when there is normal articular cartilage on the surface of a lesion with sufficient good-quality subchondral bone to support internal fixation and the absence of necrotic bone at the base. This circumstance occurs almost exclusively with acute lateral lesions and is uncommon in the typical chronic posteromedial lesions.

In some cases, the cartilage surface overlying the lesion may appear normal; however, palpation with a probe will reveal abnormal resilience of this cartilage compared to cartilage that is not overlying the lesion. In this circumstance, the surgeon must make the decision to remove the abnormal cartilage and proceed as discussed next or consider a retrograde drilling procedure.

After the decision is made to excise the lesion, it is elevated with the probe or an angled curette and the major fragments are removed with loose-body forceps. Small fragments can be removed

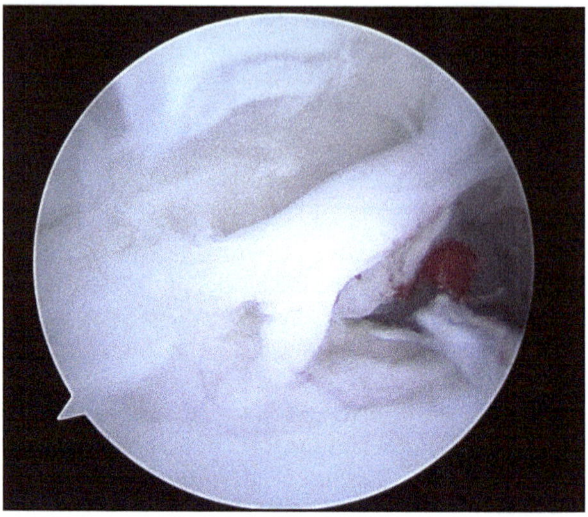

Figure 2-4. Initial arthroscopic view of a medial talar dome lesion showing irregular articular cartilage, which is attached to a loose bony fragment.

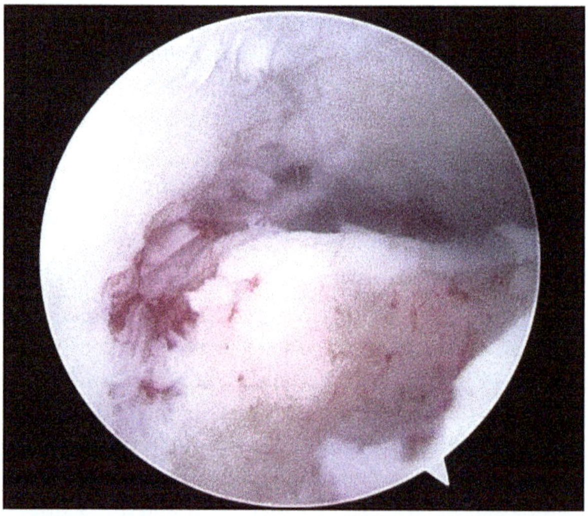

Figure 2-5. Arthroscopic view after complete debridement of the lesion. It is most important to perform a complete debridement of all loose fragments, which often include the vertical surface of the talar dome in the medial gutter. Failure to perform a complete debridement of all loose fragments will result in failure of the procedure to relieve symptoms.

using a motorized suction shaver. A selection of angled curettes is used to debride the articular cartilage at the margins of the lesion back to the point where well-attached articular cartilage with perpendicular edges is achieved. It is most important in posteromedial lesions to debride loose articular cartilage and bone not only over the horizontal surface of the talus, but also onto the vertical surface in the medial gutter. Failure to excise loose fragments of bone and articular cartilage in this location will lead to failure of the surgical procedure to relieve ankle pain (Figure 2-5).

After excising the loose fragments, the base of the lesion is scraped with an angled curette to remove loose, necrotic bone. The residual base of the lesion may then be treated with abrasion using a motorized burr, drilled with a Kirschner wire (K-wire), or "picked" with a microfracture awl. Microfracture has been proposed as a means of bringing bone marrow progenitor cells to the surface of the lesion without the heat necrosis that occurs with drilling. However, it has recently been suggested that drilling in the fluid environment may cause less damage than the pressure necrosis that may occur as a larger diameter microfracture pick is forced into the bone, which is compressed at the margins of the awl.[17] Microfracture of these talar dome lesions should be performed with small-diameter microfracture awls, which are commercially available (Figure 2-6).

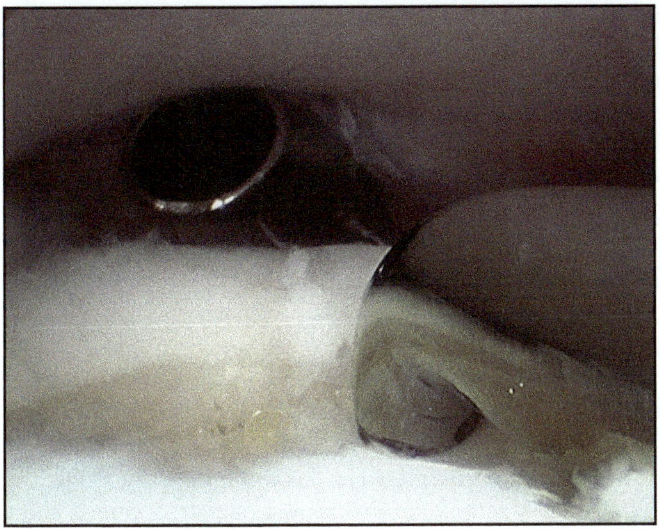

Figure 2-6. Arthroscopic view of a medial talar dome lesion with a small-diameter, right-angle microfracture awl used to perform multiple penetrations of the base of the lesion.

Posteromedial lesions may be difficult to approach using a K-wire even with maximum plantarflexion of the ankle. Some suggest that transmalleolar drilling using a drill guide is a reasonable alternative to approach these lesions,[18] but one must accept the inevitable damage to the normal articular cartilage of the medial malleolus that occurs with transmalleolar drilling. Anterolateral lesions are easier to approach for drilling with plantarflexion of the ankle.

The microfracture awls are commercially available in a variety of angulations, which allow the surgeon to approach posteromedial lesions more easily. It is important to use a sharp, small-diameter awl. The correct procedure for microfracture involves placing the awl at a right angle to the surface being penetrated. In the case of a posteromedial talar dome lesion, the right-angle awl is most useful and must be placed perpendicular to the surface for accurate placement in the lesion. The force applied to the instrument must be at the same angle as the awl point. Therefore, for a right-angle awl, the force must be applied perpendicular to the shaft of the instrument. Using a mallet on the end of the instrument is not recommended for the right-angle awl. The holes are placed at approximately 5-mm intervals to a depth of approximately 3 mm. After placement of the holes, it is important to decrease the inflow pressure (and deflate the tourniquet if it was inflated during the procedure) to observe marrow elements arising from the holes into the joint.

Drilling with a smooth K-wire (approximately 0.062-inch diameter) is an alternative to using a microfracture awl. Although the awls were initially thought to avoid potential heat necrosis due to motorized drilling, the drilling procedure may be preferred because it avoids the pressure necrosis that may occur with impaction microfracture awls. Drilling can usually be performed on anterolateral lesions as they are accessible at an appropriate angle by plantarflexing the ankle while introducing the wire through the anterolateral portal or an accessory anterolateral portal placed more proximally and directed more vertically toward the lesion. However, direct drilling may not be possible for posteromedial lesions. I recommend use of a microfracture awl for these lesions rather than transmalleolar drilling with a drill guide as this procedure unnecessarily causes injury to the otherwise normal articular cartilage of the medial malleolus.

Postoperative Protocol

A single suture is placed into each wound at the conclusion of the case and a bulky compressive dressing is applied along with a posterior plaster splint in neutral position. The wounds are checked at 7 to 10 days postoperatively and the sutures are removed. At this point, active range of motion exercises are encouraged. For small lesions less than 1 cm in diameter, weightbearing is advanced as tolerated. For larger lesions, a period of weight relief is recommended for 3 to 6 weeks while encouraging range of motion exercises. Physical therapy may begin at 3 to 6 weeks postoperatively to facilitate range of motion, perform modalities to decrease pain and swelling, and advance a strengthening and return-to-work or -sports program.

Potential Complications

The most common complication of ankle arthroscopy is injury to a superficial sensory nerve resulting in pain, numbness, or paresthesias. Adherence to proper technique of portal creation using the "nick and spread" technique along with gentle handling of the soft tissues minimizes the chances of these complications.

Complications related to the noninvasive joint distraction can be minimized by using the minimum force required to achieve sufficient distraction and by keeping operative time as short as possible. Distractor complications are rare but directly related to force and time applied.

DVT is rare after ankle arthroscopy, and routine prophylaxis for DVT is not recommended. DVT prophylaxis is recommended for patients who have a past history of DVT or pulmonary embolus or for those who have a known genetic predisposition to clotting, such as factor V Leiden deficiency.

Intraoperative monitoring of the leg by inspection and palpation should be performed at regular intervals to prevent extravasation of inflow fluid by an improperly placed cannula. Unrestricted extravasation of fluid could result in compartment syndrome, but this is a very rare complication of ankle arthroscopy.

Top Technical Pearls for the Procedure

1. Use noninvasive distraction and a small-joint arthroscope (30- and 70-degree viewing angles) to access the joint.
2. Create the posterolateral portal for dedicated inflow and to allow placement of the arthroscope or instruments when approaching posteromedial talar dome lesions.
3. For medial lesions, be certain to carry the debridement as far medially onto the vertical surface of the talus as necessary to remove all loose bone and cartilage fragments. Failure to debride the lesion completely will lead to failure of the operation to resolve symptoms of pain, clicking, and locking.
4. Use small-diameter microfracture picks when making multiple perforations in the base of the lesion after debridement.
5. When using a right-angle microfracture pick, the direction of pressure must be perpendicular to the talar dome surface, a direct downward application of force.

References

1. Berndt AL, Harty M. Transchondral fractures (osteochondritis dissecans) of the talus. *J Bone Joint Surg Am.* 1959;41A:988-1020.
2. Chuckpaiwong B, Berkson EM, Theodore GH. Microfracture for osteochondral lesions of the ankle: outcome analysis and outcome predictors of 105 cases. *Arthroscopy.* 2008;24:106-112.
3. Robinson DE, Winston IG, Harries WJ, Kelly AJ. Arthroscopic treatment of osteochondral lesions of the talus. *J Bone Joint Surg Br.* 2003;85:989-993.
4. Kumai T, Takakura Y, Higashiyama I, Tamai S. Arthroscopic drilling for the treatment of osteochondral lesions of the talus. *J Bone Joint Surg Am.* 1999;81:1229-1235.
5. Kelberine F, Frank A. Arthroscopic treatment of osteochondral lesions of the talar dome: a retrospective study of 48 cases. *Arthroscopy.* 1999;15:77-84.
6. Becher C, Thermann H. Results of microfracture in the treatment of articular cartilage defects of the talus. *Foot Ankle Int.* 2005;26:583-589.
7. Gobbi A, Francisco RA, Lubowitz JH, et al. Osteochondral lesions of the talus: randomized controlled trial comparing chondroplasty, microfracture, and osteochondral autograft transplantation. *Arthroscopy.* 2006;22:1085-1092.
8. Choi WJ, Park KK, Kim BS, Lee JW. Osteochondral lesion of the talus: is there a critical defect size for poor outcome? *Am J Sports Med.* 2009;37(10):1974-1980.
9. Scranton PE Jr, Frey CC, Feder KS. Outcome of osteochondral autograft transplantation for type-V cystic osteochondral lesions of the talus. *J Bone Joint Surg Br.* 2006;88(5):614-619.
10. Zengerink M, Struijs PA, Tol JL, van Dijk CN. Treatment of osteochondral lesions of the talus: a systematic review. *Knee Surg Sports Traumatol Arthrosc.* 2010;18(2):238-246.
11. Ferkel RD, Zanotti RM, Komenda GA, et al. Arthroscopic treatment of chronic osteochondral lesions of the talus: long-term results. *Am J Sports Med.* 2008;36:1750-1761.
12. van Bergen CJ, Kox LS, Maas M, Sierevelt IN, Kerkhoffs GM, van Dijk CN. Arthroscopic treatment of osteochondral defects of the talus: outcomes at eight to twenty years of follow-up. *J Bone Joint Surg Am.* 2013;95(6):519-525.
13. Stroud CC, Marks RM. Imaging of osteochondral lesions of the talus. *Foot Ankle Clin.* 2000;5:119-133.
14. De Smet AA, Fisher DR, Burnstein MI, et al. Value of MR imaging in staging osteochondral lesions of the talus (osteochondritis dissecans): results in 14 patients. *Am J Roentgenol.* 1990;154:555-558.
15. Verhagen RA, Maas M, Dijkgraff MG, et al. Prospective study on diagnostic strategies in osteochondral lesions of the talus. Is MRI superior to helical CT? *J Bone Joint Surg Br.* 2005;87:41-46.
16. van Dijk CN, van Bergen CJ. Advancements in ankle arthroscopy. *J Am Acad Orthop Surg.* 2008;16(11):635-646.
17. Savage-Elliott I, Ross KA, Smyth NA, Murawski CD, Kennedy JG. Osteochondral lesions of the talus: a current concepts review and evidence-based treatment paradigm. *Foot Ankle Spec.* 2014;7(5):414-422.
18. Stetson WB, Ferkel RD. Ankle arthroscopy: II. Indications and results. *J Am Acad Orthop Surg.* 1996;4:24-34.

Please visit www.routledge.com/9781617119989 to access additional material.

3

Osteochondral Lesions of the Talar Dome
Osteochondral Autologous Transplantation Treatment

Jin Woo Lee, MD, PhD and Woojin Choi, MD, PhD

Introduction

Osteochondral autologous transplantation (OAT) is a restorative procedure that substitutes the pathology with viable hyaline cartilage and subchondral bone as a whole unit.[1] For this reason, OAT has been an appealing option for osteochondral lesions of the talus (OLT) with a large size, cystic lesions, and failed bone marrow stimulation procedures (Figure 3-1). The concept of cartilage and bone unit transplantation was first reported by Wagner[2] to treat osteochondritis dissecans of the knee. OAT was then developed using multiple plugs in the knee, and favorable short- to mid-term outcome was reported.[3] Upon the success of OAT in the knee, the technique was applied to the ankle. In a preliminary report of a prospective study, Hangody et al[4] first reported OAT for the OLT in 11 patients. The promising results of this study were followed by several similar results with short- to mid-term outcomes.[1,5-8] However, previous reports lack long-term results and a high level of evidence.[9] Also, further concerns regarding donor site morbidity have increased because the technique involves the normal knee as a donor.[10,11]

Indications

When considering surgical treatment for OLT, delineating clear-cut indication between reparative and restorative technique is still a matter of controversy. For patients with lesion less than 15 mm in diameter or a lesion size of < 150 mm^2, many authors have consistently reported good or excellent outcomes with primary marrow stimulation technique.[12,13] However, considering there is only one level II study that presented no significant difference among chondroplasty, microfracture, and OAT, further studies to identify the exact role of OAT in OLT treatment are mandatory.[6]

Most orthopedic surgeons reserve OAT for more complicated cases or larger lesions because the technique is more invasive and bears the potential morbidity at the donor site.[9-11,14-16] The following is a list of generally accepted indications for OAT:

Stone JW, Kennedy JG, Glazebrook M, eds. *The Foot and Ankle: AANA Advanced Arthroscopic Surgical Techniques* (pp 19-26).

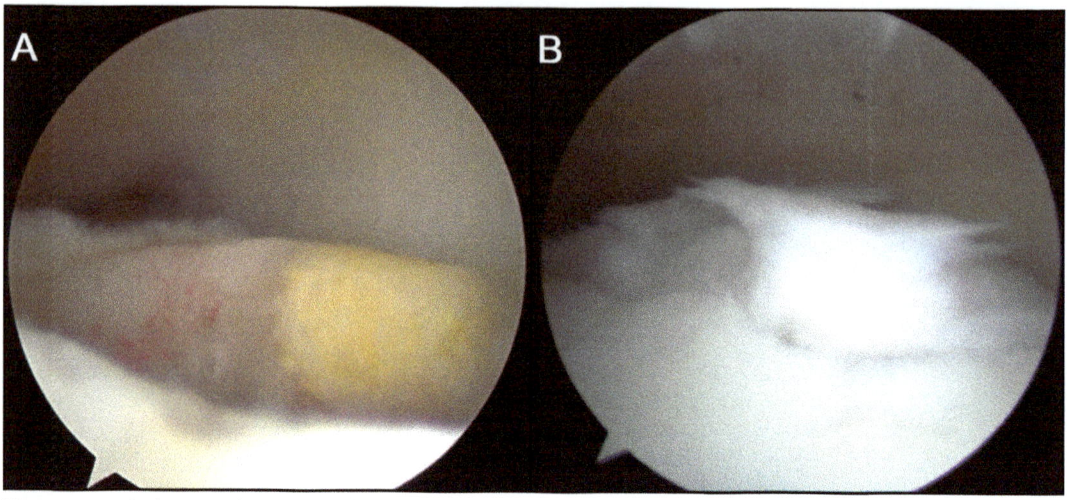

Figure 3-1. Arthroscopic images. (A) Primary arthroscopic debridement and microfracture of the osteochondral lesion with a subchondral cyst in the medial talar dome. (B) Repeat arthroscopy 2 years after primary treatment showed the lesion was covered with unstable and friable fibrocartilage, implying failed treatment.

- Secondary procedure for failed arthroscopic bone marrow stimulation technique[15]
- OLTs associated with large subchondral cysts (stage V lesions), which lacks the subchondral plate
- Large OLTs, generally considered as lesions larger than 15 mm in diameter or a lesion size of $> 150 \text{ mm}^2$
- OLTs that are located in areas with limited accessibility (tight ankle)

Contraindications

- Infection
- Malignancy
- Severe medical comorbidities

Relative Contraindications

- OLTs associated with osteoarthritis
- Ankle malalignment
- Ankle instability
- "Kissing" chondral lesions at tibial plafond
- Knee arthritis or patellofemoral symptoms
- Noncontained OLTs that include the lateral or medial wall of the talus making geometrical matching of the donor plug impossible

Surgeons should correct the accompanying malalignment and instability concomitantly or prior to OAT.

Pertinent Physical Findings

Since most physical signs and symptoms are similar to those observed in other pathologies around the ankle, a thorough physical examination of the ankle and hindfoot is mandatory to distinguish other possible causes of ankle pain and identify other associated pathologic conditions. The following are symptoms and signs of patients with OLT:

- Typical OLT patients present with ankle pain during weightbearing that is relieved by resting.
- Most patients with OLT have a history of trauma, such as inversion injury, while often associated with chronic lateral ankle instability.
- History of effusion around ankle joint
- Giving way during walking
- Limited range of motion of the ankle joint
- Author's recommended "best" test: Careful palpation over the ankle joint line elicits tenderness. Depending on the location of the lesion, deep plantarflexion of the ankle joint is necessary during palpation. Additionally, if the OLT fragment is unstable, crepitation could be examined during ankle joint motion.

Pertinent Imaging

Berndt and Harty[17] classified OLT according to plain radiographs. Several positions and different views of the ankle joint in plain radiographs have been proposed to increase the visualization of pathology.[16] However, reported detection rate could be as low as 50% as not all of the pathologic conditions in cartilage and subchondral bone are presented in plain radiographs.[18] Therefore, the author recommends the following further imaging assessment when there is suspicion of OLT:

- Computed tomography (CT) scans: Because CT scans can accurately define the cortical outlines of the bone, the exact size of the OLT could be measured without confounding bone edema. The detection rate of OLT using high-resolution CT scan (1- to 2-mm, thin-cut images) is comparable to magnetic resonance imaging (MRI) and also provides high specificity in grading a lesion.[9] Classification based on CT scans was developed by Anderson and colleagues.[19] Incorporating with radioisotopes, single-photon emission CT (SPECT) could be used to correlate with the symptoms and location of the lesion.[20]
- MRI: The author's choice of further imaging modality is MRI, which allows the detection of associated soft tissue pathology bone edema and the size of the OLT. Also, advanced imaging of cartilage status allows early-stage OLT detection. However, overestimation of the lesion due to associated bone marrow is the limitation of the MRI.

Equipment

Other than basic surgical instruments for osteotomy and exposure of the ankle joint, specially designed instruments are necessary to perform OAT. While each company provides a slightly different design and the name of the instrument set, a recipient sizer, recipient harvester, donor harvester, and tamp are 4 basic instruments for OAT.

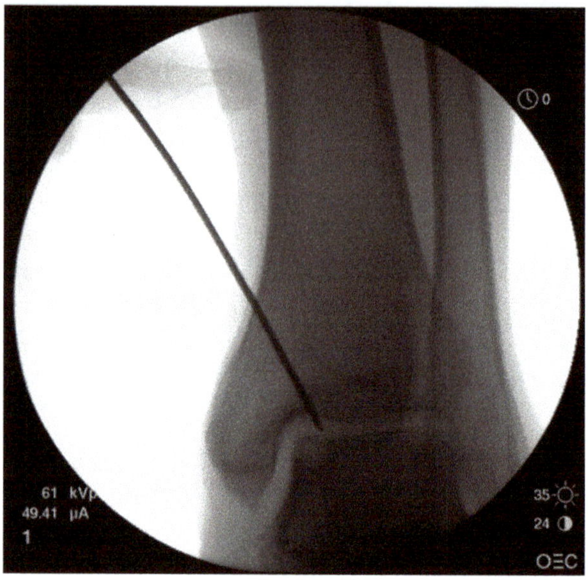

Figure 3-2. Under the guidance of fluoroscopy, the apex and direction of the medial malleolar osteotomy is determined to facilitate the approach with a clear vision of the lesion.

Positioning and Portals

Under general or spinal anesthesia, the patient is placed in the supine position on the operating table. The level of the heel is set around the edge of the table. The author prefers to use a thigh tourniquet as clear visualization of the operation field is necessary for sizing, grafting, and tampering the osteochondral graft plug. Depending on the planned osteotomy site, a bump under the ipsilateral hip aids more comfortable access to the operation field, especially for the fibular osteotomy. During the OAT procedure, change of knee flexion is necessary to gain perpendicular trajectory. Thus, a triangular-shaped support below the popliteal fossa or blanket roll should be prepared.

Step-by-Step Description of the Procedure

After positioning, preparation, and draping the patient, we recommend performing ankle arthroscopy to confirm the location and grade of the OLT and to identify other intra-articular pathologies that may be treated simultaneously.[15] The best operative approach for OAT is determined by the location of the OLT. If the lesion is located on the anterior aspect of the talar dome, all arthroscopic or mini-open arthrotomy can be used. However, surgeons should not hesitate to use osteotomy to expose the lesion because a perpendicular path to the lesion is required for implantation, especially OLTs located in the posterior talar dome.

As most of the medial OLTs are located central to posterior, a medial malleolus osteotomy is required to allow perpendicular osteochondral grafting to the talar dome. The osteotomy design could be either step- or straight-cut in oblique fashion. Step-cut osteotomy is reported to provide more intrinsic stability and resistance to rotation due to more stable interdigitation.[21] Some authors have introduced using anterior distal tibia osteotomy; however, this author has no experience with the technique.[22,23] After palpating the medial corner of the joint line, a skin incision is made over the medial malleolus. Soft tissue, including periosteum, is reflected anteriorly and posteriorly with extra care to protect the tibialis posterior tendon. Under the guidance of fluoroscopy, the apex and direction of the oblique osteotomy is determined (Figure 3-2). Before placing the osteotomy, 2 to 4 predrilled holes with Kirschner wires for lateral fixation facilitates later restoration of the osteotomized medial malleolus into the anatomic position with screws. An incomplete osteotomy using a sagittal saw is finalized with an osteotome to protect the tibialis posterior tendon. The osteotomized medial malleolus is then reflected plantarward on the deltoid ligament hinge to expose the medial aspect of the talar dome.

Because the lateral OLTs are often located in the anterior aspect of the talar dome, anterolateral arthrotomy combining deep plantarflexion of the ankle joint could sufficiently expose the lesions. The incision is placed between the extensor digitorum longus medially and peroneus tertius laterally while protecting branches of the superficial peroneal nerve. If the lesion is located in the posterolateral aspect or more wide exposure is required, then fibular osteotomy could be performed.

After procuring a good perpendicular view of the targeted OLT, debridement of the damaged cartilage is performed using a curette and rongeur. Debridement should be performed thoroughly to achieve a stable and viable cartilage rim. Also, remnants of residual fibrotic tissue should be removed from the subchondral bone of the defect. Then, the lesion size and number of grafts required are determined with a recipient sizer provided in the OAT instruments set (generally 6, 8, and 10 mm). Depending on the lesion size, 2 or more grafts could be used. After selecting the appropriate size, the recipient harvester is advanced slightly deeper than the desired length of the osteochondral graft plug in order to prevent protrusion of the graft (1 to 4 mm). It is also important to maintain the recipient harvester orientation perpendicular to the OLT during the advancement.

Osteochondral donor graft plugs could be harvested from the ipsilateral knee. The author prefers using the nonweightbearing portion of the superior lateral femoral condyle. A longitudinal skin incision is made along the lateral border of the patella with further arthrotomy. After exposing the superior aspect of the lateral femoral condyle, the donor harvester is placed on the optimal site for graft harvest. For the press-fit technique, the size of the donor harvester should be 1 mm larger than the recipient harvester. The orientation of the harvester must be maintained perpendicular to the harvest site as in the recipient site. The length of the harvested osteochondral graft plug is around 10 mm, which is slightly shorter than the recipient site.

Finally, the osteochondral graft plug is transferred to the recipient site. It is mandatory to maintain perpendicular orientation of the donor harvester over the recipient site while advancing the graft. When the graft is nearly seated at the recipient site, the donor harvester is removed and the rest of the positioning is carefully performed using a corresponding tamp. At this stage, the goal is to place the graft as flush as possible to surrounding articular cartilage. Because the osteochondral graft plug is prepared with a slightly larger diameter, press-fit at the recipient site prevents countersinking of the graft (Figure 3-3).

After OAT, the medial malleolus is reduced to the original anatomical position using the predrilled holes as a guide. Under the guidance of fluoroscopy, the congruency of the osteotomy site and the joint line is confirmed before placing three or four 4.0-mm cannulated screws. Before wound closure, final range of motion is checked to determine whether there is any impingement or incongruence in the ankle joint.

Postoperative Protocol

The ankle is immobilized in a walking boot or short-leg cast for 4 to 6 weeks until the osteotomy is adequately healed based on postoperative radiographs. If there is a delay in wound and/or osteotomy healing, the author recommends immobilization in a cast until healing is satisfactory. Generally, the initial 2- to 10-week nonweightbearing phase is recommended to prevent graft subsidence during osseous integration.[5] This period may be supported by controlled passive motion to promote cartilage metabolism and lessen soft-tissue edema around the joint. Partial weightbearing supports fibrocartilage repair among implanted cylindrical plugs, further enhancing secure graft incorporation.[1] Normal daily activity can be achieved in 8 to 10 weeks. High-demand sporting activity should be delayed until after 5 to 6 months.

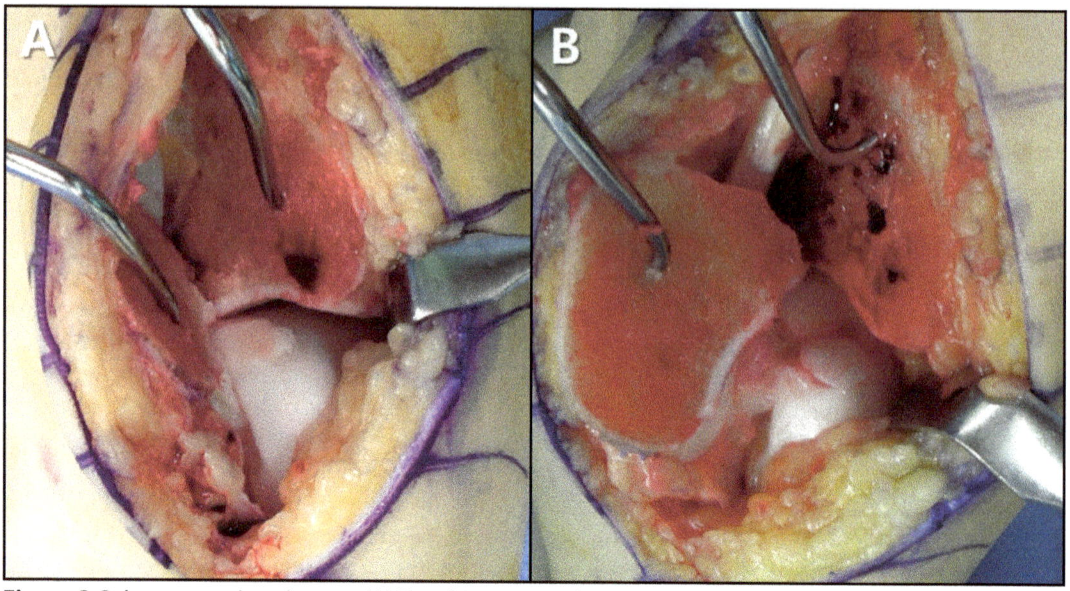

Figure 3-3. Intraoperative pictures. (A) To achieve a good perpendicular view of the targeted osteochondral lesion of medial talar dome, a medial malleolar osteotomy is usually needed. (B) After debridement and curettage of the lesion, the defect with viable cartilage rim and clean bony bed was filled with an osteochondral plug harvested from the nonweightbearing portion of the ipsilateral lateral femoral condyle.

Potential Complications

Reports of donor site morbidity varies from authors, but knee pain after OAT is the most concerning complication. Previous studies with short- to mid-term follow-up reported minimal or no donor site morbidity.[6,24] The reported cases of knee pain usually last for 6 months after the procedure, then subside within 1 year. However, some authors have reported much higher rates of donor site morbidity. Reddy et al[11] reported that 36% (4 of 11) of patients were rated as poor in the Lysholm knee scoring scale after a mean follow-up of 47 months. After a mean follow-up of 72 months, Valderrabano et al[10] reported that over 50% (7 of 12) of patients had mild or severe knee pain. The other 5 patients also had knee pain after the operation that resolved within the first year. In addition to donor site morbidity, small or large bone cyst formation after OAT is another concern. Because the subchondral bone plate is exposed to joint fluid through the gap between the osteochondral plug and the native cartilage, synovial fluid could be pumped into the subchondral bone during gait, which might lead to cyst formation.[25] Other minor complications include nonunion at the osteotomy site, infection, and impingement due to fibrous tissue formed in the ankle joint.

Top Technical Pearls for the Procedure

1. Poor regenerative capacity is expected after a failed arthroscopic marrow stimulation technique; therefore, OAT could be the first-line treatment instead of repeat arthroscopy.[15]

(continued)

2. For perpendicular access to an OLT, adequate exposure through a malleolar osteotomy is the utmost first step. Plan the osteotomy to access at the lateral margin of the medial side OLT.
3. During a medial malleolar osteotomy for medial-side OLT, the final cut should be done using an osteotome rather than a motorized saw to protect the tibialis posterior tendon.
4. Because a talar shoulder lesion lacks structural integrity of surrounding cartilage, place the harvester with special attention. The harvester should be tilted according to the slope of the talar shoulder.
5. Smooth articular surface after OAT should be achieved. In order to prevent proud osteochondral graft plug, the author routinely advances the recipient harvester 1 to 2 mm deeper than the desired osteochondral graft plug. Because the osteochondral graft plug is prepared with a slightly larger diameter, countersinking of the graft is also prevented by press-fit.

References

1. Hangody L, Fules P. Autologous osteochondral mosaicplasty for the treatment of full-thickness defects of weight-bearing joints: ten years of experimental and clinical experience. *J Bone Joint Surg Am.* 2003;85-A(Suppl 2):25-32.
2. Wagner H. Operative behandlung der osteochondrosis dissecans des kniegelenkes. *Z Orthop.* 1964;98:333-355.
3. Matsusue Y, Yamamuro T, Hama H. Arthroscopic multiple osteochondral transplantation to the chondral defect in the knee associated with anterior cruciate ligament disruption. *Arthroscopy.* 1993;9(3):318-321.
4. Hangody L, Kish G, Karpati Z, Szerb I, Eberhardt R. Treatment of osteochondritis dissecans of the talus: use of the mosaicplasty technique—a preliminary report. *Foot Ankle Int.* 1997;18(10):628-634.
5. Hangody L, Kish G, Modis L, et al. Mosaicplasty for the treatment of osteochondritis dissecans of the talus: two to seven year results in 36 patients. *Foot Ankle Int.* 2001;22(7):552-558.
6. Gobbi A, Francisco RA, Lubowitz JH, Allegra F, Canata G. Osteochondral lesions of the talus: randomized controlled trial comparing chondroplasty, microfracture, and osteochondral autograft transplantation. *Arthroscopy.* 2006;22(10):1085-1092.
7. Scranton PE, Jr., Frey CC, Feder KS. Outcome of osteochondral autograft transplantation for type-V cystic osteochondral lesions of the talus. *J Bone Joint Surg Br.* 2006;88(5):614-619.
8. Haleem AM, Ross KA, Smyth NA, et al. Double-plug autologous osteochondral transplantation shows equal functional outcomes compared with single-plug procedures in lesions of the talar dome: a minimum 5-year clinical follow-up. *Am J Sports Med.* 2014;42(8):1888-1895.
9. Savage-Elliott I, Ross KA, Smyth NA, Murawski CD, Kennedy JG. Osteochondral lesions of the talus: a current concepts review and evidence-based treatment paradigm. *Foot Ankle Spec.* 2014;7(5):414-422.
10. Valderrabano V, Leumann A, Rasch H, Egelhof T, Hintermann B, Pagenstert G. Knee-to-ankle mosaicplasty for the treatment of osteochondral lesions of the ankle joint. *Am J Sports Med.* 2009;37(Suppl 1):105S-111S.
11. Reddy S, Pedowitz DI, Parekh SG, Sennett BJ, Okereke E. The morbidity associated with osteochondral harvest from asymptomatic knees for the treatment of osteochondral lesions of the talus. *Am J Sports Med.* 2007;35(1):80-85.
12. Choi WJ, Park KK, Kim BS, Lee JW. Osteochondral lesion of the talus: is there a critical defect size for poor outcome? *Am J Sports Med.* 2009;37(10):1974-1980.
13. Chuckpaiwong B, Berkson EM, Theodore GH. Microfracture for osteochondral lesions of the ankle: outcome analysis and outcome predictors of 105 cases. *Arthroscopy.* 2008;24(1):106-112.

14. Murawski CD, Kennedy JG. Operative treatment of osteochondral lesions of the talus. *J Bone Joint Surg Am*. 2013;95(11):1045-1054.
15. Yoon HS, Park YJ, Lee M, Choi WJ, Lee JW. Osteochondral autologous transplantation is superior to repeat arthroscopy for the treatment of osteochondral lesions of the talus after failed primary arthroscopic treatment. *Am J Sports Med*. 2014;42(8):1896-1903.
16. O'Loughlin PF, Heyworth BE, Kennedy JG. Current concepts in the diagnosis and treatment of osteochondral lesions of the ankle. *Am J Sports Med*. 2010;38(2):392-404.
17. Berndt AL, Harty M. Transchondral fractures (osteochondritis dissecans) of the talus. *J Bone Joint Surg Am*. 1959;41-A:988-1020.
18. Dragoni M, Bonasia DE, Amendola A. Osteochondral talar allograft for large osteochondral defects: technique tip. *Foot Ankle Int*. 2011;32(9):910-916.
19. Anderson IF, Crichton KJ, Grattan-Smith T, Cooper RA, Brazier D. Osteochondral fractures of the dome of the talus. *J Bone Joint Surg Am*. 1989;71(8):1143-1152.
20. Leumann A, Valderrabano V, Plaass C, et al. A novel imaging method for osteochondral lesions of the talus—comparison of SPECT-CT with MRI. *Am J Sports Med*. 2011;39(5):1095-1101.
21. Amendola A, Panarella L. Osteochondral lesions: medial versus lateral, persistent pain, cartilage restoration options and indications. *Foot Ankle Clin*. 2009;14(2):215-227.
22. Sammarco GJ, Makwana NK. Treatment of talar osteochondral lesions using local osteochondral graft. *Foot Ankle Int*. 2002;23:693-698.
23. Kreuz PC, Steinwachs M, Erggelet C, et al. Mosaicplasty with autogenous talar autograft for osteochondral lesions of the talus after failed primary arthroscopic management: a prospective study with a 4-year follow-up. *Am J Sports Med*. 2006;34:55-63.
24. Baltzer AW, Arnold JP. Bone-cartilage transplantation from the ipsilateral knee for chondral lesions of the talus. *Arthroscopy*. 2005;21(2):159-166.
25. Krueger JA, Thisse P, Ewers BJ, Dvoracek-Driksna D, Orth MW, Haut RC. The extent and distribution of cell death and matrix damage in impacted chondral explants varies with the presence of underlying bone. *J Biomech Eng*. 2003;125(1):114-119.

Please visit www.routledge.com/9781617119989 to access additional material.

4

Autologous Chondrocyte Implantation

Adam F. Meisel, MD and Richard D. Ferkel, MD

Introduction

Despite advances in basic science, biologics, and surgical technique, osteochondral lesions of the talus (OLT) remain a challenging problem due to the limited healing potential of cartilage. Surgical treatment in the form of debridement, abrasion arthroplasty, microfracture, and subchondral drilling has been used for the treatment of OLT. Autologous chondrocyte implantation (ACI) has been developed as a method for treating full-thickness cartilage defects using autologous harvested, cultured, and expanded chondrocytes. ACI was developed initially for chondral defects of the knee and was based on the work of Smith, who was able to isolate and culture chondrocytes in a medium ex vivo.[1] Subsequently, Bentley and Greer transplanted isolated chondrocytes into rat tibial defects,[2] and then Grande et al developed a technique for treating full-thickness cartilage defects with expanded chondrocytes,[3] which showed viable chondrocytes and hyaline-like repair tissue on histologic examination.[4] Success with ACI in the knee[5] has led to its use in the ankle for the treatment of OLT.

ACI is a 2-stage procedure. During the first stage, healthy chondrocytes are harvested (usually arthroscopically) from nonweightbearing areas. Potential donor sites include local (ie, the periphery of the OLT, removed loose osteochondral fragments, nonweightbearing talar dome, or tibial plafond) or distant (ie, the ipsilateral intercondylar notch) sites. Candrian et al have shown decreased cartilage-forming capacity from the excised osteochondral fragment, so the authors of this chapter prefer to use the ipsilateral intercondylar notch.[6] A sample of 200 to 300 mg of cartilage is needed and is processed and stored remotely at an outside laboratory facility. The second stage involves implantation of the harvested, isolated, and expanded chondrocytes into the prepared OLT. Both stages will be discussed in further detail.

Classically, ACI involves the use of an autologous periosteal patch sutured over the transplanted chondrocytes to form a watertight seal. Advancements in the field of ACI have lead to the development of second- and third-generation techniques that do not rely on periosteal patches. Second-generation ACI involves the use of a tissue-engineered collagen graft (eg, Chondro-Gide and Bio-Gide [Geistlich Biomaterials]) held in place with suture and fibrin glue to cover the

Stone JW, Kennedy JG, Glazebrook M, eds. *The Foot and Ankle: AANA Advanced Arthroscopic Surgical Techniques* (pp 27-36).

implanted chondrocytes.[7] Third-generation ACI involves the ex-vivo implantation of chondrocytes into a collagen scaffold prior to implantation, obviating the need for a separate patch to be used to cover the graft.[8]

Indications

A patient with a symptomatic OLT who undergoes surgical treatment will usually have a diagnostic arthroscopy of the ankle joint with debridement of the lesion and marrow stimulation (ie, microfracture and/or drilling). ACI is typically used as a second-line treatment option for patients who have failed such procedures. ACI is approved by the United States Food and Drug Administration for the treatment of cartilage defects of the femoral condyle, so the use for OLT is an off-label use.

Indications for ACI for the treatment of symptomatic OLT are as follows:

- Age 15 to 55 years
- Focal lesions with an area > 1.0 cm^2
- Unipolar (ie, nonkissing lesions)
- Contained lesions
- Failure of previous surgery
- May be considered as a primary treatment for large (> 1.5 cm^2) lesions[9] or those with significant subchondral cystic changes[10]

Contraindications

- Hypersensitivity to gentamicin or other aminoglycosides[11]
- Hypersensitivity to materials of bovine origin[11]
- Osteoarthritis
- Uncorrected malalignment and/or instability

Pertinent Physical Findings

Patients presenting with OLT will present with varying amounts and combinations of the following:

- Pain
- Swelling
- Stiffness
- Mechanical symptoms related to activities

A thorough history and physical should be performed, including the following:

- Standing alignment
- Gait analysis
- Instability testing
- Review of prior surgical documentation (if applicable)

Oftentimes, patients' subjective complaints and physical exam findings will reflect the location (medial vs lateral) of an OLT.

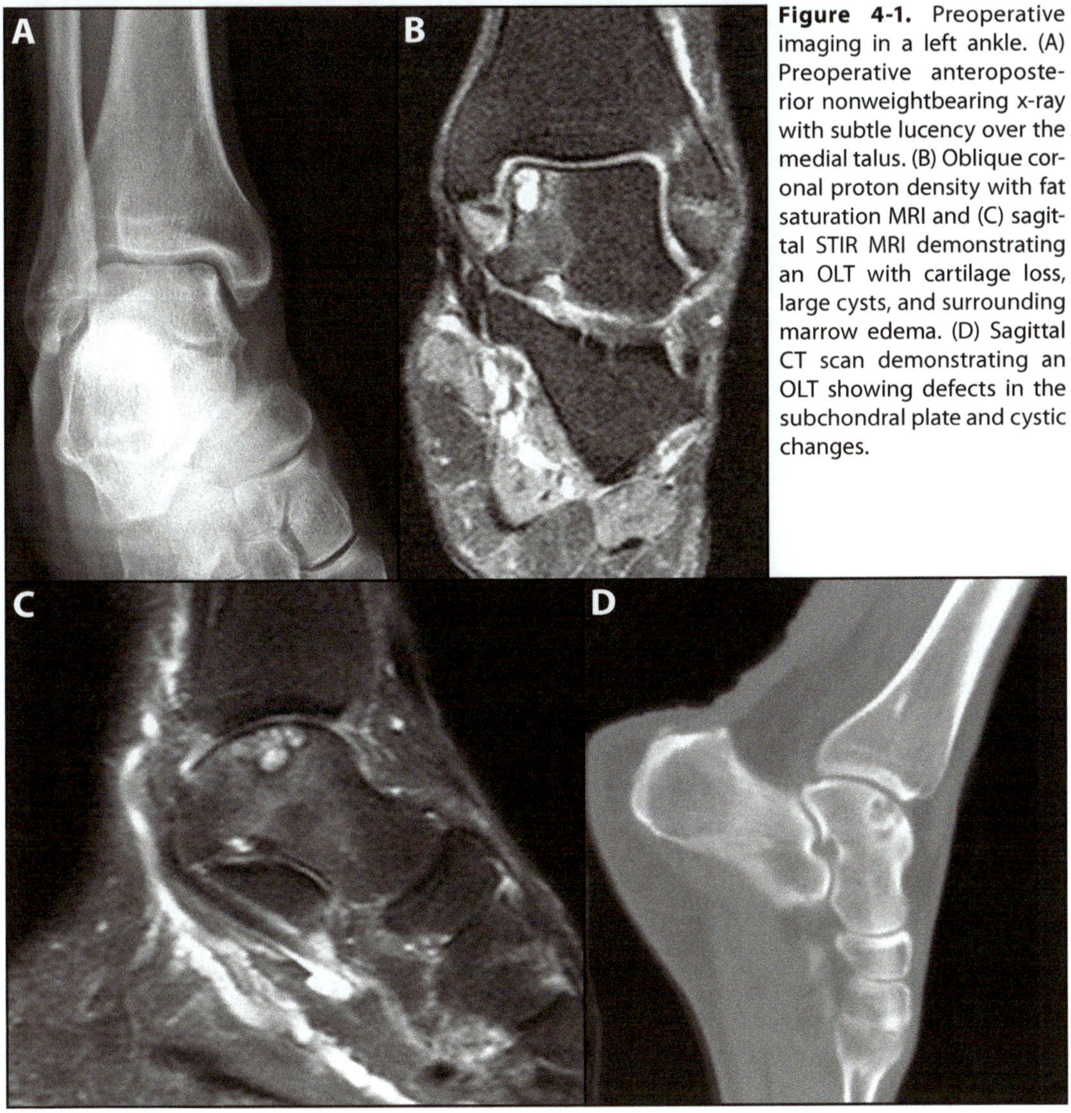

Figure 4-1. Preoperative imaging in a left ankle. (A) Preoperative anteroposterior nonweightbearing x-ray with subtle lucency over the medial talus. (B) Oblique coronal proton density with fat saturation MRI and (C) sagittal STIR MRI demonstrating an OLT with cartilage loss, large cysts, and surrounding marrow edema. (D) Sagittal CT scan demonstrating an OLT showing defects in the subchondral plate and cystic changes.

Pertinent Imaging

- Current and adequate plain radiographs (Figure 4-1A)
  - Weightbearing anteroposterior, mortise, and lateral views as well as stress radiographs if any ligamentous laxity or instability is suspected
- Magnetic resonance imaging (MRI; Figures 4-1B and C)
  - Useful for evaluating articular cartilage and periarticular soft tissues
  - May overestimate the size of the lesion[12]
- Computed tomography (CT) with coronal, axial, and sagittal views (Figure 4-1D)
  - Helpful for localizing and measuring the lesion and preoperative planning

Equipment

The first phase is done arthroscopically in both the knee and ankle joints (see next section). Ankle arthroscopy is performed through the anteromedial, anterolateral, and posterolateral portals using the 30- and 70-degree, 2.7-mm arthroscopes (a 30-degree, 1.9-mm arthroscope may be used for tight joints). Ring curettes and graspers are used in the knee joint as well as a cannula to facilitate graft harvest.[13]

The second phase as described in detail next first involves debriding the lesion to sharp margins using curettes and any other instruments needed to do so effectively. To secure the graft and patch, 6-0 undyed Vicryl suture and fibrin glue are used. An angiocatheter and saline-filled syringe will be needed to test the patch and fill the graft site. At the end of the procedure, appropriate internal fixation devices are needed to fix the osteotomy, and splint/cast materials are needed for immobilizing the ankle.[13]

Positioning and Portals

During the first phase, the ankle arthroscopy is performed in the supine position. The pad is removed from the foot of the table and the nonoperative leg is padded independently to allow greater clearance between the operative ankle and the table. The operative leg is flexed approximately 45 to 50 degrees at both the hip and knee, and the thigh is supported with the use of a Ferkel Thigh Holder (Smith & Nephew). The ankle is distracted using a sterile soft-tissue distractor (GUHL Non-Invasive Ankle Distractor, Smith & Nephew).

During the second phase, the patient positioning and approach to the ankle are dictated by the location of the lesion.

Step-by-Step Description of the Procedure

The first phase of the procedure involves a diagnostic arthroscopy of the ankle (using previously described techniques) to ensure the lesion is appropriate for treatment with ACI. Debridement of the OLT is deferred until implantation, but other areas in the ankle that will not be accessible at the second phase are debrided. The cartilage biopsy is typically taken from the lateral aspect of the intercondylar notch of the ipsilateral knee. Using standard knee arthroscopic portals, a healthy-appearing area of nonweightbearing cartilage on the lateral aspect of the intercondylar notch is identified. Using sharp ring curettes, a piece of cartilage is harvested off of the subchondral bone. The sample is not detached completely with the curette to prevent it from floating free in the knee joint. The cartilage biopsy is amputated from the donor site with a grasper using a gentle twisting motion and removed through a cannula to prevent the piece becoming entrapped in the soft tissue. Approximately 200 to 300 mg of cartilage is needed in total. The sample is stored in chilled sodium chloride in the packaging provided by, and according to the instructions of, Vericel Corporation.

The second phase of the procedure is the implantation phase. A tourniquet is used to maintain a bloodless field. Patient positioning and surgical approach is dictated by the location of the lesion to ensure adequate perpendicular access to it for preparation and implantation (Figure 4-2A). Typically, medial lesions are positioned supine with a bump under the contralateral hip and approached through a medial malleolar osteotomy. The medial malleolus is first predrilled for two 4.0-mm cancellous lag screws (Figure 4-2B), and the location of the osteotomy is confirmed with fluoroscopy. A guide pin is inserted along the osteotomy site to use as a cutting guide for the saw (Figure 4-2C). Care must be taken to ensure the osteotomy exits the tibial plafond lateral

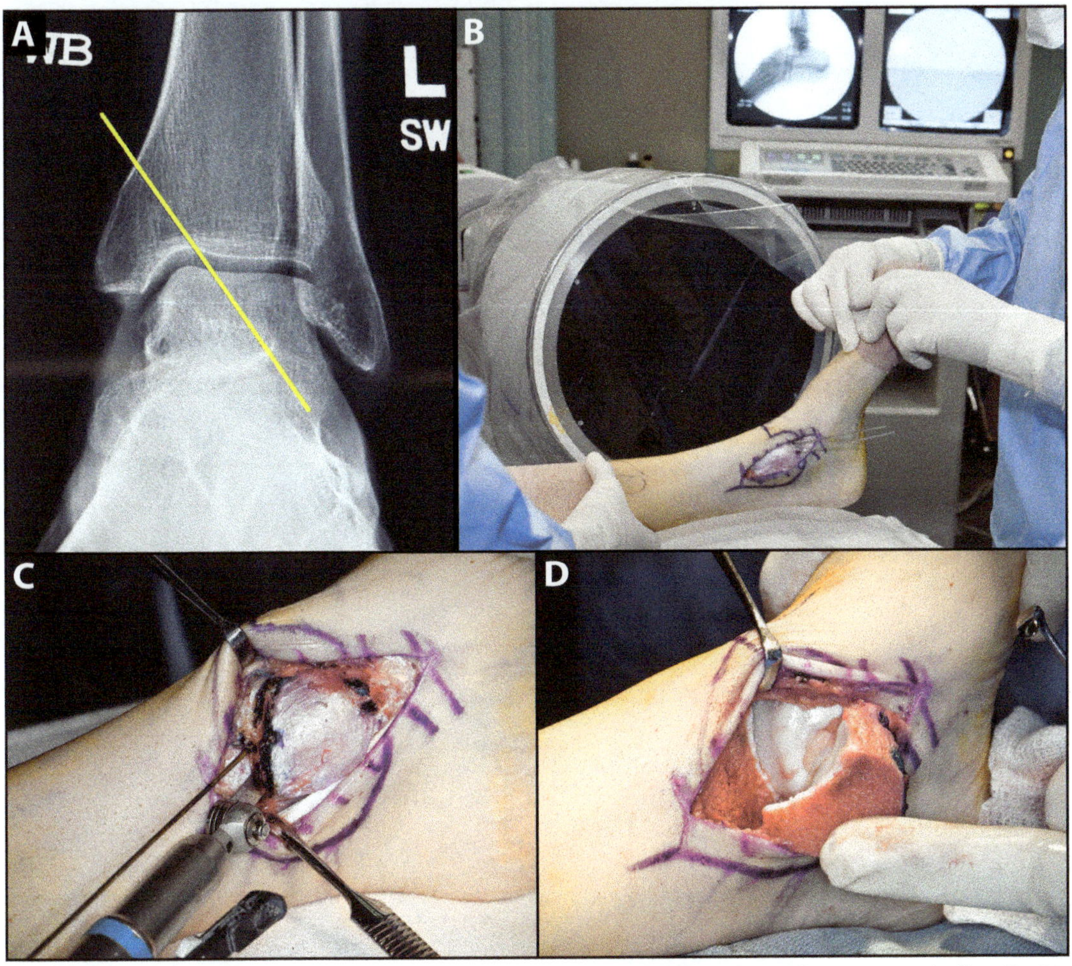

Figure 4-2. Osteotomy of the medial malleolus in a left ankle. (A) The planned osteotomy (yellow line) is templated on an anteroposterior x-ray in the operating room. Note the osteotomy exits lateral to the OLT to allow direct access to the entire lesion. (B) The guide pins are inserted under fluoroscopic guidance to predrill for the two 4.0-mm cannulated screws used to fix the osteotomy. (C) An oscillating saw is used to perform the osteotomy utilizing the pin as a cutting guide. (D) The medial malleolus is reflected inferiorly to allow direct access to the OLT.

to the extent of the OLT to allow access for suturing the periosteal patch (Figure 4-2D). Lateral lesions are accessed by first predrilling the fibula for 2 interfragmentary lag screws and then making an oblique fibular osteotomy. The anterior capsule and anterior talofibular ligament need to be released to allow the fibula to be rotated posteriorly. A cuff of tissue is left on the fibula for later repair.

Once exposure is obtained, the OLT is debrided to stable vertical margins (Figure 4-3A). The subchondral bone should be left intact to prevent bleeding. The tourniquet is then deflated, and thrombin-soaked pledgets are used to dry the lesion as needed. Once the defect is prepared, it is measured so that an appropriately sized periosteal patch or membrane can be obtained; sterile glove packaging can be used as tracing paper to make a template of the lesion (Figure 4-3B). When performing first-generation ACI, a periosteal patch is harvested from the tibia, taking care to note which side is the cambium layer as this should face the subchondral bone.[14] The harvested periosteum should be sized 1 to 2 mm larger than the defect to account for shrinkage.[15] The patch is sutured in place with 6-0 Vicryl interrupted sutures coated with mineral oil[14] (Figure 4-4A) and

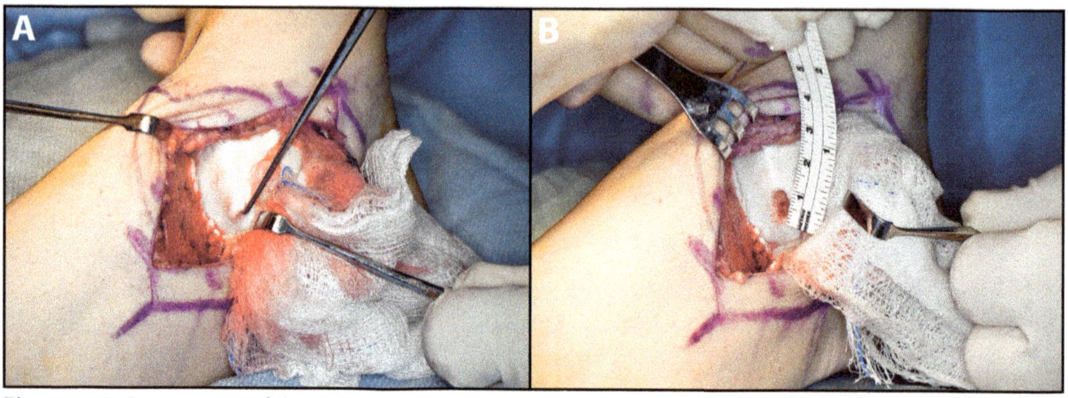

Figure 4-3. Preparation of the OLT in a left ankle. (A) Palpation of the OLT to determine the extent of the lesion. (B) The OLT is completely excised, leaving stable vertical margins, and the lesion is measured.

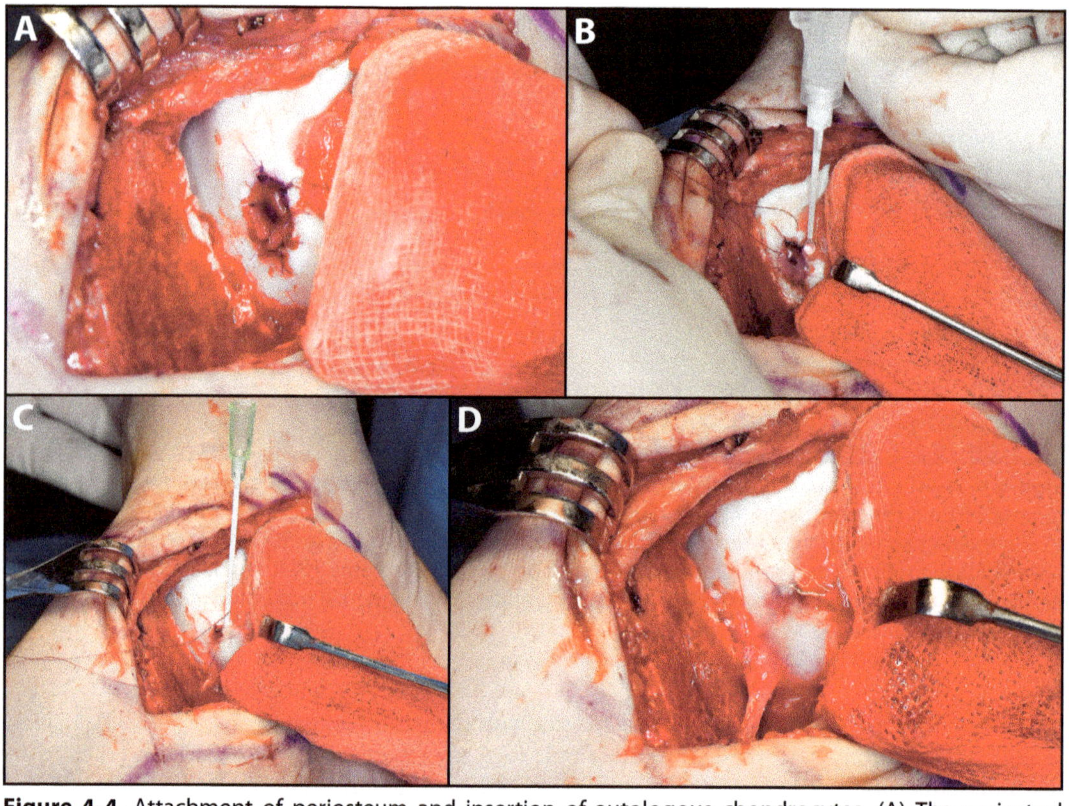

Figure 4-4. Attachment of periosteum and insertion of autologous chondrocytes. (A) The periosteal patch is sutured over the OLT bed with interrupted 6-0 Vicryl sutures. (B) The final suture is passed but not tied, and the periosteal patch is sealed with fibrin glue. (C) An angiocatheter is inserted through the remaining opening to allow delivery of the chondrocytes. (D) After implantation of the chondrocytes, the final suture is tied and the area is sealed with fibrin glue.

sealed with fibrin glue (Figure 4-4B) to ensure a watertight seal around an 18-gauge angiocatheter (Figure 4-4C). The patch is tested with saline injected through the catheter and is reinforced with fibrin glue if needed. The saline is then aspirated out and the catheter left in place. In the presence of large (≥ 8 mm) subchondral defects, the "sandwich" technique may be used.[16] To do this, the base of the defect is first drilled, microfractured, and filled with cancellous autograft,

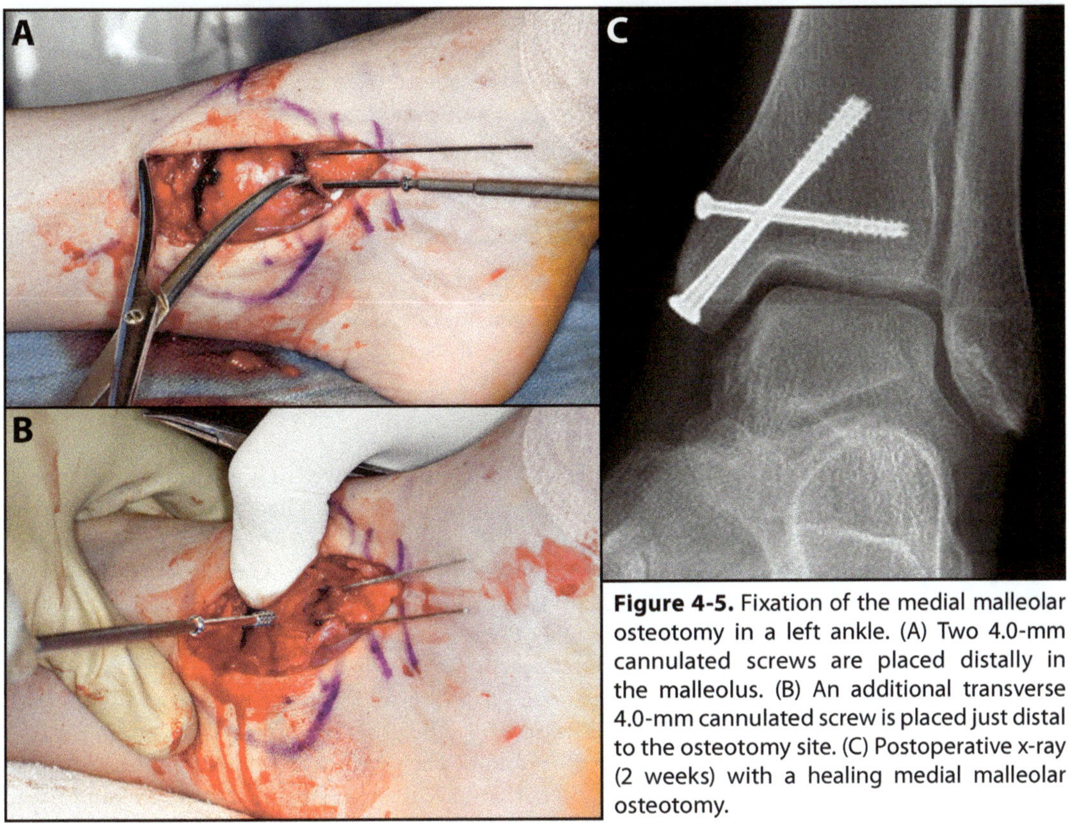

Figure 4-5. Fixation of the medial malleolar osteotomy in a left ankle. (A) Two 4.0-mm cannulated screws are placed distally in the malleolus. (B) An additional transverse 4.0-mm cannulated screw is placed just distal to the osteotomy site. (C) Postoperative x-ray (2 weeks) with a healing medial malleolar osteotomy.

then covered with an appropriately sized periosteal patch. The patch is secured over the bone graft with 6-0 Vicryl sutures and fibrin glue with the cambium layer facing away from the bone graft (toward the joint). The second periosteal patch is then sutured in place with the cambium layer facing toward the defect as described previously and tested for watertightness. The cultured chondrocytes are then injected through the catheter while moving the catheter across the defect to evenly distribute the graft. Once the catheter is removed, additional sutures and fibrin glue are placed to seal its entry site (Figure 4-4D).

Once the graft is placed and sealed, the osteotomy (or arthrotomy) is reduced and repaired. For medial malleolar osteotomies, an additional transverse screw at the proximal portion is used due to the oblique nature of the osteotomy (Figure 4-5). Lateral osteotomies are fixed with the predrilled interfragmentary compression screws and a one-third tubular plate in neutralization fashion. The incisions are closed tightly with 4-0 nylon vertical-mattress sutures, and the leg is placed in a well-padded short-leg cast that is split in the recovery room.

Postoperative Protocol

The postoperative and rehabilitation protocol is essential for avoiding complications and helping to ensure optimal outcomes after ACI. A thorough understanding of the protocol by the physician, patient, and physical therapist as well as a close working relationship with the therapist is an important part of the process.[16] The goals of the rehabilitation protocol are to ensure safe and effective healing of the surgical site and cartilage graft, as well as to return the patient to a functional and enjoyable activity level. There is little high-level direct evidence for this in the treatment of OLT[17]; therefore, parts of the protocol have been extrapolated from research in animal models, known concepts of cartilage physiology, and prior experience with ACI in the knee. While several authors have described their rehabilitation protocols, and they may vary slightly, most agree on the general concepts that will be described next as well as the need for supervision by a skilled physical therapist.[18] The rehabilitation period is divided into 4 phases[19]:

1. Phase 1 is the "healing phase," from surgery to week 6
2. Phase 2 is the "transitional phase," from 6 to 12 weeks
3. Phase 3 is the "remodeling phase," from 12 to 32 weeks
4. Phase 4 is the "maturation phase," from 32 to 52 weeks

The following protocol described is for first-generation ACI; second- and third-generation techniques may allow more rapid rehabilitation protocols as they do not rely on a periosteal patch.

Phase 1: 0 to 6 Weeks

Patients are seen in follow-up and their cast and sutures are removed at 2 weeks postoperatively. At this time, a thromboembolic deterrent compression stocking is applied, patients are placed in a controlled ankle motion (CAM) walking boot, and they are allowed to begin partial weight-bearing with a maximum of about 30 lb through the operative ankle. Gentle range of motion exercises are initiated at 2 weeks in the sagittal plane, and patients may ride a stationary bike without resistance at 4 weeks. At approximately 6 weeks, the patients are allowed to gradually increase their weightbearing toward full weightbearing in a CAM boot as long as the osteotomy is healing appropriately. They are then transitioned to a lace-up figure-of-8 brace and supportive athletic shoes, and formal physical therapy is initiated.[19] The goals of phase 1 are to recover/maintain full range of motion while balancing the need to protect the healing chondrocytes as well as provide the motion and gentle compressive forces that have been shown to stimulate chondrocyte health.[20,21]

Phase 2: 6 to 12 Weeks

During this phase, the focus is on strengthening the musculature around the ankle. Under close guidance and direction of the physical therapist, patients should begin proprioceptive exercises with continued use of the stationary bicycle; however, resistance can gradually be added, and isometric strengthening should lead into eccentric strengthening exercises.[19] During phase 2, the chondrocytes are maturing and can withstand increased compressive loads but are still softer than the final repair.[22] The goals of phase 2 are to increase strength and proprioception before progressing to higher-level activities.

Phase 3: 12 to 32 Weeks

At this point, the patients' activity levels and strengthening can be increased. Patients are encouraged to increase both their walking speed and duration as pain and swelling allow, but they should not be jogging or running yet. Additional strengthening exercises are introduced, including those in weightbearing positions. The goals of phase 3 are to increase strength and endurance, maintain range of motion, and prepare for the introduction of sport-specific activities in phase 4 while the graft continues to mature. In order to progress to sport-specific training, patients should be able to perform 30 minutes of weightbearing exercise without pain and swelling as well as demonstrate full range of motion.[19]

Phase 4: 32 to 52 Weeks

Rehabilitation can now begin to progress to cross training and return-to-sport activities. The graft site should be continuing to mature, and by 8 months should be able to tolerate higher impact and sporting activities. The intensity and duration can be increased under a therapist's guidance as symptoms (lack of pain and swelling) dictate. It is important to remember that the patient will likely be deconditioned from a general standpoint and adequate periods of rest should be afforded in between training sessions. Unrestricted high-impact activities should not be allowed until 12 months from the time of surgery. The graft site may continue to mature and remodel for 2 years postoperatively.[23]

Potential Complications

As with any foot and ankle surgery, potential complications include infection, bleeding, wound breakdown and drainage, neurovascular injury, and incomplete resolution of symptoms. The most common complication specific to ACI that has been described is hypertrophy of the graft and periosteal patch.[24] This can cause persistent pain and mechanical symptoms and has required subsequent surgery for debridement, although this can usually be done arthroscopically.[25] More recently, studies have shown a decreased incidence of patch hypertrophy when second-generation ACI using a collagen-based membrane is used in the knee, which may be beneficial in the ankle as well.[26] Other potential complications of ACI for OLT would also include nonunion of the osteotomy and pain related to the fixation devices.

Top Technical Pearls for the Procedure

1. Ensure the osteotomy site allows direct perpendicular access to the entire lesion (ie, exits the plafond lateral to a medial OLT and medial to a lateral OLT).
2. Perform a thorough debridement of all diseased tissue from the lesion and ensure stable, vertical borders.
3. The periosteal patch should be 1 to 2 mm larger than the defect to allow for shrinkage.
4. The periosteal patch must be sealed watertight, and the cambium layer should be facing toward the graft.
5. Correct any associated malalignment or instability in the ankle.

References

1. Smith A. Survival of frozen chondrocytes isolated from cartilage of adult mammals. *Nature.* 1965;(205):782-784.
2. Bentley G, Greer RB 3rd. Homotransplantation of isolated epiphyseal and articular cartilage chondrocytes into joint surfaces of rabbits. *Nature.* 1971;230(5293):385-388.
3. Grande DA, Pitman MI, Peterson L, Menche D, Klein M. The repair of experimentally produced defects in rabbit articular cartilage by autologous chondrocyte transplantation. *J Orthop Res.* 1989;7(2):208-218.
4. Brittberg M, Lindahl A, Nilsson A, Ohlsson C, Isaksson O, Peterson L. Treatment of deep cartilage defects in the knee with autologous chondrocyte transplantation. *N Engl J Med.* 1994;331(14):889-895.
5. Peterson L, Vasiliadis HS, Brittberg M, Lindahl A. Autologous chondrocyte implantation: a long-term follow-up. *Am J Sports Med.* 2010;38(6):1117-1124.
6. Candrian C, Miot S, Wolf F, et al. Are ankle chondrocytes from damaged fragments a suitable cell source for cartilage repair? *Osteoarthritis Cartilage.* 2010;18(8):1067-1076.

7. Brittberg M. Autologous chondrocyte implantation--technique and long-term follow-up. *Injury.* 2008;39(Suppl 1):S40-49.
8. Hettrich CM, Crawford D, Rodeo SA. Cartilage repair: third-generation cell-based technologies—basic science, surgical techniques, clinical outcomes. *Sports Med Arthrosc.* 2008;16(4):230-235.
9. Choi WJ, Park KK, Kim BS, Lee JW. Osteochondral lesion of the talus: is there a critical defect size for poor outcome? *Am J Sports Med.* 2009;37(10):1974-1980.
10. Kumai T, Takakura Y, Higashiyama I, Tamai S. Arthroscopic drilling for the treatment of osteochondral lesions of the talus. *J Bone Joint Surg Am.* 1999;81(9):1229-1235.
11. Genzyme. Carticel (autologous cultured chondrocytes). *U.S. Food and Drug Administration website.* http://www.fda.gov/downloads/BiologicsBloodVaccines/CellularGeneTherapyProducts/ApprovedProducts/UCM109339.pdf. Accessed August 27, 2015.
12. Verhagen RAW, Maas M, Dijkgraaf MGW, Tol JL, Krips R, van Dijk CN. Prospective study on diagnostic strategies in osteochondral lesions of the talus. Is MRI superior to helical CT? *J Bone Joint Surg Br.* 2005;87(1):41-46.
13. Coughlin MJ, Saltzman CL, Anderson RB. *Mann's Surgery of the Foot and Ankle Vol 1.* 9th ed. Philadelphia, PA: Saunders/Elsevier; 2014.
14. Nam EK, Ferkel RD, Applegate GR. Autologous chondrocyte implantation of the ankle: a 2- to 5-year follow-up. *Am J Sports Med.* 2009;37(2):274-284.
15. Kwak SK, Kern BS, Ferkel RD, Chan KW, Kasraeian S, Applegate GR. Autologous chondrocyte implantation of the ankle: 2- to 10-year results. *Am J Sports Med.* 2014;42(9):2156-2164.
16. Mandelbaum BR, Gerhardt MB, Peterson L. Autologous chondrocyte implantation of the talus. *Arthroscopy.* 2003;19(Suppl 1):129-137.
17. Hambly K, Bobic V, Wondrasch B, Van Assche D, Marlovits S. Autologous chondrocyte implantation postoperative care and rehabilitation: science and practice. *Am J Sports Med.* 2006;34(6):1020-1038.
18. Larsen NJ, Sullivan M, Ferkel RD. Autologous chondrocyte implantation for treatment of osteochondral lesions of the talus. *Oper Tech Orthop.* 2014;24(3):195-209.
19. Antkowiak T, Ferkel R, Sullivan M, Kreulen C, Giza E, Whitlow S. Rehabilitation after cartilage reconstruction. In: van Dijk CN, Kennedy JG, eds. *Talar Osteochondral Defects.* Berlin, Germany: Springer; 2014:135-144. http://dx.doi.org/10.1007/978-3-642-45097-6_16. Accessed August 27, 2015.
20. Cohen NP, Foster RJ, Mow VC. Composition and dynamics of articular cartilage: structure, function, and maintaining healthy state. *J Orthop Sports Phys Ther.* 1998;28(4):203-215.
21. Brittberg M, Peterson L, Sjogren-Jansson E, Tallheden T, Lindahl A. Articular cartilage engineering with autologous chondrocyte transplantation. A review of recent developments. *J Bone Joint Surg Am.* 2003;85-A(Suppl 3):109-115.
22. Gillogly SD, Myers TH. Treatment of full-thickness chondral defects with autologous chondrocyte implantation. *Orthop Clin North Am.* 2005;36(4):433-446.
23. Giannini S, Buda R, Vannini F, Di Caprio F, Grigolo B. Arthroscopic autologous chondrocyte implantation in osteochondral lesions of the talus: surgical technique and results. *Am J Sports Med.* 2008;36(5):873-880.
24. Zaslav K, Cole B, Brewster R, et al. A prospective study of autologous chondrocyte implantation in patients with failed prior treatment for articular cartilage defect of the knee: results of the Study of the Treatment of Articular Repair (STAR) clinical trial. *Am J Sports Med.* 2009;37(1):42-55.
25. Cole BJ, DeBerardino T, Brewster R, et al. Outcomes of autologous chondrocyte implantation in Study of the Treatment of Articular Repair (STAR) patients with osteochondritis dissecans. *Am J Sports Med.* 2012;40(9):2015-2022.
26. Gomoll AH, Probst C, Farr J, Cole BJ, Minas T. Use of a type I/III bilayer collagen membrane decreases reoperation rates for symptomatic hypertrophy after autologous chondrocyte implantation. *Am J Sports Med.* 2009;37(Suppl 1):20S-23S.

Please visit www.routledge.com/9781617119989 to access additional material.

5

Osteochondral Lesions of the Talar Dome

Matrix-Induced Autologous Chondrocyte Implantation

Alberto Gobbi, MD; Georgios Karnatzikos, MD; and Dnyanesh Lad, MD

Introduction

Osteochondral lesions of the talus (OLT) may occur due to a multitude of reasons. These include trauma (the most common cause); vascular compromise; genetic, endocrine, or morphologic abnormalities; or idiopathic phenomena.[1,2] The exact incidence remains unknown and threatens to be higher than what has been reported.[3] These defects can cause swelling, pain, and instability and lead to degenerative changes of the ankle joint. Cartilage damage following ankle fractures has been proven as an independent predictor of the development of posttraumatic osteoarthritis (OA); specifically, lesions on the anterior and lateral aspects of the talus and on the medial malleolus correlate with an unfavorable clinical outcome. In most cases, the mechanism of injury is an inversion injury to the lateral ligamentous complex. Patients typically present with chronic ankle pain along with intermittent swelling and possibly weakness, stiffness, instability, and giving way.[4,5]

Treatment options include both nonsurgical and surgical measures depending on the severity and location of the lesion. Nonsurgical treatment includes restricted weightbearing and immobilization. The aim of surgery is to repair the chondral defect and decrease or limit the premature onset of OA. Articular cartilage has limited intrinsic healing potential due to its avascular and aneural nature; therefore, it is important to restore a normal or near-normal articular cartilage. Among surgical options, the most commonly utilized are drilling (usually reserved for intact lesions), internal fixation of the fragment, cartilage debridement with curettage (shaving) or abrasion of the bone bed, microfracture, and autologous chondrocyte implantation (ACI).[1,3-9] However, a technique that can be considered as the "gold standard" has not yet been established.

First-generation ACI is a 2-step procedure requiring a mini-arthrotomy approach and periosteum harvesting from the proximal tibia as a scaffold; however, it increases the local morbidity.[10,11] Many authors demonstrated in their series satisfactory results at medium- and long-term follow-up using first-generation ACI in the ankle.[12,13] However, this technique has been considered a demanding procedure as it is very difficult to suture a periosteal patch in a narrow joint and manage a liquid culture solution in a hermetic way.[13] In second-generation ACI, periosteum was

Stone JW, Kennedy JG, Glazebrook M, eds. *The Foot and Ankle: AANA Advanced Arthroscopic Surgical Techniques* (pp 37-46).

exchanged with a resorbable membrane out of collagen. The evolution of this technique represents the third-generation ACI that consists of either chondrocytes grown on scaffold carriers or within a porous matrix. The third-generation ACI was named *matrix-induced ACI* (MACI) because of the use of a matrix seeded with chondrocytes; however, the term *MACI* should be distinguished from the MACI product (European Medicines Agency), which is the commercial name of a membrane. This technique offers the advantage of an all-arthroscopic surgery as there is no need for harvesting the periosteal flap. Complications such as graft hypertrophy and ossification are also avoided with the use of the newer scaffolds.[14,15]

Associated pathologies such as ligament insufficiency should be addressed in a concomitant procedure in order to provide an identical mechanical environment and protect the cartilage from additional damage.

Indications

- Symptomatic full-thickness cartilage defects with stable edges of the surrounding cartilage and intact subchondral plate
- Osteochondral lesions with necrotic bone or fibrous tissue base
- Focal lesions with a size > 1.0 cm^2
- Patients younger than 50 years of age
- Body mass index ≤ 35
- Compliance to follow postoperative rehabilitation protocol and weightbearing restrictions
- After failed conservative treatment (≥ 2 months)
- After failed previous surgery for cartilage repair such as drilling or microfracture

Controversial Indications

- Ankle OA/rheumatoid arthritis
- "Kissing lesions" involving both the talus and tibia
- Patients older than 50 years or younger than 15 years of age
- Axial malalignment or ligamentous insufficiency (should be corrected in a previous or concomitant procedure)

Pertinent Physical Findings

- In the acute situation, OLT often remain undistinguishable from pain and swelling associated with the lateral ligamentous complex.
- Persistence of swelling, limitation of movements, and pain on weightbearing 4 to 6 weeks after initial injury may indicate an OLT.
- Locking and catching may indicate a displaced osteochondral fragment.
- Chronic lesions present with pain after activity, lack of localized tenderness, and reduced range of motion; reactive swelling and stiffness are the key findings in this situation that suggest OLT.
- Joint laxity may be noted on anterior drawer testing and should be compared with the contralateral ankle.

- Talar tilt testing may also be positive.
- Tenderness may be elicited behind the medial malleolus when the ankle is dorsiflexed, indicating a posteromedial lesion.
- Anterolateral lesions are tender when the anterolateral ankle joint is palpated with the joint in maximal plantarflexion.
- Despite advances in the field of medicine, OLT still poses a diagnostic and therapeutic dilemma.

Pertinent Imaging

- Plain film
  - In case of a large lesion, the initial radiographs (mortise and lateral views) may show an area of radiolucency.
  - X-rays may detect a displaced fragment.
  - Radiographs are insensitive in grading lower-stage lesions and are inadequate in predicting stability.
- Computed tomography (CT)
  - CT is easily able to detect displaced defects.
  - CT is required when the definition of a bone fragment is desired.
- Bone scintigraphy may show increased radionuclide uptake in the talar dome.
- Magnetic resonance imaging (MRI)
  - MRI is generally considered the modality of choice with high sensitivity and specificity for the detection of separation of the osteochondral fragment.
  - MRI is useful for the diagnosis of concomitant soft tissue pathology and lesion affecting only the cartilage and not underlying osseous structure.
  - T1-weighted imaging may show a variable signal with an intermediate to low signal adjacent to fragment and variable fragment signal.
  - T2-weighted images show a high-intensity signal (rim sign) demarcating the fragment from bone.
    - This usually indicates an unstable lesion; however, false positives can result from edema.
    - Loose bodies usually show a low-intensity signal outlined by high signal fluid. Donor defect is filled with high intensity fluid, and subchondral cysts may be evident.
  - Delayed gadolinium-enhanced MRI of cartilage at 3 T has been proven feasible to assess the thin cartilage layers of the ankle and evaluate the quality of repair tissue after cartilage surgery.[16]

Equipment

- Noninvasive Ankle Distractor Set (Smith & Nephew; distractor head, distractor post, bed rail clamp, ankle distractor case, and ankle distraction strap)
- Small joint limb holder

- 5-mm cannula and obturator
- 2.7-mm and 4.5-mm arthroscopic trocar and cannula (30-degree angled scope)
- Curette, angled ring, straight shaft, 100 mm
- Curette, straight ring, straight shaft, 100 mm
- Grasper, pointed straight tip, 2.75 mm, straight shaft
- Small joint osteotome, angled up
- Small joint osteotome, straight standard arthroscopic equipment
- Noninvasive ankle distractor

Scaffolds

The criteria for the design of cartilage repair scaffold[17] are as follows:

- Biocompatibility: Both the intact scaffold and its degradation products must produce "friendly" break-down products.
- Porosity: Sufficiently porous to allow in-growth of host tissue
- Mechanical strength: To withstand implantation procedure and mechanical forces at joint surface
- Retainability: If easily dislodged, delivery of cells or growth factors is of little use.

Among the natural and synthetic materials that have been investigated, few have been used in ankle lesions, probably due to the lack of studies in the field of ankle tissue regeneration.

- Hyaluronan (hyaluronic acid, HA) is a naturally occurring and highly conserved glycosaminoglycan that is widely distributed in the body. It has proven to be an ideal molecule for tissue-engineering strategies in cartilage repair given its impressive multifunctional activity through its structural and biological role. Hyaluronan-based scaffolds are entirely based on the benzylic ester of hyaluronic acid and consist of a network of 15- to 20-µm–thick fibers, with interstices of variable sizes, which has been demonstrated to be a good physical support to allow cell-to-cell contacts, cluster formation, and extracellular matrix deposition.

  Specifically, scaffold based on hyaluronan-based biomaterial (Hyaff-11), a derivative of HA, has been shown to provide successful tissue-engineered repair of cartilage in a 2-step MACI procedure (Hyalograft C, Anika Therapeutics)[14,15] or a 1-step procedure (Hyalofast, Anika Therapeutics), utilizing bone marrow–derived mesenchymal stem cells (MSCs).[18]
- Bioseed C (BioTissue Technologies) scaffold is composed of fibrin, polyglycolic/polylactic acid, and polydioxanone.
- Neocart (Histogenics Corporation) consists of a 3-dimensional (3D) type I collagen scaffold seeded with autologous chondrocytes that then undergo development in a bioreactor.
- Novocart 3D (B. Braun-Tetec) comprises autologous chondrocytes embedded in a 3D collagen-chondroitin sulphate scaffold.
- CaReS (Ars Arthro) consists of autologous chondrocytes seeded on 3D type I collagen gel. The cells are isolated and mixed with collagen and, after complete gelling and 2 weeks of culturing, the chondrocyte-loaded gel is available for transplantation.
- Chondron (Sewon Cellontech Co) is another gel-type ACI.
- MaioRegen (Fin-Ceramica Faenza) is an osteochondral nanostructured biomimetic scaffold with a porous, tri-layered structure that can reproduce the cartilaginous layer, tide mark, and subchondral bone.

Positioning and Portals

Positioning of the patient is the same as a standard arthroscopy of the ankle in a supine straight-leg position. A thigh tourniquet is applied and the leg is prepared and draped. A thigh holder is used to secure the femur in approximately 60 degrees. Noninvasive distraction of the ankle joint is applied with the use of a sterile clamp attached to a bar and ankle strap, which is placed around the heel and midfoot.

Step-by-Step Description of the Procedure

The first step is a conventional ankle arthroscopy for evaluation and debridement of the lesions and cartilage biopsy.

- In the ankle joint, the cartilage is very thin, so harvesting a sufficient amount of cartilage tissue would result in a large cartilage lesion likely to cause symptoms.
- Cartilage is harvested from the nonweightbearing areas of the joint (anterior part of the talus). Peripheral superolateral medial or lateral femoral condyle or the intercondylar notch of the ipsilateral knee might be used for harvesting chondrocytes as well. Damaged cartilage from the talus can be used as a reliable source for chondrocyte cell harvesting.[19]
- Sufficient amounts of cartilage are obtained depending on the size of the defect to be repaired: 2 or 3 cartilage cylinders of 3-mm diameter are harvested, placed in a medium at 5°C to maintain the cold chain, and transported to the manufacturer of the scaffold.
- After enzymatic breakdown of the matrix and isolation of the chondrocytes, the cells are cultured and seeded on a scaffold until the desired cell population is achieved, which normally takes 2 to 3 weeks.
- The quality of the chondrocytes at the time of implantation is crucial for the outcome; the number of morphological abnormal cells is correlated with a poor clinical outcome.[20]

The second step is cell-scaffold composite implantation, either using an arthroscopic or mini-arthrotomy technique. A thorough understanding of ankle anatomy and biomechanics is important to reduce complications and obtain good surgical outcomes.[21]

- Arthroscopic technique offers several advantages, the most important being reduction of the surgical trauma.
- A mini-arthrotomy might be required to access the lesion. A medial or lateral incision can be performed in a tourniquet-controlled bloodless field depending on the location of the defect. In some medial and posterior lesions, a malleolar osteotomy could be necessary to obtain access to the defect.
- The defect is then debrided in order to obtain stable and vertical edges down from the surface to the subchondral bone while avoiding damage on the subchondral bone (Figures 5-1A through D).
- A template of the lesion is prepared and the cell-scaffold composite is fashioned for accurate fit and no leakage of cells.
- The graft is then implanted into the defect area (Figures 5-1E and F).
- Fibrin glue is used to achieve "watertight" closure. The wound is then closed in layers.
- Bony defects or the pathologic involvement of the subchondral bone deeper than 5 to 6 mm require concomitant bone grafting to recreate the subchondral bone architecture.
- Any ligamentous instability may jeopardize the mechanical properties of the graft. Therefore, reconstruction of the ligaments is advised to achieve a stable joint.

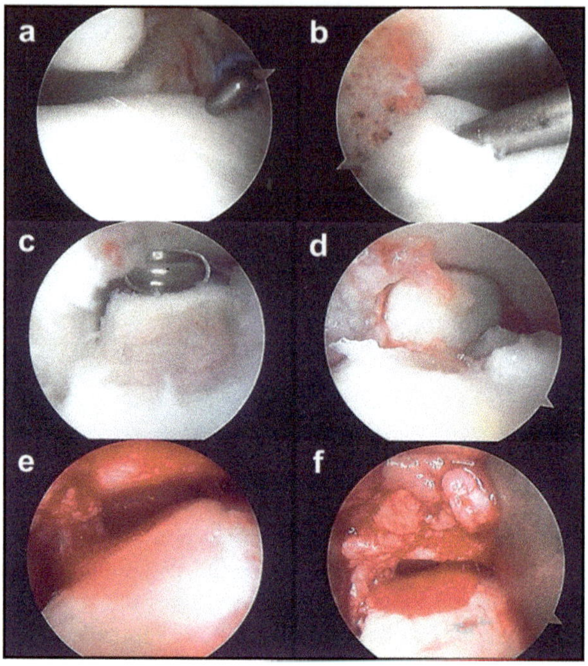

Figure 5-1. MACI technique. (A through D) Evaluation and debridement of the cartilage defect and (E, F) cell-scaffold composite implantation into the defect area.

Postoperative Protocol

Second-generation cephalosporin antibiotic is given for 48 hours and a pharmacological thromboprophylaxis for 3 weeks.

A brace is placed and calibrated to allow motion of 15 degrees plantarflexion and 15 degrees dorsiflexion for 6 weeks. Continuous passive motion is begun 6 to 8 hours after surgery and is used intermittently throughout the hospitalization, usually for 2 to 3 days. The patient is then encouraged to continue with active range of motion exercises.

Consequently, the patient is allowed to use crutches with limited weightbearing (20 kg) for the first 6 weeks. Gradual increase in weightbearing is then commenced every week until full weightbearing is achieved in week 8 to 10.

Once the brace is removed, pool exercises are encouraged. As full weightbearing is reached, gait training is started along with long-distance walking and bicycling.

Functional exercises in closed chain are also incorporated into the rehabilitation program.

Motion and proprioceptive training is continued throughout the rehabilitation; running and plyometric exercises are allowed only after 6 months.

Potential Complications

In rare cases, the harvested chondrocytes are not suitable for culture. Typical causes are avital cells or contamination. In addition, delayed union in the malleolar osteotomy is possible. Major complications include disturbed fusion of the regenerative cartilage and the healthy surrounding cartilage, insufficient regenerative cartilage, and delamination.

Postsurgery pain may persist. The source of pain remains ill-defined and the success of cartilage resurfacing procedures is not 100%.

General surgical complications such as deep venous thrombosis, wound healing problems, or infection can occur.

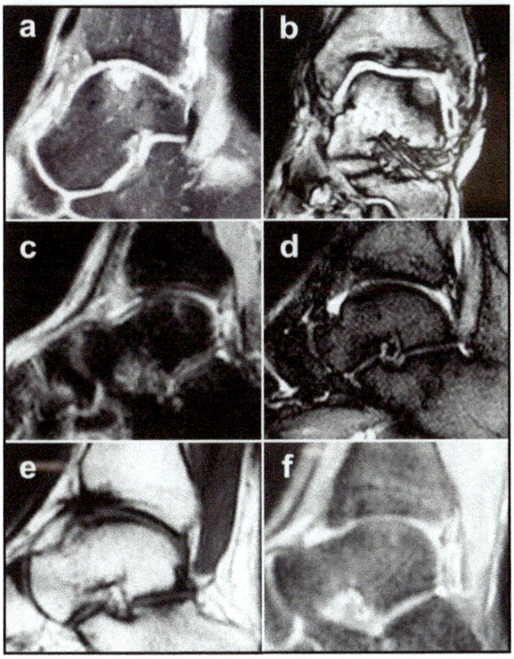

Figure 5-2. MRI after MACI technique. (A, B) Preoperative images and results at (C) 6, (D) 12, and (E, F) 24 months postoperatively.

Results and Future Directions: One-Step Surgery With Mesenchymal Stem Cells

MACI is a safe procedure for the treatment of OLT and can be performed arthroscopically with overall good clinical and MRI results (Figure 5-2). Significant improvement in pain and function has been reported after MACI over medium-term follow-up.[22-26] However, the need of 2 operations and the high cost for chondrocyte culture remain the major problems in performing MACI technique.

Evolution in tissue engineering and regenerative medicine provided new approaches in cartilage repair and the possibility to perform one-step surgery.[27,28] In this regard, the use of MSCs and growth factors offer the possibility to avoid the first surgery (biopsy) and subsequent chondrocyte cultivation. MSCs have a high proliferation and multilineage differentiation potential into adipogenic, osteogenic, and chondrogenic cells. Once MSCs are cultured in the appropriate microenvironment, they can differentiate to chondrocytes and form cartilage.[29,30]

Surgical Technique

Positioning of the patient is of a standard arthroscopy of the ankle (supine straight-leg position). A conventional ankle arthroscopic evaluation is initially performed to evaluate the condition of the joint and confirm the MRI findings with regard to the size and location of the lesions. Bone marrow is harvested from the ipsilateral iliac crest using a dedicated aspiration kit and centrifuged using a commercially available system (Arthrex Angel System) to obtain a concentration of bone marrow cells. With the use of Batroxobin enzyme (Plateltex Act), the bone marrow concentrate is activated to produce a sticky clot material. Next, the ankle is approached either using an arthroscopic or mini-arthrotomy technique depending on the location of the lesions (similarly to the second step of MACI technique), and the chondral defects are prepared. A 3D Hyaff-11 scaffold (Hyalofast) is fashioned according to the defect size. Finally, the prepared clot is implanted into the prepared cartilage defect and covered with a pre-sized scaffold, which is sealed with fibrin glue (Tissucol, Baxter Spa).

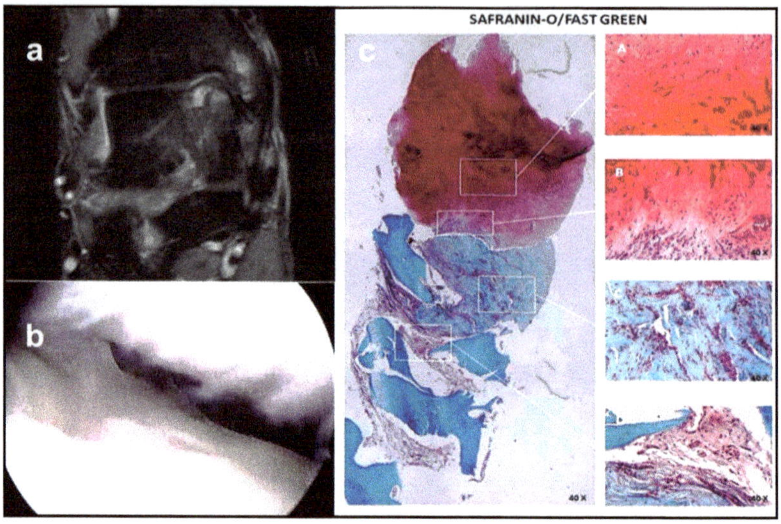

Figure 5-3. (A) Osteochondral lesion of talar dome treated with MSC implantation. (B) Second-look arthroscopy and (C) histologic findings at 12-month follow-up.

Preliminary results are promising and the treatment shows good clinical outcomes at early- and medium-term follow-up.[31,32] MSCs implantation is a new technique with potential advantages including a single-step surgery, no need of cartilage biopsy, and cell cultivation, thus reducing the total cost (Figure 5-3).

Top Technical Pearls for the Procedure

1. Bone marrow-derived MSCs implantation is a single-step surgical technique with potential advantages.
2. An accurate debridement is essential in order to establish a stable lesion rim.
3. Special attention should be paid to the preparation of the shoulder of the lesion.
4. Ensure the clot and scaffold are well secured.
5. Postoperative rehabilitation with early motion is paramount.

References

1. Stone JW. Osteochondral lesions of the talar dome. *J Acad Orthop Surg.* 1996;4:63-73.
2. Takao M, Ochi M, Uchio Y, Naito K, Kono T, Oae K. Osteochondral lesions of the talar dome associated with trauma. *Arthroscopy.* 2003;19(10):1061-1067.
3. Giannini S, Vannini F. Operative treatment of osteochondral lesions of the talar dome. *Curr Concepts Rev Foot Ankle Int.* 2004;25:168-175.
4. Murawski CD, Kennedy JG. Operative treatment of osteochondral lesions of the talus. *J Bone Joint Surg Am.* 2013;95(11):1045-1054.
5. Van Dijk CN, Reilingh ML, Zengerink M, Van Bergen CJA. Osteochondral defects in the ankle: why painful? *Knee Surg Sports Traumatol Arthrosc.* 2010;18(5):570-580.
6. Hannon CP, Murawski CD, Fansa AM, Smyth NA, Do H, Kennedy JG. Microfracture for osteochondral lesions of the talus: a systematic review of reporting of outcome data. *Am J Sports Med.* 2013;41(3):689-695.

7. van Bergen CJ, Kox LS, Maas M, Sierevelt IN, Kerkhoffs GM, van Dijk CN. Arthroscopic treatment of osteochondral defects of the talus: outcomes at eight to twenty years of follow-up. *J Bone Joint Surg Am.* 2013;95(6):519-525.
8. Ferkel RD, Zanotti RM, Komenda GA, et al. Arthroscopic treatment of chronic osteochondral lesions of the talus: long-term results. *Am J Sports Med.* 2008;36(9):1750-1762.
9. Gobbi A, Ramces F, Lubowitz J, Allegra F, Canata G. Osteochondral lesions of the talus: randomized controlled trial comparing chondroplasty, microfracture, and osteochondral autograft transplantation. *Arthroscopy.* 2006;22(10):1085-1092.
10. Brittberg M, Lindahl A, Nilsson A, Ohlsson C, Isaksson O, Peterson L. Treatment of deep cartilage defects in the knee with autologous chondrocyte transplantation. *N Engl J Med.* 1994;331(14):889-895.
11. Peterson L, Vasiliadis HS, Brittberg M, Lindahl A. Autologous chondrocyte implantation: a long-term follow-up. *Am J Sports Med.* 2010;38(6):1117-1124.
12. Giannini S, Battaglia M, Buda R, Cavallo M, Ruffilli A, Vannini F. Surgical treatment of osteochondral lesions of the talus by open-field autologous chondrocyte implantation: a 10-year follow-up clinical and magnetic resonance imaging T2-mapping evaluation. *Am J Sports Med.* 2009;37(Suppl 1):112S-118S.
13. Kreuz PC, Steinwachs M, Erggelet C, et al. Classification of graft hypertrophy after autologous chondrocyte implantation of full-thickness chondral defects in the knee. *Osteoarthritis Cartilage.* 2007;15(12):1339-1347.
14. Marcacci M, Berruto M, Brocchetta D, et al. Articular cartilage engineering with Hyalograft C: 3-year clinical results. *Clin Orthop Relat Res.* 2005;435:96-105.
15. Gobbi A, Kon E, Berruto M, et al. Patellofemoral full-thickness chondral defects treated with Hyalograft-C: a clinical, arthroscopic, and histologic review. *Am J Sports Med.* 2006;34:1763-1773.
16. Domayer SE, Trattnig S, Stelzeneder D, et al. Delayed gadolinium-enhanced MRI of cartilage in the ankle at 3 T: feasibility and preliminary results after matrix-associated autologous chondrocyte implantation. *J Magn Reson Imaging.* 2010;31(3):732-739.
17. Frenkel S, Di Cesare P. Scaffolds for articular cartilage repair. *Ann Biomed Eng.* 2004;32(1):26-34.
18. Gobbi A, Chaurasia S, Karnatzikos G, Nakamura N. Matrix-induced autologous chondrocyte implantation versus multipotent stem cells for the treatment of large patellofemoral chondral lesions: a nonrandomized prospective trial. *Cartilage.* 2015;6(2):82-97.
19. Kreulen C, Giza E, Kim J, Campanelli V, Sullivan M. Viability of talus osteochondral defect cartilage for chondrocyte harvesting: results of 151 patients. *Foot Ankle Int.* 2014;35(4):341-345.
20. Pietschmann MF, Horng A, Niethammer T, et al. Cell quality affects clinical outcome after MACI procedure for cartilage injury of the knee. *Knee Surg Sports Traumatol Arthrosc.* 2009;17(11):1305-1311.
21. Frank RM, Hsu AR, Gross CE, Walton DM, Lee S. Open and arthroscopic surgical anatomy of the ankle. *Anat Res Int.* 2013;2013:182650.
22. Aurich M, Bedi HS, Smith PJ, et al. Arthroscopic treatment of osteochondral lesions of the ankle with matrix-associated chondrocyte implantation: early clinical and magnetic resonance imaging results. *Am J Sports Med.* 2011;39(2):311-319.
23. Dixon S, Harvey L, Baddour E, Janes G, Hardisty G. Functional outcome of matrix-associated autologous chondrocyte implantation in the ankle. *Foot Ankle Int.* 2011;32(4):368-374.
24. Anders S, Goetz J, Schubert T, Grifka J, Schaumburger J. Treatment of deep articular talus lesions by matrix associated autologous chondrocyte implantation—results at five years. *Int Orthop.* 2012;36(11):2279-2285.
25. Magnan B, Samaila E, Bondi M, Vecchini E, Micheloni GM, Bartolozzi P. Three-dimensional matrix-induced autologous chondrocytes implantation for osteochondral lesions of the talus: midterm results. *Adv Orthop.* 2012;2012:942174.
26. Apprich S, Trattnig S, Welsch GH, et al. Assessment of articular cartilage repair tissue after matrix-associated autologous chondrocyte transplantation or the microfracture technique in the ankle joint using diffusion-weighted imaging at 3 Tesla. *Osteoarthritis Cartilage.* 2012;20(7):703-711. Epub 2012 Mar 21. Erratum in: *Osteoarthritis Cartilage.* 2012;20(9):1056. Sokolwski, M [corrected to Sokolowski, M].
27. Correia SI, Pereira H, Silva-Correia J, et al. Current concepts: tissue engineering and regenerative medicine applications in the ankle joint. *J R Soc Interface.* 2013;11(92):20130784.
28. Gobbi A, Karnatzikos G, Nakamura N, Mahajan V. Next generation cartilage solutions. In: Doral MN, ed. *Sports Injuries: Prevention, Diagnosis, Treatment and Rehabilitation.* Berlin, Germany: Springer Verlag; 2012:739-749.

29. Caplan A. Mesenchymal stem cells. The past, the present, the future. *Cartilage*. 2010;1(1):6-9.
30. Cavallo C, Desando G, Cattini L, et al. Bone marrow concentrated cell transplantation: rationale for its use in the treatment of human osteochondral lesions. *J Biol Regul Homeost Agents*. 2013;27(1):165-175.
31. Gobbi A, Karnatzikos G, Scotti C, Mahajan V, Mazzucco L, Grigolo B. One-step cartilage repair with bone marrow aspirate concentrated cells and collagen matrix in full-thickness knee cartilage lesions: results at 2-year follow-up. *Cartilage*. 2011;2(3):286-299.
32. Gobbi A, Karnatzikos G, Sankineani SR. One-step surgery with multipotent stem cells for the treatment of large full-thickness chondral defects of the knee. *Am J Sports Med*. 2014;42(3):648-657.

Please visit www.routledge.com/9781617119989 to access additional material.

6

Stem Cells and Platelet-Rich Plasma in the Treatment of Osteochondral Lesions of the Talus

Ethan J. Fraser, MD, MBBS; John G. Kennedy, MD, MCh, FRCS;
Arianna L. Gianakos, BS; and Youichi Yasui, MD

Introduction

The ankle is one of the most commonly injured joints in recreational and competitive athletes, with lateral ankle sprains being commonly associated with osteochondral lesions of the talus (OLT).[1] In addition, acute trauma, chronic microtrauma, endocrine or metabolic factors, genetic predisposition, joint displacement, osteoarthritis, and avascular necrosis may also contribute to the development of OLT.[2-4]

Surgical techniques for treating OLT can be divided into reparative (eg, bone marrow stimulation [BMS]) or replacement (eg, autologous osteochondral graft [AOTS] or allograft) strategies. These techniques have shown favorable clinical outcomes; however, there are concerns over the dedifferentiation of type II collagen to type I collagen over time, resulting in loss of the mechanical properties of regenerative tissue. Further, poor graft interface integration and cyst formation has been noted in autograft and allograft procedures. This has prompted investigation of the use of biological adjuncts in the form of platelet-rich plasma (PRP) and concentrated bone marrow aspirate (BMC) in the repair and regeneration of cartilage. Although earlier basic scientific evidence and clinical trials show promising results, further high-level evidence is required to substantiate these findings.[5-7]

PRP contains a milieu of over 1400 growth factors with synergistic activity, including transforming growth factor beta, fibroblast growth factor, platelet-derived growth factor, and vascular endothelial growth factor.[8,9] In vitro studies have shown that these growth factors are able to inhibit catabolic cytokines, including interleukin-1 beta (IL-1 β), IL-6, IL-8, and tumor necrosis factor alpha, while also upregulating chondrogenesis, leading to improved cartilage repair tissue. Clinical studies have also shown PRP to improve outcomes when used as an adjunct in focal osteochondral lesions and global joint arthritis.[10,11]

Several reports and case series and one randomized, controlled trial have indicated that PRP is useful in OLT, while some case series have shown BMC to be useful in reparative and replacement

Stone JW, Kennedy JG, Glazebrook M, eds. *The Foot and Ankle: AANA Advanced Arthroscopic Surgical Techniques* (pp 47-56).

procedures as well.[12-23] The fundamental difference between PRP and BMC is the presence of mesenchymal stem cells (MSCs) in BMC. This percentage is so low that the cells may not be involved directly in the repair process. Therefore, at this stage, there is no evidence to suggest BMC is a more chondrogenic adjunct than PRP. Currently, BMC and PRP are used interchangeably as a biologic adjunct, the choice often based on surgeon preference or cost rather than biologic advantage.

Indications

- PRP
  - Conservative treatment: Improved outcomes (pain and function) in OLT treated conservatively with serial injection of PRP (level II evidence)[15]
  - BMS: Improved outcomes when used as an adjunct in microfracture surgery of OLT (level II evidence)[16]
  - Autologous osteochondral autograft: Evidence in AOTS showed improved graft-host integration and more hyaline-like repair at graft borders (level V evidence).
- An animal model showed increased graft-host cartilage integration when PRP was used at the time of AOTS surgery.
  - Matrix-induced autologous chondrocyte implantation (MACI)/scaffolds: Poorer outcomes were seen in one study using MACI and PRP and one study using biomimetic scaffold with PRP (level of evidence V). PRP-seeded scaffolds have been used in joints other than the ankle with good results (level IV/V evidence).
- BMC
  - BMS techniques: Evidence for use as an adjunct in the ankle and knee (level IV/V evidence)
  - Autologous osteochondral autograft: Use of BMC as an adjunct to AOTS improved clinical outcomes (level V evidence).
  - MACI/scaffolds: Similar to PRP, BMC has been used in conjunction with scaffolds and in a one-step MACI repair with good outcomes (level IV evidence).[22]

Controversial Indications

- Indications for PRP and BMC in cartilage repair are not well defined and remain controversial.
- Further characterization and standardization of cellular and molecular components of BMC and PRP for cartilage repair is needed.
- Further high-level evidence and long-term outcome studies are required to support the use of biologic adjuncts in all operative and conservative measures for ankle cartilage repair.

Contraindications

- General contraindications for the use of PRP include the following:
  - Hematologic dyscrasias, particularly with platelet dysfunction
  - Constitutional symptoms or signs of systemic infection
  - Known allergy to additive in PRP preparation, including thrombin or other platelet-activating factors
  - Overlying skin compromise if percutaneous injection indicated
  - Severe anemia (usually a hemoglobin level < 10 dL)

- General contraindications for the use of BMC include the following:
  - Hematologic dyscrasias (eg, lymphoma, leukemia, myeloma)
  - Constitutional symptoms or signs of systemic infection
  - Anatomic abnormality of iliac crest/pelvis (eg, from previous trauma or surgery)

Pertinent Physical Findings

- Pain of the ankle joint line on palpation
- Pain on weightbearing
- May have associated lateral ligament instability
  - No solid end-point of anterior talofibular ligament
  - Positive anterior drawer test
  - Functional instability
- Swelling of joint line, particularly after activity
- Locking is rare but may occur if free osteochondral body in joint
- Persistent deep joint pain; often associated with cystic change in subchondral bone
- Associated peroneal tendon pathology can be present in chronic instability

Pertinent Imaging

- Plain radiograph (anteroposterior, lateral, and mortise views): First-line imaging. Low sensitivity for detecting OLT
- Magnetic resonance imaging
  - Most valuable imaging modality for assessment of chondral layer, subchondral bone, and concomitant pathology
  - T2-mapping and delayed gadolinium-enhanced magnetic resonance imaging of cartilage give further quantitative information about cartilage morphology and biochemical structure. May be useful in assessing early degenerative change and cartilage repair
- Computed tomography: Good in assessing extent of subchondral bone involvement and cystic change
- Ultrasound: Can be used for guiding injection in some cases

Equipment

- PRP
  - Alcohol swabs/chlorhexidine swabs
  - Simple dressing (venipuncture site)
  - 30-mL syringe (for whole blood collection)
  - 10-mL syringe (for final PRP product)
  - 16- to 20-gauge standard or butterfly needle
  - Spinal needle (for injection of PRP in arthroscopic microfracture)

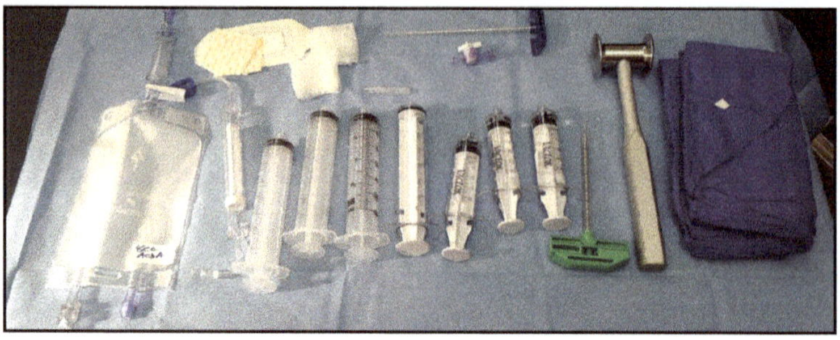

Figure 6-1. Equipment for BMC.

  - Anticoagulant citrate dextrose solution (ACD-A), solution A, United States Pharmacopeia (USP) (2.13% free citrate ion)
  - Automated centrifuge system
  - Spinal needle (for PRP injection)
- Concentrated BMC (Figure 6-1)
  - Sterile drapes
  - Alcohol swabs/chlorhexidine swabs
  - Simple dressing and steri-strips (BMC site)
  - Two 30-mL syringes
  - 10-mL syringe (for final BMC product)
  - ACD-A, solution A, USP (2.13% free citrate ion)
  - 1.0% lidocaine and 0.5% marcaine
  - Jamshidi needle (CareFusion)
  - Spinal needle (for BMC injection)
  - Mallet
  - Automated centrifuge system: System-specific requirements as per manufacturer information

Positioning and Portals

Initially, the correct limb must be identified and marked by the surgeon and confirmed with the patient. In the case of BMC, the ipsilateral hip must also be identified and marked.

Patient positioning is determined by the location of the OLT as well as surgeon preference. For most OLT surgery, including reparative and replacement techniques, the patient will be in the supine position on the operating table. A towel or padded "bump" is placed under the ipsilateral buttock, which brings the orientation of the foot into a position perpendicular to the floor. A thigh holder may be used in microfracture surgery to position the hip so that it is flexed at 60 degrees with the knee positioned at 90 degrees. A noninvasive distractor can also be used to gain improved access to the anterior talar dome.

If a posterior approach is to be used for the treatment of posterior OLT, the patient will be placed in the prone position. An ankle distractor is not typically used for the posterior approach, and the ankle is positioned so it overhangs the end of the operating table.

For PRP production, a sample of whole blood must be taken from a peripheral vein at the beginning of the procedure. The choice of the venipuncture site is dependent on many patient factors and positioning; however, the antecubital fossa veins are typically used. In the prone position, the antecubital fossa is often difficult to access; therefore, a more distal peripheral vein of the upper extremity may be used for procuring the whole blood sample.

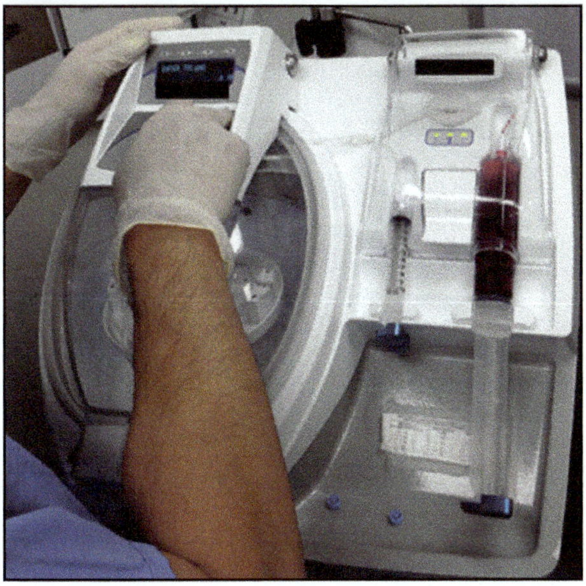

Figure 6-2. Centrifuge system.

For BMC, as with PRP, patient positioning is determined by the requirement of access to the OLT. In contrast to PRP, however, the initial collection of BMC is a more invasive procedure. Various sites have been described to obtain BMC, but the most common site used is the iliac crest. Other sites for aspiration have been described and include the tibia in children, the greater trochanter, and the sternum (particularly in very obese patients). Sternal and other aspiration sites, however, should not be used for the purposes of cartilage repair procedures given the increased risk to surrounding structures. In the supine position, adequate exposure of the ipsilateral hip is required so the landmarks for the procedure can be easily palpated. The key landmark is the anterior superior iliac spine (ASIS) and the anterior portion of the iliac crest.

In the prone patient, approaching the medullary cavity of the pelvis requires adequate access to the posterior aspect of the iliac crest, lateral to the posterior superior iliac spine (PSIS). The surgeon needs to be able to visualize the lumber spine, sacrum, PSIS, and medial portion of the iliac crest.

Step-by-Step Description of the Procedure

Platelet-Rich Plasma Harvest

The patient's antecubital vein is prepped and sterilized, and a tourniquet is placed on the upper arm. Prior to drawing blood, 4 mL of ACD-A is drawn up into a 30-mL syringe. Making sure the syringe is kept sterile, a hypodermic needle is attached and a person trained in venipuncture will obtain a 26-mL sample of whole blood into the syringe with the anticoagulant. The needle should be capped and then inverted 1 to 2 times to ensure adequate mixing of the blood with the ACD-A to prevent clotting. The venipuncture site is dressed with a simple dressing after removal of the tourniquet. After collection, the blood sample is centrifuged using a commercially available centrifuge system (Figure 6-2). There are typically 2 phases to centrifugation process: the initial slow spin (1200 to 1500 rpm) to separate the plasma and platelets from the red and white cells, followed by a second fast spin phase (4000 to 7000 rpm). The second phase further concentrates the platelets, giving the final product a higher number of platelets per unit volume. There is controversy regarding the optimum platelet concentration for tissue healing; however, it is likely that the concentration response curve is not linear with a threshold for platelet concentration, after

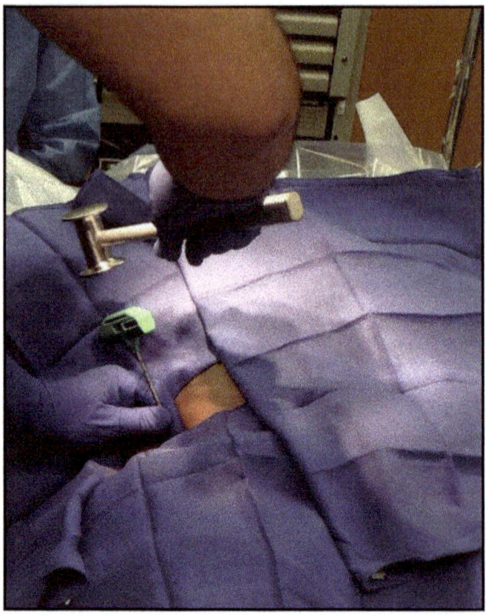

Figure 6-3. Jamshidi needle being gently tapped into the medullary cavity of the ilium, directed in a craniocaudal direction and angulated posteriorly and toward the midline.

which increased concentrations may become detrimental.[24] The final volume of PRP produced is dependent on the system in use, but it typically ranges from 2 to 5 mL. Once the final PRP sample is obtained, it is brought to the operating table and transferred into a labelled, sterile container until needed for the injection.

In BMS surgery, PRP is injected under arthroscopic guidance after the lesion has been debrided and the subchondral plate breached to allow for migration of host MSCs. PRP facilitates MSC migration to the defect site itself. Confirmation of adequate microfracture can be obtained with arthroscopic visualization of bleeding and fat droplets at the lesion site.

The PRP is then injected onto the lesion base using a spinal needle, which often needs to be angulated to approximately 45 degrees to allow for perpendicular access to the talar dome lesion. A dry scope technique is often used. The exposed collagen at the debrided site binds the factors within PRP. Fibrin or thrombin may be used to hold the PRP at the surgical site, although this has not been proven to be of additional benefit. Prior to closing the joint, the remaining PRP is injected into the joint space to affect change in the biological environment of the entire joint. This part of the process is integral in reducing proinflammatory cytokines and increasing chondrocyte production of aggrecan and other matrix products. PRP therefore acts not just at a local level, but throughout the joint, reducing inflammation, reversing the catabolic process, and promoting an anabolic environment.

Bone Marrow Aspirate Harvest

BMC is obtained from the ipsilateral hip at the time of surgery. The hip must be prepped and draped in a sterile fashion with the ASIS and anterior aspect of the iliac crest exposed. An entry point is marked approximately 3 to 5 cm posterior to the ASIS on the outer table of the iliac crest to ensure the lateral femoral cutaneous nerve is protected. A Jamshidi needle directed posteromedially and inferiorly (in the direction of the perineum) is tapped into the medullary cavity of the ilium using a mallet. It is important to carefully advance the Jamshidi needle with controlled taps of the mallet, avoiding plunging of the needle (Figure 6-3). Once the cortex is breached and the fenestrations are within the medullary cavity, no further advancement of the needle is required initially. The trocar is then removed from the inside of the cannulated Jamshidi needle, allowing a syringe to be directly attached and bone marrow drawn up (Figure 6-4). After aspirating 2 to 5 mL, the needle should be slowly and carefully advanced to the next 1-cm marking and rotated

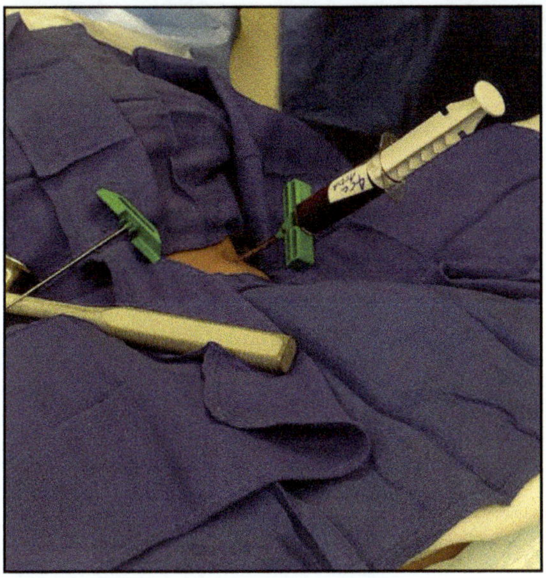

Figure 6-4. Trocar removed and syringe attached directly onto the needle for BMC.

through 90 degrees. A further 3 to 5 mL is then aspirated, and this process is repeated until the full sample is collected. This process ensures maximum biologic potential of the aspirate. Often, adequate quantities of aspirate may not be possible with initial needle position. If this is the case, the needle should be repositioned using the same entry site by directing in a more medial or lateral plane or rotating the needle 90 degrees. In the prone patient, access is gained via the posterior table on the posterior aspect of the iliac crest. The PSIS must be palpated initially, and then palpation continues laterally until the posterior table of the ilium is felt. The site for insertion of the Jamshidi needle is then marked using a sterile surgical pen. This is typically located 3 finger widths from the midline and 2 finger widths below the iliac crest, on the posterior table. Once marked, the needle is gently tapped in the direction of the ASIS. This will ensure the needle is directed into the medullary cavity of the ilium.

Once the aspirate has been obtained, it is processed using one of the commercially available systems. Often, the aspirate will require filtering prior to centrifugation with the specific filter required being dictated by the manufacturer of the centrifuge system (Figure 6-5). The quantity produced is dependent on the specific system used; however, similar to PRP, this varies from 2 to 7 mL.

In AOTS procedures, the trephine harvested from the ipsilateral knee is bathed in PRP or BMC prior to being inserted at the lesion site (Figure 6-6). It is similarly injected into the lesion site prior to insertion of graft. Following press-fit insertion, the remaining biologic adjunct (PRP or BMC) is injected around the rim of the graft to promote increased integration of the graft with the native cartilage and into the joint space, prior to closure of the joint capsule, to promote a chondrogenic and anabolic joint environment.

Postoperative Protocol

Postoperatively, all patients undergo a structured rehabilitation program based on the type of surgical procedure performed and a thorough understanding of the phases of osteochondral healing. Mithoefer et al described 3 phases of rehabilitation after cartilage repair in the knee, the principles of which are applicable to ankle cartilage repair.[25] Initially, a phase of joint protection and activation is required to allow for preliminary stages of osseous and chondral integration while ensuring ongoing passive movement of the ankle to mitigate any scar tissue and decreased

Figure 6-5. Filtering of BMC prior to centrifuge.

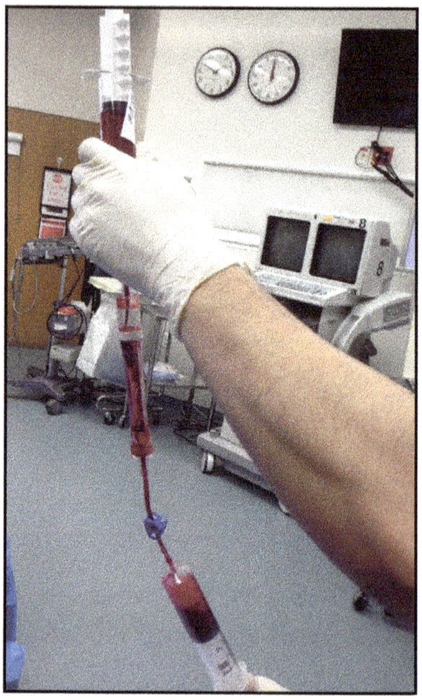

Figure 6-6. The osteochondral graft is bathed in PRP or BMC prior to being inserted at the lesion site.

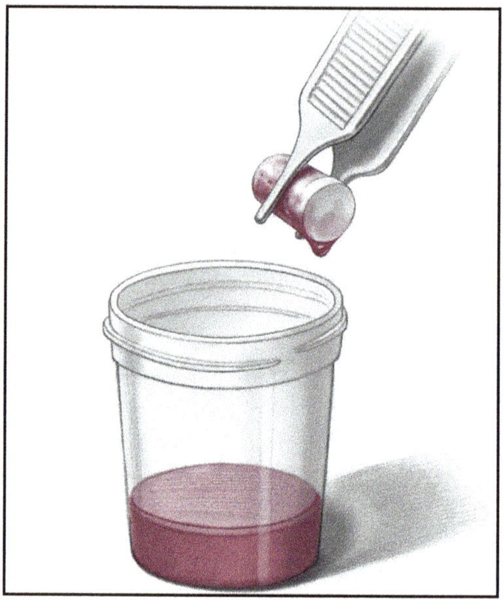

joint motion. During the initial phase, the repair tissue is vulnerable to overloading; therefore, weightbearing should be restricted for the first 10 to 14 days following surgery. During this time, the addition of biological adjuncts reduces joint inflammation through their action on nuclear factor kappa-light-chain enhancer of activated B cells transactivation and reduction in IL-1 β.[26] BMC introduces MSCs in addition to growth factors, increasing the chondrogenic potential and producing repair tissue with biomechanical properties more similar to the native cartilage.

The following phase introduces increased joint loading, starting from 2 weeks with 10% of the patient's body weight and progressing over 2 weeks so that the patient is fully weightbearing by 6 weeks. Functional training also commences at this time, working on joint range of motion and proprioception. Once the patient is fully weightbearing (6 weeks following surgery), physical therapy is focused on strengthening and continued proprioceptive training followed by sport-specific training.

Potential Complications

Complications associated with the use of PRP and BMC are relatively rare. With BMC, the main complications encountered include donor site morbidity at the ipsilateral hip, bleeding, infection, and neuralgia. In a recent study of 523 bone marrow aspirations, the authors reported a 1% incidence of early donor site pain, which reduced to 0.04% at 1 year.[27] In the same study, neuralgia was seen in 0.02% of patients, and 2% had minor complications including hematoma formation, superficial infection, or seroma formation. PRP is advantageous in that it avoids the donor site complications associated with BMC. Potential complications with PRP are those associated with venipuncture and include infection, hematoma, and bleeding risk.

Top Technical Pearls for the Procedure

1. BMC: Advance and rotate the Jamshidi needle every 3 to 5 mL to ensure the maximum biologic potential of aspirate is achieved.
2. PRP: Be aware that all systems are not the same. Use a low white cell–based system for cartilage repair procedures (based on current evidence).
3. Bathe the graft in biologic solution prior to insertion to ensure maximum delivery of MSC and/or growth factors.
4. The joint is a system of which the OLT is a part. Inject the entire joint to enhance the anti-inflammatory effects of the biologic milieu.
5. Ensure all staff are well versed in the use and protocols involved with the processing system being used, including the amount to be drawn and the final amount of biologic produced. This will ensure maximum concentration of growth factors and platelets.

References

1. Saxena A, Eakin C. Articular talar injuries in athletes: results of microfracture and autogenous bone graft. *Am J Sports Med*. 2007;35:1680-1687.
2. Berndt AL, Harty M. Transchondral fractures (osteochondritis dissecans) of the talus. *J Bone Joint Surg Am*. 1959;41-A:988-1020.
3. Guettler JH, Demetropoulos CK, Yank KH. Osteochondral defects in the human knee: influence of defect size on cartilage rim stress and load redistribution to surrounding cartilage. *Am J Sports Med*. 2004;32:1451-1458.
4. Mullet H, Kennedy JG, Quinlan W. Subchondral talar cyst following open reduction and internal fixation of an ankle fracture. *Foot Ankle Surg*. 1999;5:147-149.
5. Smyth NA, Murawski CD, Haleem AM, et al. Establishing proof of concept: platelet-rich plasma and bone marrow aspirate concentrate may improve cartilage repair following surgical treatment for osteochondral lesions of the talus. *World J Orthop*. 2012;3(7):101-108.
6. Valderrabano V, Leumann A, Rasch H, Egelhof T, Hintermann B, Pagenstert G. Knee-to-ankle mosaicplasty for the treatment of osteochondral lesions of the ankle joint. *Am J Sports Med*. 2009;37(Suppl 1):105S-111S.

7. Smyth NA, Haleem AM, Murawski CD, Do HT, Deland JT, Kennedy JG. The effect of platelet-rich plasma on autologous osteochondral transplantation: an in vivo rabbit model. *J Bone Joint Surg Am.* 2013;95(24):2185-2193.
8. Fortier LA, Barker JU, Strauss EJ, McCarrel TM, Cole BJ. The role of growth factors in cartilage repair. *Clin Orthop Relat Res.* 2011;469(10):2706-2715.
9. Miller Y, Bachowski G, Benjamin R, Eklund DK, Hibbard AJ, Lightfoot T. *Practice Guideline for Blood Transfusion: A Compilation From Recent Peer-Reviewed Literature.* 2nd ed. Washington, DC: American Red Cross; 2007:56.
10. Abrams GD, Frank RM, Fortier LA, et al. Platelet-rich plasma for articular cartilage repair. *Sports Med Arthrosc Rev.* 2013;21(4):213-219.
11. Chubinskaya S, Segalite D, Pikovsky D, et al. Effects induced by BMPs in cultures of human articular chondrocytes: comparative studies. *Growth Factors.* 2008;26:275-283.
12. Milano G, Sanna Passino E, Deriu L, et al. The effect of platelet rich plasma combined with microfracture on the treatment of chondral defects: an experimental study in a sheep model. *Osteoarthritis Cartilage.* 2010;18:971-980.
13. Smyth NA, Haleem AM, Murawski CD, Do HT, Deland JT, Kennedy JG. The effect of platelet-rich plasma on autologous osteochondral transplantation: an in vivo rabbit model. *J Bone Joint Surg Am.* 2013;95(24):2185-2193.
14. Patel S, Dhillon MS, Aggarwal S, et al. Treatment with platelet-rich plasma is more effective than placebo for knee osteoarthritis: a prospective, double-blind, randomized trial. *Am J Sports Med.* 2013;41:356-364.
15. Mei-Dan O, Carmont MR, Laver L, Mann G, Maffulli N, Nyska M. Platelet-rich plasma or hyaluronate in the management of osteochondral lesions of the talus. *Am J Sports Med.* 2012;40(3):534-541.
16. Guney A, Akar M, Karaman I, Oner M, Guney B. Clinical outcomes of platelet rich plasma (PRP) as an adjunct to microfracture surgery in osteochondral lesions of the talus. *Knee Surg Sports Traumatol Arthrosc.* 2015;23(8):2384-2389.
17. Filardo G, Madry H, Jelic M, et al. Mesenchymal stem cells for the treatment of cartilage lesions: from preclinical findings to clinical application in orthopedics. *Knee Surg Sports Traumatol Arthrosc.* 2013;21:1717-1729.
18. Wilke MM, Nydam DV, Nixon AJ. Enhanced early chondrogenesis in articular defects following arthroscopic mesenchymal stem cell implantation in an equine model. *J Orthop Res.* 2007;25:913-925.
19. Fortier LA, Potter HG, Rickey EJ, et al. Concentrated bone marrow aspirate improves full-thickness cartilage repair compared with microfracture in the equine model. *J Bone Joint Surg Am.* 2010;92:1927-1937.
20. Kim YS, Park EH, Kim YC, et al. Clinical outcomes of mesenchymal stem cell injection with arthroscopic treatment in older patients with osteochondral lesions of the talus. *Am J Sports Med.* 2013;41:1090-1099.
21. Becher C, Driessen A, Hess T, Longo UG, Maffulli N, Thermann H. Microfracture for chondral defects of the talus: maintenance of early results at midterm follow-up. *Knee Surg Sports Traumatol Arthrosc.* 2010;18:656-663.
22. Giannini S, Buda R, Battaglia M, et al. One-step repair in talar osteochondral lesions: 4-year clinical results and t2-mapping capability in outcome prediction. *Am J Sports Med.* 2013;41(3):511-518.
23. Hannon CP, Ross KA, Murawski C, et al. Arthroscopic bone marrow stimulation and concentrated bone marrow aspirate for osteochondral lesions of the talus: a case-control study of functional and magnetic resonance observation of cartilage repair tissue outcomes. *Arthroscopy.* 2015 Sep 19. pii: S0749-8063(15)00633-7. doi: 10.1016/j.arthro.2015.07.01
24. Yin Z, Yang X, Jiang Y, et al. Platelet-rich plasma combined with agarose as a bioactive scaffold to enhance cartilage repair: an in vitro study. *J Biomater Appl.* 2014;28:1039-1050.
25. Mithoefer K, Hambly K, Logerstedt D, Ricci M, Silvers H, Della Villa S. Current concepts for rehabilitation and return to sport after knee articular cartilage repair in the athlete. *J Orthop Sports Phys Ther.* 2012;42(3):254-273.
26. Bendinelli P, Matteucci E, Dogliotti G, et al. Molecular basis of anti-inflammatory action of platelet-rich plasma on human chondrocytes: mechanisms of NF-κB inhibition via HGF. *J Cell Physiol.* 2010;225:757-766.
27. Hernigou P, Desroches A, Queinnec S, et al. Morbidity of graft harvesting versus bone marrow aspiration in cell regenerative therapy. *Int Orthop.* 2014;38(9):1855-1860.

7

Synthetic Plug

Francesco Allegra, MD

Introduction

Several surgical procedures have been described in the literature for treating osteochondral lesions of the talus (OLT) including transfer and implantation of autologous mature tissue, seeding of mature engineered cells, migration of undifferentiated cells from bone covered by a biological membrane, and seeding of harvested undifferentiated cells using a biologic scaffold. When the lesion includes a subchondral cyst, an additional surgical procedure such as bone grafting may be required. Any ideal procedure to treat these lesions would lead to coverage with hyaline cartilage. Most of these procedures are limited to the young, active population. The aging process is accompanied by a diminished capacity for bone healing, cartilage healing, and tissue integration. For patients who are older but still active, treatment of a symptomatic talar dome osteochondral lesion using a biomimetic composite plug may be a reasonable option.

Three different types of products have been developed by different companies; all have a porous 3-dimensional (3D) composite multilayered structure that mimics the original osteochondral anatomical tissue.

The first scaffold, Tru-fit (Smith & Nephew), is a biphasic osteochondral biodegradable substitute for the treatment of a bone defect. The osseous substitute consists of a matrix of calcium triphosphate ($CaSO4^{3}$) and the cartilaginous substitute of poly(DL-lactide-co-glycolide) (PLGA). The use of this product for OLT or for backfill of osteochondral donor sites in the knee is off label in the United States due to new Food and Drug Administration guidelines instituted in 2012. As of the date of this printing, this product, licensed only for the treatment of bone voids, has been retired from the market.

The second one, BioMatrix CRD (Kensey Nash Corp), is a sterile, biphasic, bioresorbable scaffold. The superficial phase is a collagen sponge derived from bovine hide and composed predominantly of type I collagen (P1076 Collagen Sponge, Kensey Nash), whereas the deep phase is made from Porous Tissue Matrix (DSM Biomedical) material, integrated onto a subchondral bone construct composed of a mixture of D,D-L,L-polylactic acid (D-L PLA) and beta tricalcium phosphate (β-TCP) that has been fabricated into an open-cell, 3D architecture simulating

Stone JW, Kennedy JG, Glazebrook M, eds. *The Foot and Ankle: AANA Advanced Arthroscopic Surgical Techniques* (pp 57-64).

cancellous bone (OPLA, Kensey Nash). Both phases of the scaffold and the interface between them are porous. The interface where these biomaterials are joined functions as a barrier to passage of fluids to facilitate cell migration across it. The device is resorbed over a period of approximately 18 months, is cylindrical in shape, and is offered in diameters ranging from 4 to 15 mm with a 15-mm length.

The third product, Maioregen (Fin-Ceramica Faenza SpA), is another osteochondral biomimetic scaffold with a porous, 3D composite, trilayered structure that mimics the native osteochondral anatomy. The superficial layer, consisting of type I collagen, has a smooth surface. The intermediate layer tide mark–like consists of a combination of type I collagen (60%) and hydroxyapatite (40%), whereas the lower layer consists of a mineralized blend of type I collagen (30%) and hydroxyapatite (70%) reproducing the subchondral bone layer. It is supplied as a 40x40-mm square, which can be easily sized to fit round or irregularly shaped lesions. Currently, these 2 products are not present in the United States market. Few studies have been published on the use of these second-generation scaffolds. Among them, one study demonstrated improvements over 6 to 18 months postoperatively with a decrease in the size of the bony defects as bone remodeling occurred during resorption of the implants.[1] Histological examination performed at 12 to 18 months postoperatively suggested that the repair tissue was both durable and sustainable in the animal model.

An ex vivo biomechanical testing study evaluated the scaffold capability to repair osteochondral defects: once implanted, it produces a tissue that exhibits biomechanical properties similar to unoperated articular tissue, evident as early as 6 months postoperatively and maintained through 18 months. These authors demonstrated that the repair tissue in the recipient site integrated with biomechanical properties similar to native bone.[2]

Indications

- Symptomatic bony defects of the talar dome consisting of a well-circumscribed defect with normal surrounding articular cartilage
- Absence of generalized degenerative changes of the ankle joint
- Failure to respond to traditional treatment including excision of the lesion with stimulation of the base using abrasion, drilling, or microfracture
- Middle-aged or older patient who desires an active lifestyle
- Absence of inflammatory arthropathy, infection, or synovial proliferative disorder
- Absence of hindfoot malalignment

Controversial Indications

The biomimetic porous composite plug is an artificial biodegradable scaffold with characteristics and composition similar to an autologous plug thanks to several layers replicating the original structure. Each layer is designed to match the physical and mechanical properties of the adjacent tissue, thus replicating physical and mechanical properties of host tissue.

Compared to the osteochondral autograft transfer system procedure, this plug does not require a donor site from another healthy joint. Furthermore, small differences in contouring with surrounding cartilage can be leveled removing superficial proud tissue as needed without damaging the plug, which is not possible in a traditional osteochondral autograft transfer system procedure.

Some authors have shown average to poor results using first-generation materials.[3] In contrast, the second-generation products appear to integrate without any local bone marrow reaction healing with new tissue with similar mechanical properties as the native bone.[4] Some authors evidenced repair tissue in a bony defect treated with a resorbable second-generation scaffold (β-TCP/PLA/collagen) exhibiting biomechanical properties more similar to healthy bone compared to first-generation scaffold (PLGA/CaSO4).[4] No systemic or local inflammation occurred in response to this device, demonstrating that it can be implanted in vivo without causing an adverse long-lasting response, present in the first-generation scaffold.[5]

Patient Evaluation

A patient with a symptomatic osteochondral lesion of the talar dome will generally complain of ankle joint pain that tends to be worse with increasing activity. Pain severity may depend upon ankle position and whether weightbearing or nonweightbearing. The location of the pain does not necessarily correlate with the side of the lesion medially or laterally and may be perceived to be greater anteriorly or posteriorly. Although the patient may complain of instability of the ankle, objective signs of joint laxity are absent unless there is coexisting ankle ligament pathology, perhaps related to the development of the osteochondral lesion.

Pertinent Physical Findings

Physical examination should include a careful assessment of the following:

- Lower limb alignment
- Muscle mass
- Joint range of motion
- Fixed hindfoot varus or valgus must be noted since successful treatment of the osteochondral lesion may depend on correction of misalignment in addition to local treatment of the lesion itself.
- Tenderness may be present on the side of the lesion and intensity may depend on the position of the ankle in dorsi- or plantarflexion and whether the palpation is performed anterior or posterior to the involved malleolus.
- Assessment of ligament laxity including lateral ligaments, medial ligament, and syndesmosis

Pertinent Imaging

- Anteroposterior, lateral, and mortise plain x-ray views should be obtained on every patient.
- These may be supplemented with standing radiographs to assist in the evaluation of hindfoot alignment.
- Computed tomography is the most accurate means of assessing the bony defect to evaluate the size of the lesion, amount of bone attached to the lesion, and precise location on the talar dome.
- Magnetic resonance imaging (MRI) may overestimate lesion size because of the degree of bony edema noted on T2 images. However, the MRI may assist in assessing the presence of a fluid layer between the lesion and the underlying bone.
- The condition of overlying articular cartilage is evaluated with MRI using T2 fat-suppressed and spin echo-weighted sequences, also useful to evaluate graft incorporation over time.

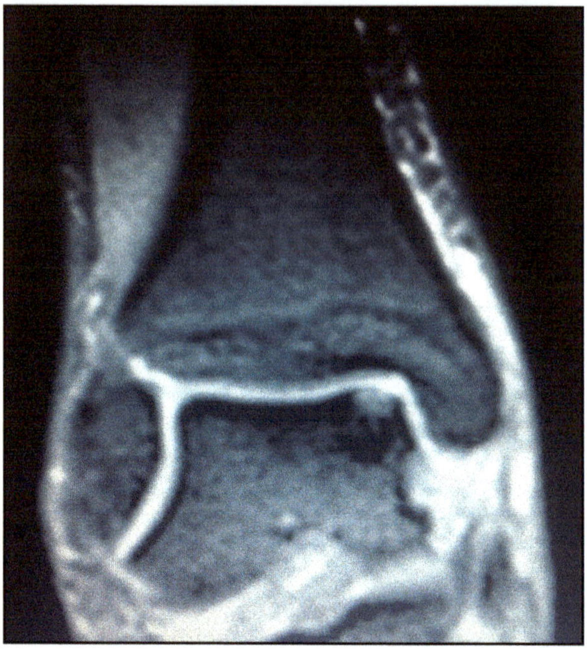

Figure 7-1. The control MRI in T2-weighted scans.

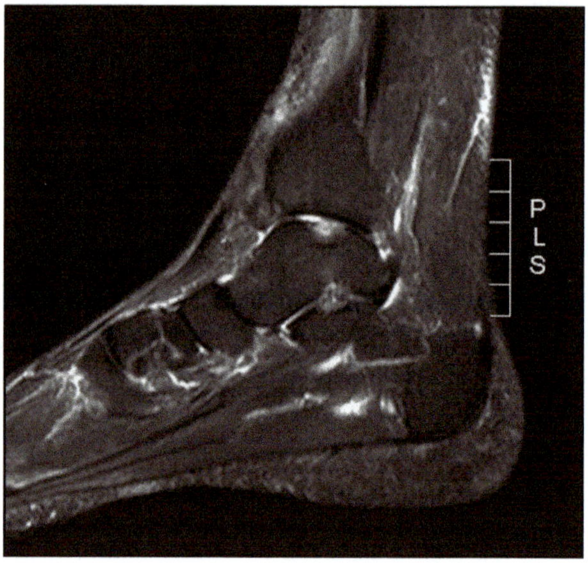

Figure 7-2. The 6-month image shows (sagittal view) an uncompleted repair with the presence of new tissue inside the defect and some edema around the plug.

Persistence of bony edema on the MRI or the development of bone cysts may indicate failure of graft incorporation. In 30% to 35% of cases treated by the author, the PLGA/CaSO4 scaffold device did not show resorption on the MRI obtained at 24 months postoperatively despite the fact that the patients were generally happy with surgical result as their pain had diminished significantly. This lack of correlation between the MRI findings and the clinical success of the procedure has led the author to discontinue obtaining the 24-month postoperative MRI unless otherwise clinically indicated. In contrast, the β-TCP/PLA/collagen scaffold has shown complete resolution of bony edema on MRI examinations obtained at 12 months postoperatively (Figures 7-1 through 7-3).

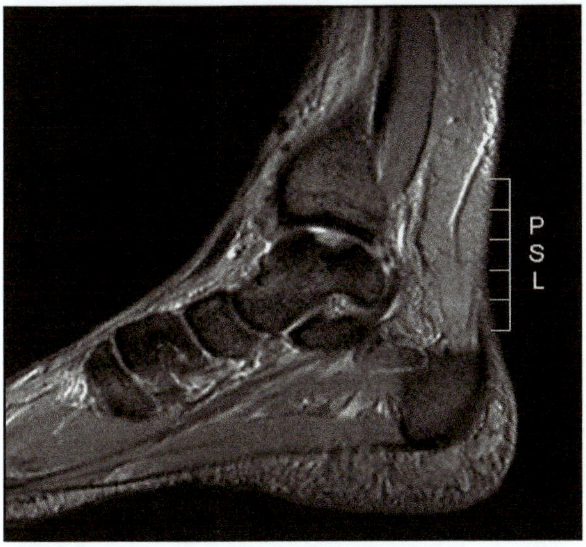

Figure 7-3. The 12-month scan (same sagittal view) shows a more mature repair tissue, the disappearance of bony edema, and the reconstruction of the articular space between the 2 tibial and talar surfaces.

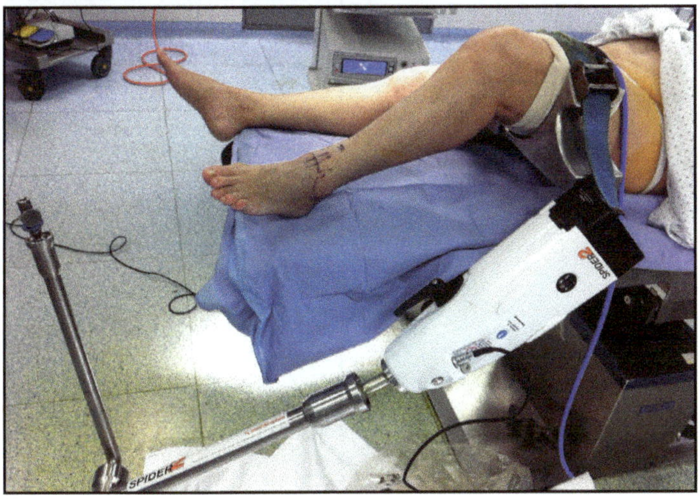

Figure 7-4. The patient assessment on surgical bed: the ankle is put in traction using an arm device with the leg in countertraction.

Equipment

- A standard 4-mm, 30-degree arthroscope along with a 3.5-mm, full radius shaver blade and a 4-mm, radiofrequency wand
- A 2.7-mm, 30-degree arthroscope can be utilized in cases of narrow joint space

Positioning and Portals

The patient is positioned supine on the operating table with a thigh tourniquet and the calf secured in a leg holder, maintaining 30 to 40 degrees of flexion at the hip and knee (Figure 7-4). Noninvasive distraction is applied to the ankle joint using a commercially available distraction strap. Routine anteromedial and anterolateral portals are established for initial arthroscopic examination. A posterolateral portal may be added at the surgeon's discretion for dedicated inflow or for instrumentation.

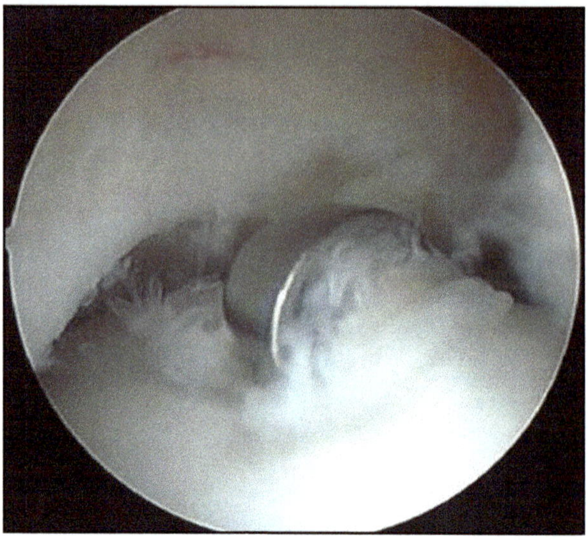

Figure 7-5. The curette exposes the defected area removing the instable cartilage layer.

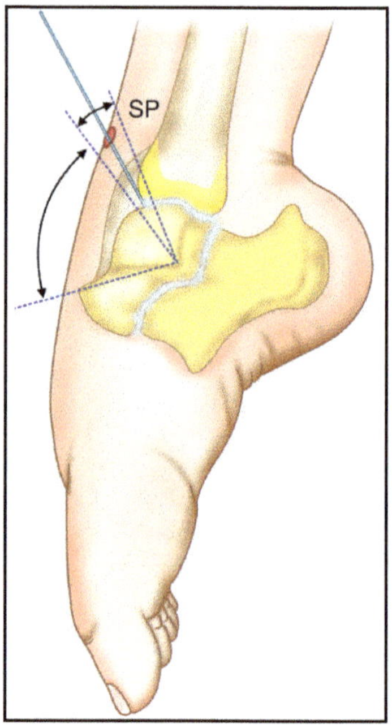

Figure 7-6. The visualization of the talar dome central area is made easy by removing the dorsal capsule and by forcing the foot in maximum plantarflexion. Removing some bone with a burr blade from the Harty's notch is possible to gain 15 degrees of further exposition. SP, superior portal.

Step-by-Step Description of the Procedure

A comprehensive, diagnostic arthroscopic examination is performed to evaluate for associated intra-articular pathology such as loose bodies or osteophytes.

The osteochondral talar defect is evaluated with a probe and debrided using a combination of elevators, curettes, and loose body forceps, in addition to a shaver or burr (Figure 7-5). Medial or lateral lesions less than 100 to 120 mm^2 located on the anterior half of the talus can be approached arthroscopically by placing the ankle in maximal plantarflexion after an anterior capsulotomy on the tibial side (Figure 7-6). A perpendicular approach to the lesion may be achieved by establishing an accessory anterosuperior portal either medially or laterally depending on the side of the defect.

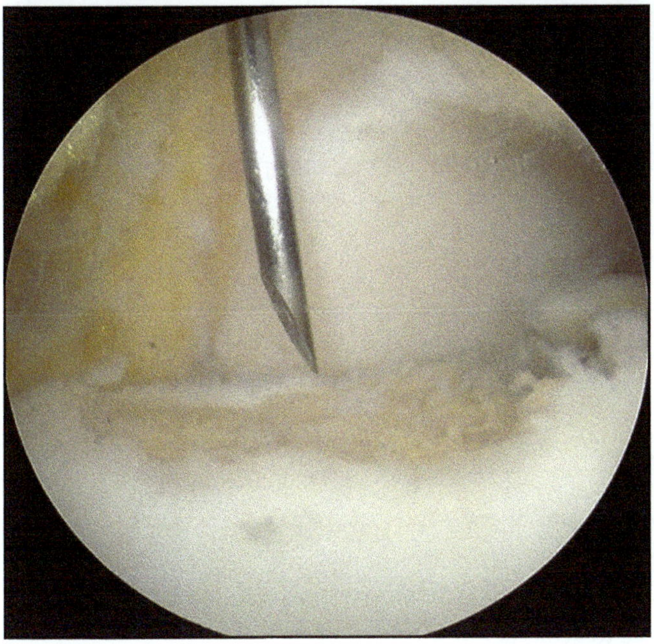

Figure 7-7. The ancillary anterosuperior portal is opened following the direction of a spinal needle inserted along the anterior tibial shaft, taking care to target the defected area as vertical as possible.

The location of the portal is determined using a spinal needle to optimize the vertical approach to the lesion (Figure 7-7). The portal is made by the nick and spread technique using a blunt trocar to approach the lesion initially. The approach may be enhanced by using a burr to remove a small amount of bone at the notch of Harty medially or in the area of the anteroinferior tibiofibular ligament laterally. Resection of even a small amount of bone in this area can significantly improve the approach to the lesion.[6]

If the lesion is on the posterior talar dome, then prone posterior arthroscopy is performed using the technique of van Dijk et al[7] without traction with the ankle maximally dorsiflexed to expose the posterior dome of the talus. If the size or location of the lesion precludes comfortable access using arthroscopic techniques, then the procedure is converted to open surgery using a malleolar osteotomy medially or fibular osteotomy laterally to obtain exposure.

A coring reamer of a size appropriate for the diameter of the lesion is introduced and advanced to a depth appropriate for the plug, which is available in multiple sizes depending on the size of the lesion. The plug is then inserted into the defect and gently tamped into place. The plug must be placed accurately in the vertical position inside the recipient socket. It should be positioned 1 mm below the native cartilaginous surface. When hydrated with blood, it expands to become level with the surrounding cartilage. The author prefers a biphasic scaffold consisting of type I collagen with a composite of β-tricalcium phosphate and polylactic acid, which may be hydrated with autologous bone marrow aspirate prior to being press-fit into the defect. The portals are closed with sutures.

Postoperative Protocol

A bulky postoperative dressing is applied. At suture removal 7 to 10 days after surgery, the patient is allowed to increase weightbearing as tolerated using crutches or a walker. Physical therapy may be utilized as necessary to help regain range of motion, strength, and overall proprioception.

Potential Complications

Ankle arthroscopy is a procedure with a very low risk of complications. The author has not encountered any complications particular to this technique. The use of an ancillary portal has not represented an increased risk of neurovascular injury. Careful attention to portal creation using the nick and spread technique will minimize the chance of iatrogenic neurovascular injury. In case of osteotomy, the major complication is malleolar nonunion; in this case, an accurate examination of all possible causes can help to reach complete recovery.

Top Technical Pearls for the Procedure

1. Use the technique for isolated focal symptomatic bony talar lesions in patients older than 50 years.
2. Use an accessory medial or lateral portal placed superiorly to achieve a perpendicular approach to the lesion.
3. Use joint distraction and maximal plantarflexion to reach most lesions on the talar dome.
4. Use the nick and spread technique to avoid neurovascular injury.
5. Place the implant 1 mm below the normal articular surface to accommodate the small amount of swelling that occurs with hydration after implantation.

References

1. Ahern BJ, Underwood C, Bradica G, et al. Single site osteochondral resurfacing. An in vivo caprine study. Poster presented at 56th Annual Meeting of the Orthopaedic Research Society; March 6-9, 2010; New Orleans, LA.
2. Maher SA, Chen D, Deng XH, et al. Biomechanical evaluation of a biphasic scaffold for the repair of osteochondral defects by ex vivo indentation testing. Poster presented at 49th Annual Meeting of the Orthopaedic Research Society; February 2-5, 2003; New Orleans, LA.
3. Pearce CJ, Gartner LE, Mitchell A, Calder JC. Synthetic osteochondral grafting of ankle osteochondral lesions. *Foot Ankle Surg.* 2012:18:114-118.
4. Kon E, Delcogliano M, Filardo G, et al. Novel nano-composite multilayered biomaterial for osteochondral regeneration. A pilot clinical trial. *Am J Sports Med.* 2011;39:1180-1190.
5. Saska RA, Castiglione E, Bradica G, Kronengold RT. Performance of a novel bone void filler in restoring the mechanical integrity of bone in the rabbit model. A comparative analysis. Poster presented at 55th Annual Meeting of the Orthopaedic Research Society; February 22-25, 2009; Las Vegas, NV.
6. Allegra F, Amelina A. Osteochondral autograft of the talus. In: McGinty JB, ed. *Operative Arthroscopy.* 3rd ed. Philadelphia, PA: Lippincot, Williams & Wilkins; 2004:930-943.
7. van Dijk CN, Scholten PE, Krips R. A 2-portal endoscopic approach for diagnosis and treatment of posterior ankle pathology. *Arthroscopy.* 2000;16(8):871-876.

Please visit www.routledge.com/9781617119989 to access additional material.

8

Osteochondral Allograft Transplantation for Osteochondral Lesions of the Talar Dome

Gokhan Meric, MD and William Bugbee, MD

Introduction

Osteochondral lesions of the talus (OLT) are commonly associated with traumatic injuries and ligamentous laxity or instability.[1] These lesions frequently cause significant pain, functional limitations, and disability of the ankle.[2] Treatment of these lesions is challenging, especially in young patients.[3] Conservative treatment, arthroscopic debridement, curettage with or without bone grafting, autologous chondrocyte transplantation, and osteochondral autograft transplantation have all been reported as treatment options for OLT.[3-6] Many of these techniques are limited to smaller lesions and the outcome appears to be related to lesion size with failure rates increasing for lesions greater than 1.5 cm^2.[7]

Fresh osteochondral allografting (OCA) of the talar dome has been shown to be an excellent treatment option for large, complex talar defects not optimally appropriate for other cartilage restoration procedures.[8-11] The survival rates of talar OCA are in the range of 66% to 83% at 1 to 3.1 years follow-up. El-Rashidy et al[12] reported on 38 patients implanted with fresh OCA plugs at an average 38 months follow-up. Four patients out of the 38 were found to have a poor outcome (10.5% failure rate), all of which were noted to have had a prior operation or additional pathology. Gross et al[13] reported 9 patients who were treated with large talar OCA. The average age of the patients was 38 years (range, 22 to 47). Graft survival was 6 out of 9 at a mean of 11 years (range, 4 to 19) follow-up. Three patients required ankle arthrodesis.[13] Berlet et al[14] reported 17 patients who received frozen OCA for OLT. The patients had an average age of 34.7 years and a mean defect area of 2 cm^2. All patients had failed prior surgical treatment, and average follow-up was 2.1 years (minimum 1 year). In their study, one graft (5.9%) failed due to fragmentation and was revised with a single osteoarticular transfer system plug for a contained flap lesion at 2.7 years. Raikin[15] reported 6 patients who underwent OCA transplantation for large osteochondral talus lesions. Four grafts were frozen and 2 were fresh. Average follow-up was 21 months (range, 6 to 39). In his report, one patient underwent ankle arthrodesis after 17 months, 2 patients showed some degree of graft collapse, and all patients were pleased with their results.[15] Gortz et al[11]

Stone JW, Kennedy JG, Glazebrook M, eds. *The Foot and Ankle: AANA Advanced Arthroscopic Surgical Techniques* (pp 65-74).

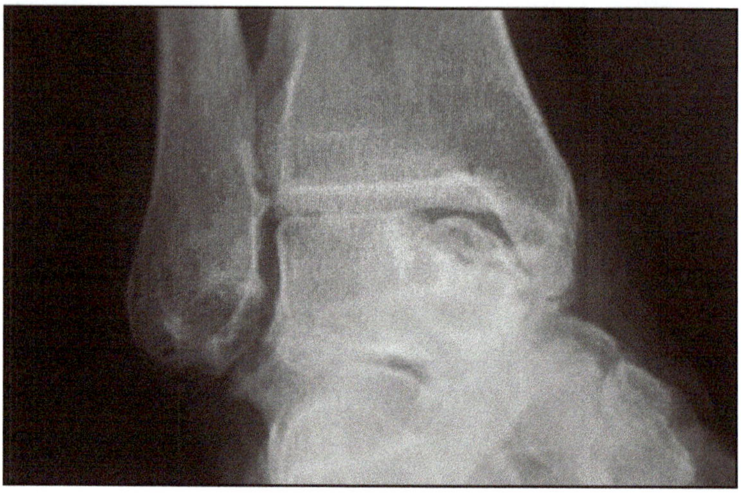

Figure 8-1. Large, cystic OLT of the medial talus. OCA is ideal for this lesion.

reported fresh OCA of 12 ankles in 11 patients. The patients' mean age was 35.5 years (range, 26 to 57). The average graft size was 3.6 cm^2 (range, 1.7 to 6.0). Mean follow-up was 38 months (range, 24 to 107). Two patients failed, with one undergoing revision allografting and one undergoing arthrodesis. The survival rate was 83%.[11]

The disadvantages of the fresh allografting technique include the difficulty in obtaining donor tissue and the technically demanding nature of the procedure. However, fresh OCA allows defective tissue (both bone and cartilage) to be anatomically reconstructed through transplantation. Size-matched fresh OCAs resolve each of these issues by having matching anatomic contours and a volume to match that of the host talus. The ability to transplant mature hyaline cartilage with viable chondrocytes that can sustain its surrounding collagen matrix, along with structural bone to restore osseous deficiency to recreate a congruent joint, is attractive.[11,16,17]

This chapter will review the processes of fresh OCA of the talus, reviewing techniques for implantation and potential complications of OCA transplantation procedures.

Indications

- The most common indications for allograft surgery are as follows:
  - OLT
  - Avascular necrosis
  - In both cases, allograft can be used where lesions are either large or have failed previous surgical treatments (Figure 8-1).[11,12,16]
- Unusual indications include the following:
  - Fracture malunion
  - Focal posttraumatic arthritis or benign tumors
  - In addition, bipolar tibiotalar allografts have been used to treat advanced arthritis but will not be covered in this chapter.

Contraindications

- Inflammatory arthritis
- The presence of active infection

- Deformity or instability of the ankle that is correctable
- High body mass index is not considered an absolute contraindication.

Pertinent Physical Findings

- Symptoms associated with OLT include the following:
  - Activity-related ankle pain and dysfunction. Mechanical symptoms may be present.
  - The examination should focus on demonstration of site(s) of tenderness and on a systematic search for other pathology such as instability or deformity.
- The best test is reproduction of pain with deep palpation over the site of the lesion (medial or lateral).

Pertinent Imaging

In order to obtain an appropriate talus graft for implantation, size matching is required for the chondral and subchondral lesion dimensions.

- Standing anteroposterior, mortise, and lateral ankle radiographs should be obtained routinely before surgery.
- Preoperatively, the size of the donor talus is matched to the patient using standard radiographs and direct measurements of the allograft. A match is considered to be a size difference of 1 mm or less.
- Magnetic resonance imaging and computed tomography are also used to identify the size and location of the lesion.
- Computed tomography in axial and coronal planes can be helpful in demarcating the subchondral extent of osteochondral fragment to aid in preoperative planning.

Equipment

- OCA transfer system (Arthrex)
- Plug sizes (8 to 20 mm)
- Rigid unipolar external fixator (Vision Unilateral Fixator [Biomet])
- Reciprocating and oscillating saws
- Metallic compression screws (< 3 mm and/or > 3 mm [Synthes])
- Poly-L-lactic acid chondral darts (Arthrex)
- Fluoroscopy

Special equipment that may be necessary includes an OCA transfer system specially designed for the ankle or an osteochondral autograft transfer instrument set more typically used for the knee. Available plug sizes should range from 8 to 20 mm. A rigid unipolar external fixator that is capable of providing distraction of the ankle is useful for the anterior approach. Reciprocating and oscillating saws are necessary to resect the talus and prepare a shell onlay graft if that technique is chosen. Small 3-mm or less metallic compression screws or several small poly-L-lactic acid chondral darts should be available for fixation of the graft. In cases where malleolar osteotomy is used, larger screws should be available for fixation. Fluoroscopy is essential for the procedure.

Fresh allograft tissue is obtained from healthy donors between the ages of 16 and 40 years who meet the criteria of the American Association of Tissue Banks.[18] Donor tissue is recovered within 24 hours after donor death and then processed and maintained fresh at 4°C until the time of implantation, which is between 10 and 28 days from tissue recovery. Because the graft tissue is avascular and relatively immunoprivileged, no blood group matching or tissue typing is performed and no immunosuppressive therapy is used. The graft should be inspected prior to surgical incision to ensure its acceptability for implantation.

Positioning and Portals

Surgery is performed with the patient in the supine position with a thigh tourniquet under general anesthesia with popliteal and saphenous block augmentation. It is useful to place a bump under the buttock or tilt the table to resist the tendency for the leg to externally rotate.

Step-by-Step Description of the Procedure

Talus Plug Allograft Technique

The localization of the lesion is important to determine the approach. Medial talar lesions need to be approached through a medial malleolar osteotomy to access the osteochondral lesion. Lateral lesions can usually be approached through an anterolateral incision (lateral to the peroneus tertius tendon). Access to the lesion can usually be gained by plantarflexing the ankle joint. If perpendicular access cannot be obtained through this technique, a lateral tibial plafondplasty can be performed. It is important to ensure that perpendicular access to the talar dome lesion is obtained to guarantee appropriate removal and reproducible donor plug implantation into the defect.

The medial malleolar osteotomy is performed with a Kirschner wire, which is drilled under image intensification guidance from the medial distal tibial flare in order to exit the plafond just lateral to the lateral border of the osteochondral lesion. This wire is used to plan the malleolar osteotomy. The steep chevron-shaped osteotomy is performed to access the talar dome. It is technically important to predrill the proposed fixation holes for the osteotomy prior to making the cuts to aid in the post-procedure anatomic replacement of the osteotomy fragment. In addition to the 2 standard oblique screws inserted from the tip of the malleolus, a horizontal screw should be planned and subsequently inserted to prevent the malleolus from sliding proximally during reduction and insertion of the oblique screws. Additionally, care must be taken to prevent injury to the saphenous vein and nerve anterior to the malleolus and the posterior tibial tendon behind the malleolus while making the saw cuts. Once completed, the osteotomy is hinged medially around the deltoid ligament, which must be kept intact. This will allow full visualization of the medial talar dome (Figure 8-2). The osteochondral lesion size is measured with measuring guides, which can be used to measure the optimal size plug required for transplantation. Because of the dense nature of the talar bone, it is preferable to use an instrument system that requires power tools to prepare the recipient site and allograft rather than instruments that rely on direct impaction. Once the lesion is identified and a size has been determined, a guide wire is driven through the sizing guide and into the talus. A reamer is then placed over the guide wire and reaming of the lesion is performed. Care must be taken not to ream too deeply as a depth of 6 to 10 mm is generally adequate to extirpate the diseased bone and allow enough surface area for press-fit graft fixation (Figure 8-3). Depth measurements are made in the recipient site to be used for preparing the allograft.

Once the recipient site is prepared, the donor graft must be harvested from the talus allograft (Figure 8-4). Great care should be taken to clearly define the orthotopic site and angle of reaming

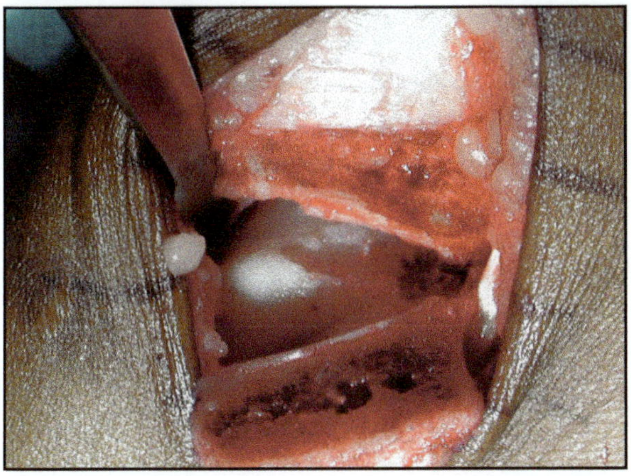

Figure 8-2. OLT of the medial talus exposed through a medial malleolar osteotomy. Note the predrilled screw paths in the medial malleolus.

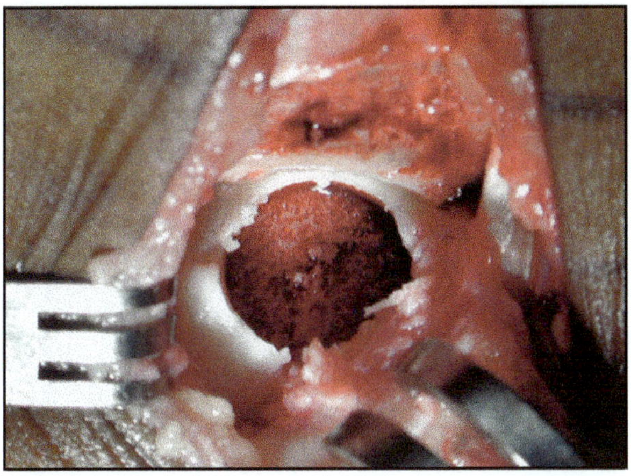

Figure 8-3. The recipient site has been prepared with a cannulated reamer.

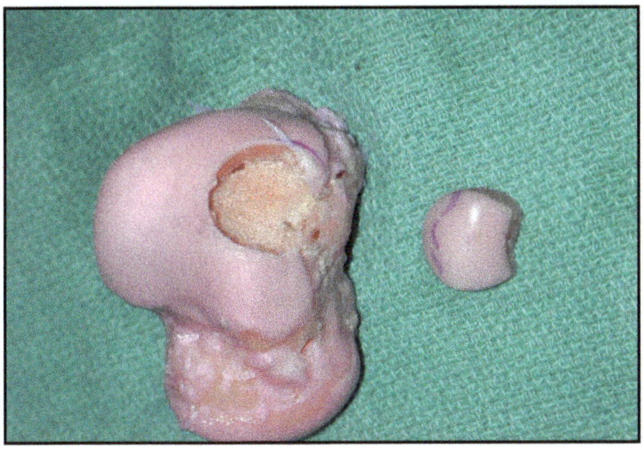

Figure 8-4. The allograft plug is harvested from the donor talus. Note the relationship of the plug to the shoulder of the talus, which must match the prepared recipient site.

necessary to create a matched graft. This can be extremely difficult on the shoulder of the talus. The graft should be held firmly while the donor graft is harvested. The appropriate-sized (matched) graft harvester (coring reamer) is then utilized to harvest the plug from the matching portion of the talus. Excess bone is then removed from the graft after transferring the depth measurements of the recipient site. The graft is copiously pulse lavaged to remove debris and marrow elements to decrease the immunogenicity of the graft. Often, beveling the bony edge of the graft will aid in insertion and reduce the potentially harmful impact force of insertion.

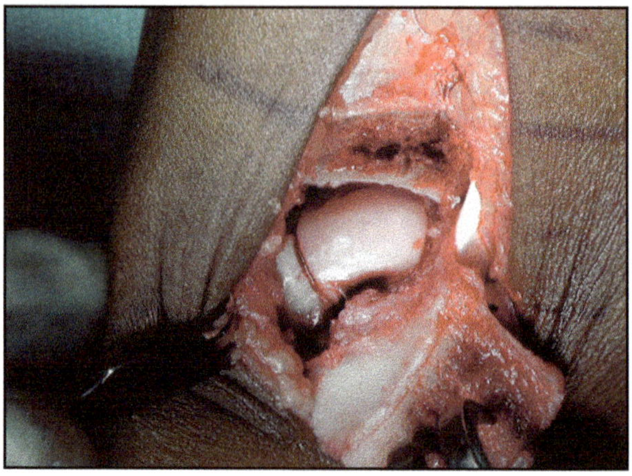

Figure 8-5. The allograft plug is in place prior to fixation of the malleolar osteotomy.

The donor plug is carefully and gently impacted down into the recipient site to obtain a flush articular edge match on the articular surface of the talar dome (Figure 8-5). Rarely, it is necessary to place 2 plug grafts; if required, care should be taken not to dislodge the first graft. Temporary fixation of the first graft with a Kirschner wire may be advisable. At this point, the osteotomy is reduced and fixed, utilizing the preplanned screws and starting with the horizontal malleolar screws. Routine wound closure is performed and the ankle is placed in a bulky cotton elastic bandage.

Partial (Shell) Talus Allograft Technique

The partial talus or "shell" technique is used for large or cystic lesions that require reconstruction of 20% or more of the talar dome. This is the authors' preferred method for OCA of the talus as it avoids the morbidity of the malleolar osteotomy and is amenable to larger lesions.

After skin preparation, a temporary unipolar external fixator is placed across the ankle medially with pins placed in the talar neck, calcaneus, and tibia with use of fluoroscopy (Figure 8-6). The purpose of this external fixator is used for intraoperative distraction of the ankle joint. An anterior approach through the interval between the extensor hallucis longus and the tibialis anterior tendons is made, centered over the tibiotalar joint. The neurovascular bundle is mobilized laterally and the joint is entered. Deep dissection is carried out depending on whether the lesion is medial or lateral. The tibiotalar joint is carefully distracted 4 to 8 mm and confirmed by fluoroscopy. Distraction is engaged to allow visualization and inspection of the tibiotalar joint as well as insertion of the saw. The position of the talus is optional. Plantarflexion allows better visualization of the lesion, but distraction in the neutral position may allow for easier estimation of the appropriate saw angle. Removal of osteophytes or a small plafondplasty is performed. The lesion is inspected and the extent of the damaged talus is marked. Using a small oscillating saw, the damaged articular portion is resected in a geometric manner using a single-sided reciprocating saw to first make a vertical cut of about 6- to 10-mm depth. A horizontal cut is then made with a small oscillating saw, taking care to avoid neurovascular, tendon, or malleolar injury (Figure 8-7). This cut invariably starts at the margin of the articular cartilage anteriorly and should be parallel to the axis of the talar dome, exiting posteriorly at the articular margin. The resected fragment is inspected and retained to serve as a template for preparation of the allograft. A ruler or depth gauge is used to measure the dimensions of the resection site, which is usually a few millimeters bigger than the resected fragment. These measurements are transferred to the allograft and used as a guide for resection. Similar vertical and horizontal saw cuts are made in the allograft to remove the desired fragment (Figure 8-8). It is important to be conservative when cutting the graft as it can be trimmed smaller but not made bigger (Figure 8-9). Generally, multiple trial fittings are performed and graft modification with either the saw, a burr, or a rasp is performed. Congruency of less than 1 mm should be obtained.

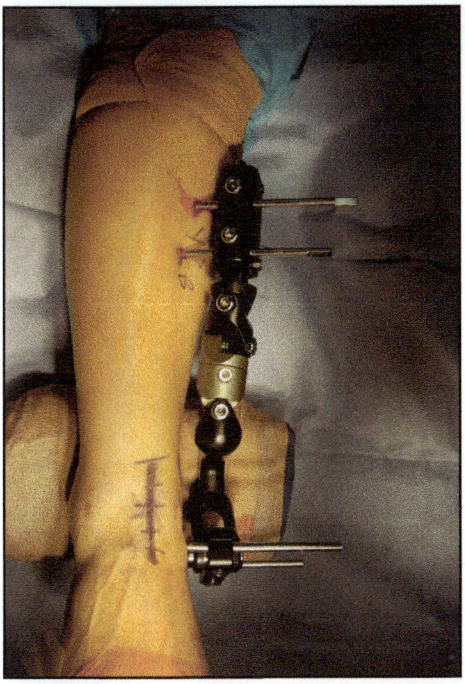

Figure 8-6. A unipolar external fixator placed across the ankle joint provides temporary distraction that facilitates surgical exposure.

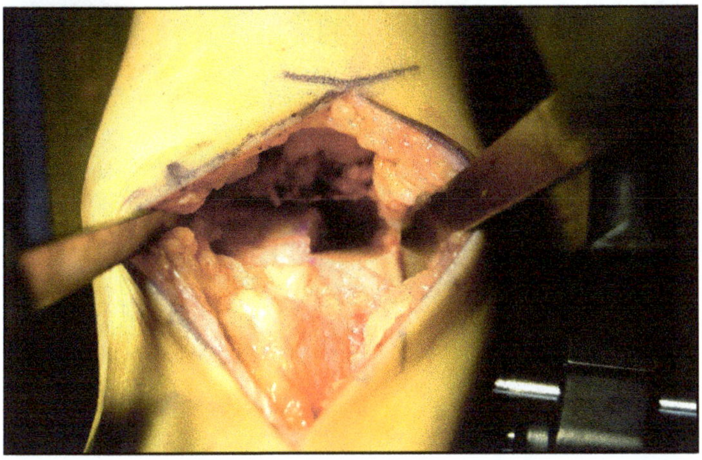

Figure 8-7. Preparation of the recipient site after completion of both the vertical and horizontal cuts.

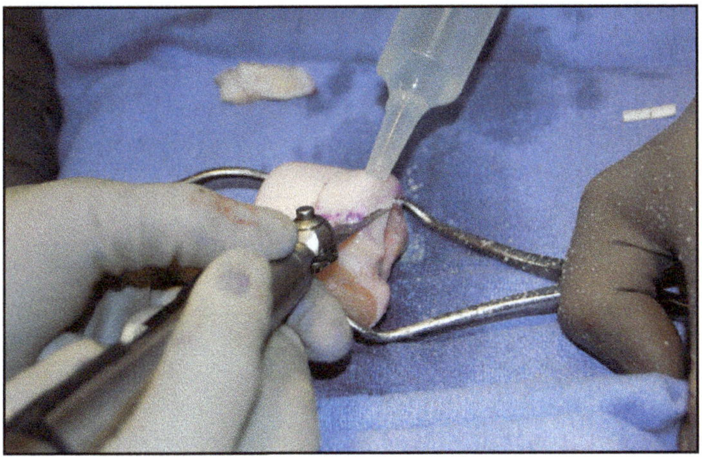

Figure 8-8. The allograft is removed from the donor talus following similarly performed resection along the measured and marked dimensions of the recipient site.

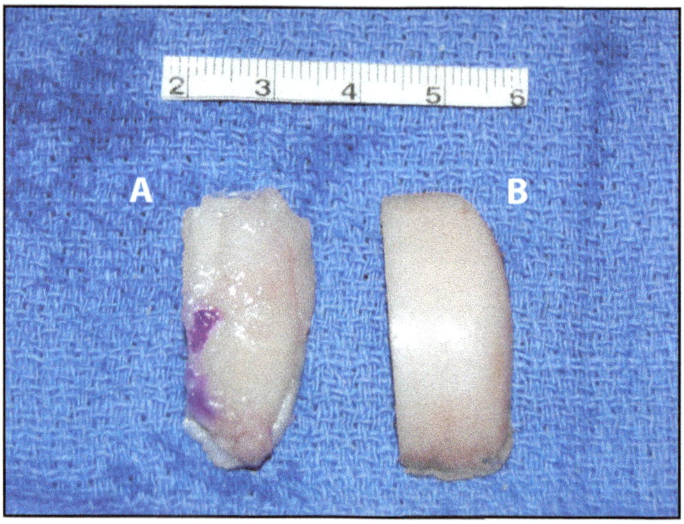

Figure 8-9. (A) The resected fragment and (B) prepared allograft fragment. Note the similar shape but slightly larger size of the allograft.

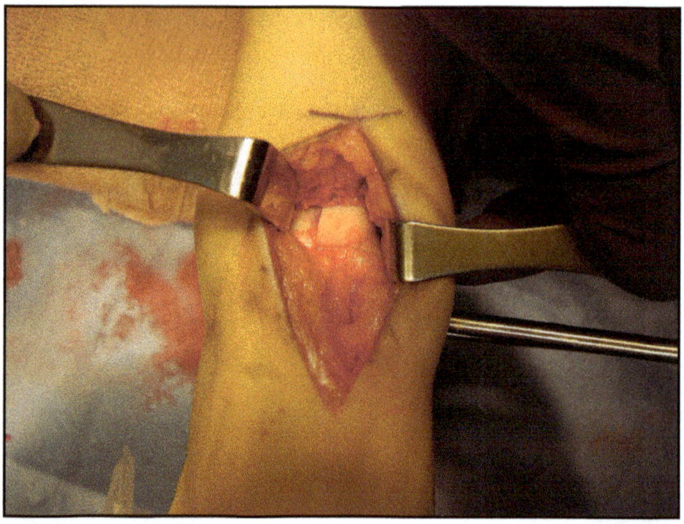

Figure 8-10. The allograft is placed into the ankle and distraction is released. Note the congruent fit of the allograft to the native talus.

Prior to final insertion of the allograft, cystic and sclerotic lesions in the patient's talus extending beyond the depth of resection level can be curetted, drilled, or grafted. The graft is copiously pulse lavaged to remove debris and marrow elements to decrease the immunogenicity of the graft. The fixator distraction is then released and the ankle is brought through a range of motion to check graft stability and position (Figure 8-10). Fluoroscopic images should be obtained at this point. Because the graft is an onlay graft, adjunct fixation should be used that allows some degree of compression. These are usually less than 3-mm diameter metal or bioabsorbable screws, which can be inserted along the shoulder of the graft. At this point, the external fixator is removed, routine wound closure is performed, and the ankle is placed in a bulky cotton splint.

Postoperative Protocol

Postoperative care includes protection in a nonweightbearing short leg splint until suture removal at 2 weeks, followed by transition to a controlled ankle motion walker to permit early ankle motion exercises. Patients are nonweightbearing for 6 weeks and then progressed to partial weightbearing (25% to 50% of body weight) in the boot with functional rehabilitation for a period of at least 6 weeks. During that time, active range of motion and isometric muscle strengthening are progressively advanced. Pool exercises and no-impact, closed-chain exercises, such as cycling without resistance, can be introduced 6 weeks postoperatively. A gradual return to full weightbearing is permitted once graft incorporation is confirmed radiographically, usually at 12 weeks. The patient is generally allowed to incrementally return to recreational activities and sports around 6 months. Complete recovery can take 12 months or longer.

Potential Complications

Complications of fresh OCA of the talus include intraoperative fracture of the fibula or medial malleolus, neurovascular, or tendon injury.[3] Skin compromise and superficial or deep infection are possible but rare in these generally healthy individuals.[19] Long-term issues include delayed or nonunion of the graft or fracture, resorption, or recurrent cyst formation in the talus.[8,9,20]

Top Technical Pearls for the Procedure

1. The plug or shell technique can be used for many lesions, but consider the shell onlay technique for lesions involving 20% or more of the talus.
2. Careful size matching of the donor and recipient is important, as congruity is essential to surgical success. Inspect the allograft before making the surgical incision.
3. Posteromedial neurovascular structures are at risk in this procedure when making the osteotomy or talar resections.
4. Making the same cut or drill angle in the recipient and donor is paramount to fitting the graft properly. Unequal cut or drill angles are nearly impossible to resolve.
5. Be prepared to perform repeated trial fittings and small graft or recipient site modifications to obtain proper fit of the allograft.

References

1. Aktas S, Kocaoglu B, Gereli A, Nalbantodlu U, Guven O. Incidence of chondral lesions of talar dome in ankle fracture types. *Foot Ankle Int.* 2008;29(3):287-292.
2. Christensen JC, Driscoll HL, Tencer AF. Contact characteristics of the ankle joint. Part 2. The effects of talar dome cartilage defects. *J Am Podiatr Med Assoc.* 1994;84(11):537-547.
3. Giannini S, Buda R, Faldini C, et al. Surgical treatment of osteochondral lesions of the talus in young active patients. *J Bone Joint Surg Am.* 2005;87(Suppl 2):28-41.
4. Schachter AK, Chen AL, Reddy PD, Tejwani NC. Osteochondral lesions of the talus. *J Am Acad Orthop Surg.* 2005;13(3):152-158.
5. Schottle PB, Oettl GM, Agneskirchner JD, Imhoff AB. Operative therapy of osteochondral lesions of the talus with autologous cartilage-bone transplantation. *Der Orthopade.* 2001;30(1):53-58.
6. Shearer C, Loomer R, Clement D. Nonoperatively managed stage 5 osteochondral talar lesions. *Foot Ankle Int.* 2002;23(7):651-654.
7. Cuttica DJ, Smith WB, Hyer CF, Philbin TM, Berlet GC. Osteochondral lesions of the talus: predictors of clinical outcome. *Foot Ankle Int.* 2011;32(11):1045-1051.

8. Kim CW, Jamali A, Tontz W Jr, Convery FR, Brage ME, Bugbee W. Treatment of post-traumatic ankle arthrosis with bipolar tibiotalar osteochondral shell allografts. *Foot Ankle Int.* 2002;23(12):1091-1102.
9. Meehan R, McFarlin S, Bugbee W, Brage M. Fresh ankle osteochondral allograft transplantation for tibiotalar joint arthritis. *Foot Ankle Int.* 2005;26(10):793-802.
10. Tontz WL Jr, Bugbee WD, Brage ME. Use of allografts in the management of ankle arthritis. *Foot Ankle Clin.* 2003;8(2):361-373, xi.
11. Gortz S, De Young AJ, Bugbee WD. Fresh osteochondral allografting for osteochondral lesions of the talus. *Foot Ankle Int.* 2010;31(4):283-290.
12. El-Rashidy H, Villacis D, Omar I, Kelikian AS. Fresh osteochondral allograft for the treatment of cartilage defects of the talus: a retrospective review. *J Bone Joint Surg Am.* 2011;93(17):1634-1640.
13. Gross AE, Agnidis Z, Hutchison CR. Osteochondral defects of the talus treated with fresh osteochondral allograft transplantation. *Foot Ankle Int.* 2001;22(5):385-391.
14. Berlet GC, Hyer CF, Philbin TM. Successful use of fresh-frozen osteochondral allograft for the management of osteochondral lesions of the talus: a prospective study. Paper presented at: AOFAS Summer Meeting; June 25-28, 2008; Denver, CO.
15. Raikin SM. Stage VI: massive osteochondral defects of the talus. *Foot Ankle Clin.* 2004;9(4):737-744, vi.
16. Raikin SM. Fresh osteochondral allografts for large-volume cystic osteochondral defects of the talus. *J Bone Joint Surg Am.* 2009;91(12):2818-2826.
17. Gortz S, Bugbee WD. Allografts in articular cartilage repair. *Instr Course Lect.* 2007;56:469-480.
18. McAllister DR, Joyce MJ, Mann BJ, Vangsness CT Jr. Allograft update: the current status of tissue regulation, procurement, processing, and sterilization. *Am J Sports Med.* 2007;35(12):2148-2158.
19. Kainer MA, Linden JV, Whaley DN, et al. Clostridium infections associated with musculoskeletal-tissue allografts. *N Eng J Med.* 2004;350(25):2564-2571.
20. Jeng CL, Kadakia A, White KL, Myerson MS. Fresh osteochondral total ankle allograft transplantation for the treatment of ankle arthritis. *Foot Ankle Int.* 2008;29(6):554-560.

Please visit www.routledge.com/9781617119989 to access additional material.

9

Osteochondral Lesions of the Tibial Plafond

Steven M. Raikin, MD and Masato Takao, MD, PhD

Introduction

Osteochondral lesions of the distal tibial plafond (OLTP) are uncommon, and there are a few references detailing the incidence, etiology, locations, size, or distribution of these lesions. A previous report showed a frequency of 2.6%,[1] and it is far less frequent than osteochondral lesions of the talus (OLT) with a ratio of 1 OLTP for every 14 to 20 OLT.[2,3] The etiology of the lesion is also varied, including high-energy trauma, an ankle inversion or eversion injury, chronic ankle instability, and no specific etiology.[4]

Although methods of treatment for OLTP previously described include arthroscopic curettage, drilling, open bone grafting of the defect with autologous bone graft or allograft, or use of a synthetic osteochondral plug,[2,5-9] effective treatment remains uncertain, especially in advanced cases.

In treating the osteochondral lesions, the healthy condition of the subchondral bone in the meaning of there being enough viable stem cells is essential for good clinical results.[10] Actually, OLT with large subchondral lesions of the ankle, including subchondral cyst, is known as being difficult to treat.[11] Malinin and Ouellette[12] performed 2 types of osteochondral autograft in nonhuman primates: one was placed into vascularized viable cancellous bone well, and another in an identical bone well but coated with methyl methacrylate to prevent direct contact between the autograft and the host bone. Three years later, the former showed healthy articular cartilage with viable subchondral bone, but the latter showed degenerative articular cartilage with nonviable subchondral bone. Accordingly, to keep the subchondral bone in viable condition is important for regenerating the morbid articular cartilage.

The osteochondral autograft transplantation from the knee is one of the choices for treating such lesions, and several authors reported good short- to mid-term clinical results.[11,13,14] However, there remain several apprehensions including the risk of malleolar osteotomy,[15] risk of donor site complications,[16] and incompatibility of an osteochondral fragment because of the different characteristics of the articular cartilage between the knee and ankle joints.[17]

Autologous bone graft is also one of the candidates in the meaning of the reconstruction of the morbid subchondral bone.[18-20] For the advanced lesions of the ankle with either deficient or absent overlying cartilage above subchondral lesions, poor functional outcome was reported in

Stone JW, Kennedy JG, Glazebrook M, eds. *The Foot and Ankle: AANA Advanced Arthroscopic Surgical Techniques* (pp 75-82).

one-half of the cases with open anterograde autologous bone grafting, requiring further surgery.[21] The authors believe that the reasons for such poor results may be caused by malleolar osteotomy similar to that of osteochondral transplantation.

To overcome these problems, the reconstruction of the morbid subchondral lesions and supplying of sufficient mesenchymal stem cells from the patient's pelvis, without osteotomy and without injuring the knee joint, should be beneficial for regeneration of the lesions. The author introduced retrograde autologous cancellous bone transplantation (RACT) under arthroscopic assistance for the reconstruction of the morbid subchondral bone,[22] especially in cases of advanced OLTP with large subchondral lesions and/or subchondral cyst formation.

Indications

- Symptomatic OLTP that is more than 150 mm^2 areas and/or subchondral cyst in preoperative magnetic resonance imaging (MRI)
- Difficult to treat with bone marrow stimulating techniques[23]

Pertinent Physical Findings

- Complaints of pain, catching, or grinding in the ankle accompanied by intermittent episodes of swelling
- The findings from physical examination of patients with OLTP are often nonspecific.

Pertinent Imaging

- MRI is obtained using a 1.5 to 3.0 T superconducting MR scanner using an extremity coil. A section thickness of 3 mm is used with a 0.5-mm intersection gap. The coronal and sagittal planes with the plane examination protocol consisted of T2-weighted fast-spin-echo-sequences are obtained (Figure 9-1).
- A computed tomography with a section thickness of 2 mm is also useful for clarifying the subchondral cyst (Figure 9-2).
- If the area of the osteochondral lesion is equal to or greater than 150 mm^2 and/or subchondral cyst formation, it is regarded as the indication of the RACT.

Equipment

- Narrow arthroscopy system (2.7-mm ankle arthroscope)
- Irrigation system
- Distraction device (ankle distraction board)
- Small instruments for surgery (probe, graspers, rasp, ring and sharp curettes)
- Motorized shaver system
- Motorized cannulated drill (6.5 mm in diameter)
- Guide wire for cannulated drill
- 6.5-mm Tubular chisel of Mosaicplasty (Smith & Nephew)

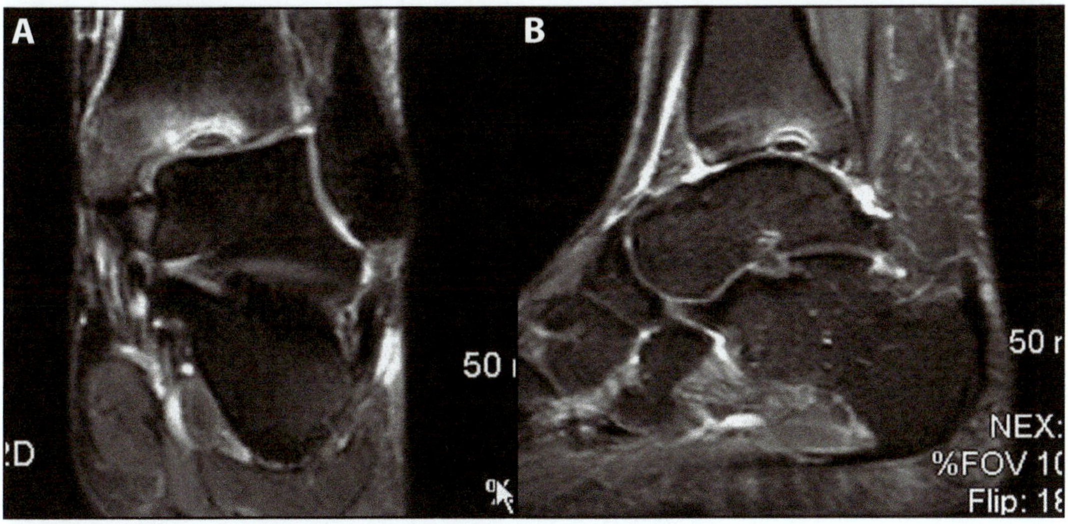

Figure 9-1. The (A) coronal and (B) sagittal planes of MRI of the left ankle.

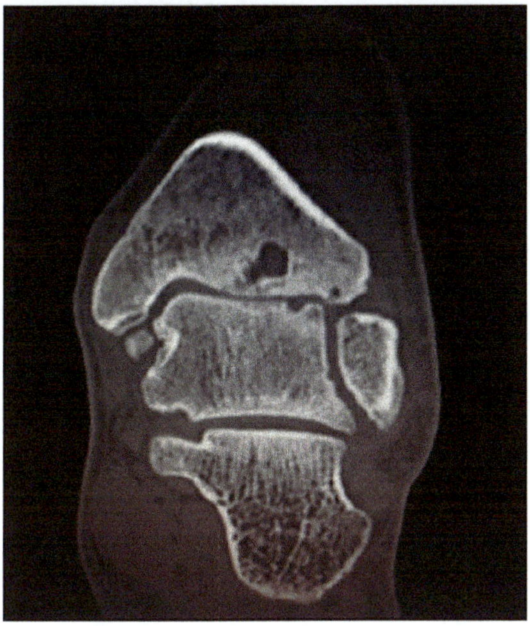

Figure 9-2. Coronal plane of the computed tomography of the left ankle (a different patient from Figure 9-1).

- Fluoroscopy
- Television monitor and recording system

Positioning and Portals

Ankle arthroscopy is performed under spinal lumbar anesthesia. The patient is placed in a supine position on an operating table. The leg is put on an ankle distraction board by means of the bandage distraction technique with a force of 6 kg (Figure 9-3).[24]

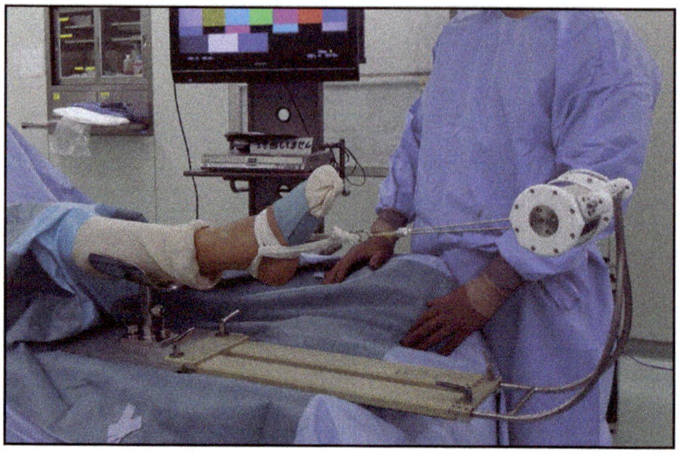

Figure 9-3. Position after putting a bandage distraction on the ankle distraction board.

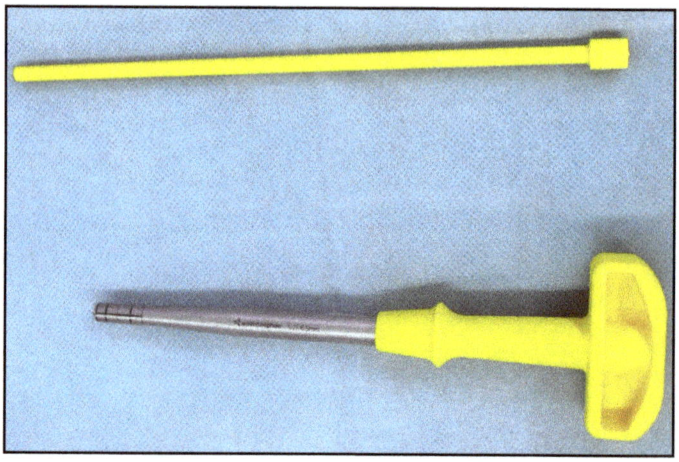

Figure 9-4. A tubular chisel of Mosaicplasty.

Step-by-Step Description of the Procedure

- Step 1—Harvesting the cancellous bone plug of the ipsilateral iliac crest: A 1.5-cm straight skin incision is initiated at the iliac crest, and bony surface is exposed. A cancellous bone plug with a 6.5-mm diameter and 30-mm length is harvested using a 6.5-mm tubular chisel of Mosaicplasty (Figure 9-4) at the exposed iliac crest.
- Step 2—Arthroscopic curettage of the degenerated cartilage: An arthroscope 2.7 mm in diameter is inserted at the anterolateral and anteromedial portals. Because the remaining degenerative cartilage disrupts the regeneration of the cartilage,[25] it should be removed using a ring curette and arthroscopic rasp (Figure 9-5).
- Step 3—Making a bone tunnel: A 2-cm longitudinal straight skin incision is initiated at the medial tibia, which is about 40 mm proximal from the tip of the medial malleolus, using a pneumotourniquet inflated to a pressure of 300 mm Hg. After exposing the bone surface, a guide wire is inserted through the medial tibia toward the lesion under fluoroscopy (Figure 9-6A and B). Through arthroscopy, the tip of the wire should be certified to penetrate the center of the tibial lesion (Figure 9-6C). A drill hole with a diameter of 6.5 mm is created toward the lesion using a cannulated drill. Care should be taken via arthroscopy never to injure the talar articular surface. If a cystic lesion remains, a curette is inserted into the hole for curettage of the cyst.

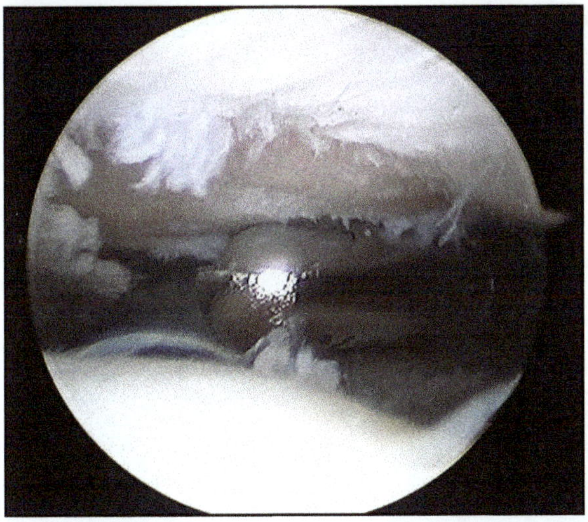

Figure 9-5. Arthroscopic photograph to remove the degenerative cartilage with a motorized shaver.

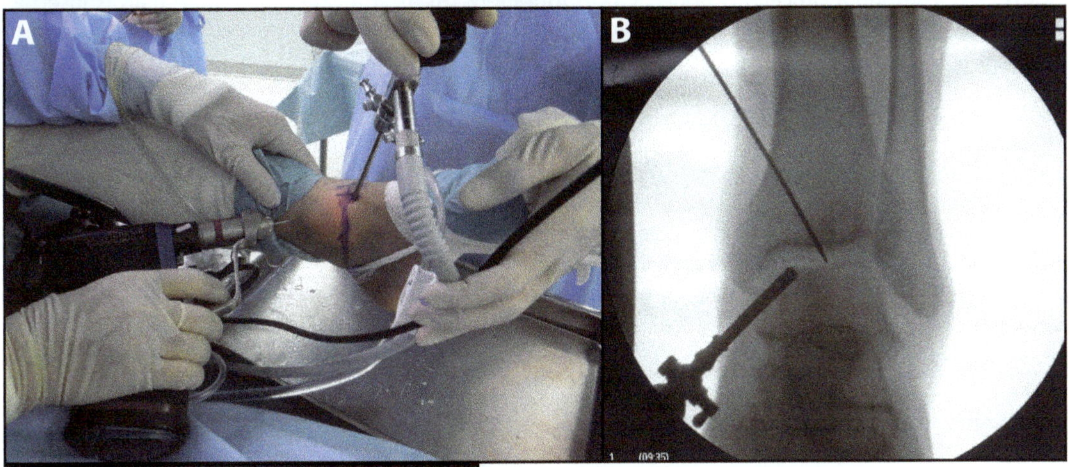

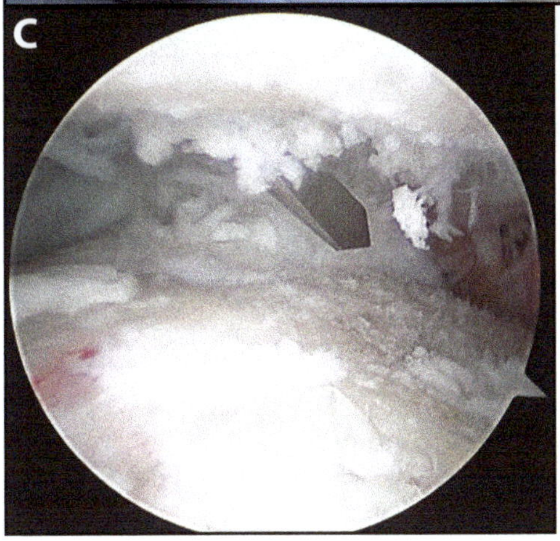

Figure 9-6. Penetrating a guide wire through the medial tibia toward the lesion. (A) Actual photograph. (B) Fluoroscopic photograph. (C) Arthroscopic photograph. *In the present case, there was a kissing lesion at the talar dome that was also treated with RACT.

- Step 4—Inserting the cancellous bone plug: Through the arthroscopic view, the cancellous bone plug is driven to protrude through the level of the articular surface (Figure 9-7A), and the surface of the graft is then leveled to the same level of the subchondral bone with forceps (Figure 9-7B).

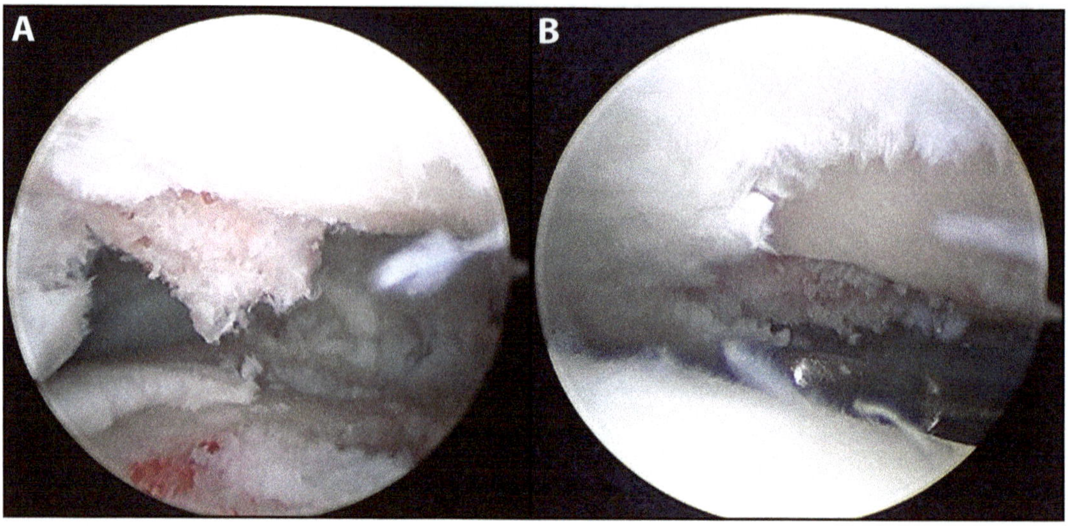

Figure 9-7. Inserting a cancellous bone plug retrogradely. (A) After a cancellous bone plug is inserted over the level of the subchondral bone surface, (B) it is then leveled to the same level of the subchondral bone with forceps.

Postoperative Protocol

The ankle is immobilized with a soft ankle orthoses for 2 weeks. Active range of motion is allowed 1 day after surgery and passive range of motion is allowed 4 weeks after surgery. Partial weightbearing is allowed at 4 weeks postsurgery and full weightbearing is allowed at 8 weeks postsurgery.

Potential Complications

Complications including superficial or deep infection, osteonecrosis of the distal tibia, skin trouble, and the lateral femoral cutaneous nerve injury during bone harvesting may happen, but there was no such case in the authors' approximately 100 experiences. Because the reproduced cartilage after RACT is not a hyaline cartilage but a fibrous cartilage, prospective osteoarthrosis of the ankle may occur.

Top Technical Pearls for the Procedure

1. Before surgery, transcript the size and location of the lesion from the MRI to anteroposterior and lateral views of the standard x-ray (Figure 9-8). It is helpful to penetrate the lesion certainly under fluorography during surgery.
2. The remaining degenerative cartilage should be removed because it may obstruct the regeneration of the cartilage.
3. If there is a subchondral cyst, it should be curettaged using ring and sharp curettes via the drill hole.

(continued)

4. A single bone graft is enough in most cases, even if the diameter of the lesion and/or subchondral cyst is larger than that of grafted bone.
5. If there is a lateral instability of the ankle, it should be treated simultaneously. The authors' recommendation is arthroscopic repair or reconstruction using the remnant of the lateral ligaments or autologous gracilis tendon graft.

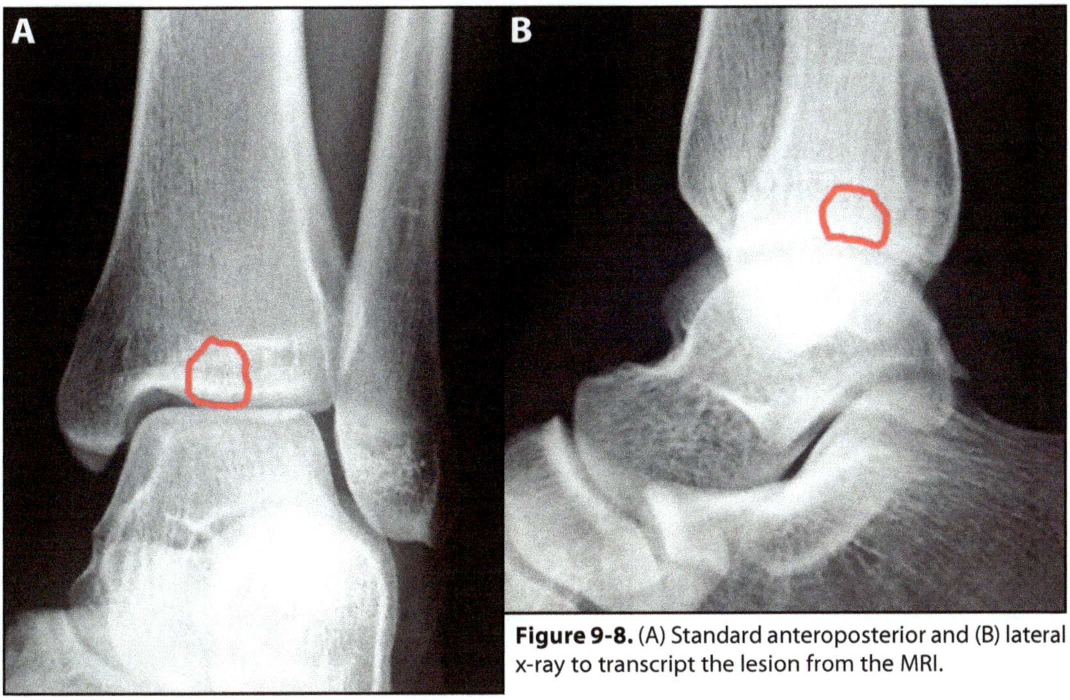

Figure 9-8. (A) Standard anteroposterior and (B) lateral x-ray to transcript the lesion from the MRI.

References

1. Mologne TS, Ferkel RD. Arthroscopic treatment of osteochondral lesions of the distal tibia. *Foot Ankle Int.* 2007;28:865-872.
2. Bui-Mansfield LT, Kline M, Chew FS, Rogers LF, Lenchik L. Osteochondritis dissecans of the tibial plafond: imaging characteristics and a review of the literature. *Am J Roentgenol.* 2000;175:1305-1308.
3. Elias I, Raikin SM, Schweitzer ME, Besser MP, Morrison WB, Zoga AC. Osteochondral lesions of the distal tibial plafond: localization and morphologic characteristics with an anatomical grid. *Foot Ankle Int.* 2009;30:524-529.
4. Cuttica DJ, Smith WB, Hyer CF, Philbin TM, Berlet GC. Arthroscopic treatment of osteochondral lesions of the tibial plafond. *Foot Ankle Int.* 2012;33:662-668.
5. Canosa J. Mirror image osteochondral defects of the talus and distal tibia. *Int Orthop.* 1994;18:395-396.
6. Chapman CB, Mann JA. Distal tibia osteochondral lesion treated with osteochondral allografting: a case report. *Foot Ankle Int.* 2005;26:997-1000.
7. Crotty JM, Brogdon BG. Posttraumatic osteochondral defect of the distal tibia. *Emergency Radiol.* 1998;5;438-441.
8. Ferkel RD, Field J, Scherer WP, Bernstein ML, Kasimian D. Intraosseous ganglion cysts of the ankle: a report of three cases with long-term follow-up. *Foot Ankle Int.* 1999;20:384-388.

9. Peace CJ, Lutz MJ, Mitchell A, Calder JD. Treatment of a distal tibial osteochondral lesion with a synthetic osteochondral plug: a case report. *Foot Ankle Int.* 2009;30:900-903.
10. Gomoll AH, Madry H, Knutsen G, et al. The subchondral bone in articular cartilage repair: current problems in the surgical management. *Knee Surg Sports Traumatol Arthrosc.* 2010;18:434-447.
11. Scranton PE Jr, Frey CC, Feder KS. Outcome of osteochondral autograft transplantation for type-V cystic osteochondral lesions of the talus. *J Bone Joint Surg Br.* 2006;88:614-619.
12. Malinin T, Ouellette EA. Articular cartilage nutrition is mediated by subchondral bone: a long-term autograft study in baboons. *Osteoarthritis Cartilage.* 2000;8:483-491.
13. Gautier E, Kolker D, Jakob RP. Treatment of cartilage defects of the talus by autologous osteochondral grafts. *J Bone Joint Surg.* 2002;84B:237-244.
14. Hangody L, Kish G, Modis L, et al. Mosaicplasty for the treatment of osteochondritis dissecans of the talus: two seven year results in 36 patients. *Foot Ankle Int.* 2001;22:552-558.
15. Angermann P, Jensen P. Osteoarthritis dissecans of the talus: long-term results of surgical treatment. *Foot Ankle.* 1989;10:161-163.
16. Kreuz PC, Steinwachs M, Erggelet C, Lahm A, Henle P, Niemeyer P. Mosaicplasty with autogenous talar autograft for osteochondral lesions of the talus after failed primary arthroscopic management: a prospective study with a 4-year follow-up. *Am J Sports Med.* 2005;33:1-9.
17. Buckwalter JA, Saltzman CL. Ankle osteoarthritis: distinct characteristics. *Instr Course Lect.* 1999;48:233-241.
18. Draper SD, Fallat LM. Autogeneous bone grafting for the treatment of talar dome lesions. *J Foot Ankle Surg.* 2000;39:15-23.
19. Greenspoon J, Rosman M. Medial osteochondritis of the talus in children: review and new surgical treatment. *J Pediatr Orthop.* 1987;7:705-708.
20. Lee CK, Mercurio C. Operative treatment of osteochondritis dissecans in situ by retrograde drilling and cancellous bone graft. *Clin Orthop.* 1981;158:129-136.
21. Kolker D, Murray M, Wilson M. Osteochondral defects of the talus treated with autologous bone grafting. *J Bone Joint Surg.* 2004;86B:521-526.
22. Takao M, Innami K, Komatsu F, Matsushita T. Retrograde cancellous bone plug transplantation for the treatment of advanced osteochondral lesions with large subchondral lesions of the ankle. *Am J Sports Med.* 2010;38:1653-1660.
23. Choi WJ, Lee JW. Osteochondral lesion of the talus: prognostic factors affecting the clinical outcome after arthroscopic marrow stimulation technique. *Foot Ankle Clin.* 2013;18:67-78.
24. Takao M, Ochi M, Shu N, et al. Bandage distraction technique for ankle arthroscopy. *Foot Ankle Int.* 1999;20:389-391.
25. Takao M, Uchio Y, Kakimaru H, Kumahashi N, Ochi M. Arthroscopic drilling with or without debridement of remaining cartilage for osteochondral lesions of the talar dome in unstable ankles. *Am J Sports Med.* 2004;32:332-336.

Please visit www.routledge.com/9781617119989 to access additional material.

SECTION II

Ankle Stabilization

10

ArthroBroström

Peter Mangone, MD and Jorge I. Acevedo, MD

Introduction

Since the advent of arthroscopy, orthopedic surgeons have successfully performed increasingly complex procedures through minimally invasive techniques. Initial knee and shoulder arthroscopy focused on purely diagnostic visualization followed by open procedures to treat the pathology. As surgeons improved their skills, these limited diagnostic procedures began to be modified to treat the underlying pathology through the smaller arthroscopic portals. Over the last 25 years, surgical stabilization of knee and shoulder instability has successfully evolved from large open procedures to small arthroscopic techniques. Foot and ankle surgeons are currently experiencing the same phenomenon in regard to ankle arthroscopy.

Traditional surgical methods to stabilize the lateral ankle rely on open incisions with either repair or reconstruction. Overall, results are satisfactory.[1-5] Biomechanical studies have also been published.[6-9]

Ankle arthroscopy is an accepted treatment option for loose bodies, exostosis, soft tissue impingement, and osteochondral lesions that have failed nonoperative management. The increased use of arthroscopy prior to open lateral ankle ligament reconstruction has resulted in the discovery of a high incidence of concomitant intra-articular pathology.[2,3,10-12] Based on the evolution of arthroscopic stabilization witnessed in knee and shoulder surgery, surgeons are now developing more successful procedures for arthroscopic lateral ankle ligament reconstruction.[13-19] An anatomic safe zone has been well defined.[20,21] Recent data examining the open modified Broström technique also indicate that satisfactory lateral ankle ligament stabilization can occur without calcaneofibular ligament repair.[5,7] With this in mind, an arthroscopic technique becomes more feasible as the anterior talofibular ligament (ATFL) and lateral capsular structures are easily visualized through the standard arthroscopic portals.

Initial attempts at lateral ankle arthroscopic stabilization using staples and thermal shrinkage techniques showed limited success.[22-24] Over the last 5 years, multiple techniques for arthroscopic lateral ankle ligament reconstruction have been published in the literature, demonstrating significant clinical efficacy.[13-19] These techniques vary in terms of the number of anchors used, the number of sutures used, the type of anchors used, and how the sutures are passed through

Stone JW, Kennedy JG, Glazebrook M, eds. *The Foot and Ankle: AANA Advanced Arthroscopic Surgical Techniques* (pp 85-93).

the lateral ankle structures. None of these methods have undergone biomechanical testing. One group published anatomic and biomechanical data on a technique, but there are no clinical data demonstrating its efficacy.[25] The ArthroBroström (Arthrex) is the only technique for which studies have now been completed that reveal clinical, anatomic, and biomechanically equivalent results between traditional open modified Broström ligament reconstruction and the arthroscopic technique.[13,17,20,26] The ArthroBroström technique described in this chapter was developed with the concepts of simplicity, reproducibility, and reliability. Although simple in design, it must be emphasized that this technique requires a surgeon who is experienced in arthroscopy and ankle anatomy. The authors' results in 93 patients were reviewed recently and demonstrate a reliable technique with only one patient who experienced recurrent instability. In addition, the authors have experienced a decreased amount of time in the operating room after the initial learning curve.

Indications

- Chronic recurrent ankle instability secondary to insufficiency of the lateral ligament complex
- Failed nonoperative treatment methods including a physical therapy program that utilizes such elements as proprioceptive training and bracing

Controversial Indications

- Severe (> 15 degrees) talar tilt documented on stress radiographs
- High-demand patients or heavier patients (these patients might be a better candidate for a tendon augmentation type of procedure for ankle stabilization)
- Patients with failed previous open Broström procedure
- Patients with congenital ligament laxity

Pertinent Physical Findings

- Lateral ankle ligament attenuation demonstrated by positive anterior drawer and positive talar tilt tests on examination. In the authors' experience, this is the "best test" to identify ankle instability. In the office setting, patient pain and guarding can make these tests less reliable. The most accurate findings will occur with an examination under anesthesia, which is performed after induction of anesthesia and before initiating the arthroscopic evaluation.
- Tenderness in the anterolateral gutter with palpation
- Tenderness or fullness of the peroneal tendon complex may suggest peroneal tendon tearing, which may need to be addressed at surgery.
- Weakness of the peroneal tendon complex. Although this could indicate a tear in the tendon complex, it could also represent general weakness leading to increased subjective instability. This weakness should be addressed with a physical therapy program prior to a surgical stabilization procedure.
- It is important for the surgeon to assess the patient closely for additional physical findings that may increase the risk of recurrent instability including obesity, congenital ligament laxity syndrome, cavovarus or hindfoot varus, and tibia vara. If these underlying problems exist, then the patient may require a different ligament reconstruction technique procedure to adequately stabilize the joint, concomitant procedures with an ArthroBroström technique to address the malalignment, or staged procedures to address the malalignment with a subsequent ArthroBroström reconstruction.

Pertinent Imaging

- Stress radiographs (either manual or with a mechanical stress device). These images are not an absolute requirement but can play a role in the decision making regarding whether to perform an ArthroBroström procedure vs an open tendon augmentation type of lateral ankle ligament stabilization. If the patient cannot relax to allow for these views to be reliable, consideration can be given to an intra-articular lidocaine injection to help decrease pain and guarding. Alternatively, intraoperative fluoroscopic stress views under anesthesia can be obtained as well.
- Magnetic resonance imaging or computed tomography scan may be needed to assess for additional intra-articular or extra-articular pathology such as osteochondral lesion, exostosis, and peroneal tendon tear. The need for these additional tests rests with the judgment of the surgeon depending on the patient's history and physical examination.

Equipment

The arthroscopy as well as the arthroscopic ligament repair is performed with 2.7-mm arthroscopic instruments. Although the 70-degree scope can facilitate visualization into the lateral gutter, the 30-degree scope will suffice for most ankles. A noninvasive ankle distractor should always be available on the back table but is only used according to surgeon preference or need. The authors currently use a commercially available kit containing two 3.0-mm suture anchors, an arthroscopic drill guide, a 2.4-mm cannulated drill, and a suture passer. Additional instruments for debridement of the joint include a 2.5-mm shaver, thermal ablation device, and small arthroscopic biter and grabber devices. An arthroscopic ring grasper, arthroscopic suture cutter, and arthroscopic knot pusher may also be used.

Positioning and Portals

The patient is positioned on a standard operating table with a well-padded tourniquet on the proximal thigh. While in the supine position, a bump or sandbag is placed under the ipsilateral buttocks to internally rotate the leg and facilitate access to the lateral ankle. A towel roll placed underneath the ankle allows access to the anterior ankle joint unless a noninvasive ankle distractor is preferred. If the distractor is utilized, then the arthroscopic knee or thigh holder is placed to keep the hip flexed 60 degrees. It is important to assure that the thigh holder does not cause pressure in the popliteal fossa as this may result in occlusion of the popliteal vein, increasing intraoperative bleeding, making arthroscopic visualization more difficult, and possibly increasing the risk of deep vein thrombosis.

Step-by-Step Description of the Procedure

Technique Overview

In the majority of cases, patients can have a regional popliteal block with monitored anesthesia care. Some patients may require a general anesthesia. If a regional popliteal block is performed, the surgeon or anesthesiologist must perform a separate local block for the saphenous nerve to cover the anteromedial portal sensation.

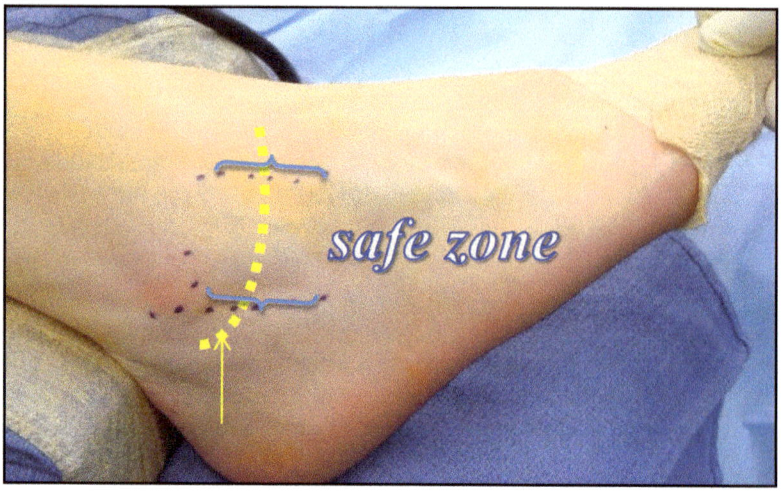

Figure 10-1. "Safe zone." Arrow points to inferior extensor retinaculum (IER) represented by yellow dashes. Dotted indelible pen markings (purple) represent the superior peroneal tendon margin (inferiorly) and the intermediate branch of the superficial peroneal nerve (superiorly).

Prior to starting the arthroscopic portion of the procedure, a stress anterior drawer and talar tilt exam under anesthesia should be performed both manually and under fluoroscopy. This allows a better assessment of the degree of instability that may not be appreciated in the awake patient. Although the standard ArthroBroström has been proven stable in the majority of cases, the stress exam may provide an indicator of whether augmentation is necessary.

Preoperative drawing of the anatomic landmarks is critical for success and involves marking the "safe zone" in the lateral ankle region (Figure 10-1). The surgeon should mark the superior margin of the peroneal tendons, the distal fibular tip, and the intermediate branch of the superficial peroneal nerve. The location of the inferior extensor retinaculum (IER) is estimated and drawn using the lateral calcaneal tubercle to help identify the margin of this tissue (usually located 1.5-cm from the tip of fibula with the ankle in neutral dorsiflexion).

Standard anteromedial and anterolateral arthroscopic portals are used throughout the procedure. Care should be taken to avoid placing the lateral portal too close to the fibula as this will make suture passage more difficult. Perform an initial diagnostic arthroscopy and address any intra-articular pathology prior to the ligamentous repair. An extensive debridement of the lateral gutter is necessary for 2 reasons: first, to remove pathologic fibrotic tissue, which may cause impingement, and second, to allow adequate visualization of the anterior aspect of the fibula. Once cleared, the medial, lateral, and inferior borders of the distal fibula should be easily probed.

At this point, the anterolateral portal is used as the working portal for anchor placement and passage of sutures while the scope is maintained in the anteromedial viewing portal. The first anchor is drilled through the arthroscopic drill guide and placed 1 cm above the distal tip of the fibula with sutures brought out through the standard anterolateral portal (Figure 10-2). Fluoroscopy is optional but may be helpful to assure appropriate distal anchor placement. Shuttling of the suture limbs is then accomplished with the sharp-tipped suture passer using either an "inside-out" or "outside-in" technique (see next sections; Figure 10-3). With either method, the sutures exit the capsular tissue a minimum of 1.5 cm from the distal tip of the fibula to ensure capture of the IER. The first suture limb (from first anchor) is passed just superior to the peroneal tendons, and the second suture limb (from first anchor) is passed 1 cm dorsal/anterior to the first suture along the arc of the IER. This set of sutures is intended to capture the inferior capsule, ATFL, and part of the IER.

After passing the first set of sutures, the second anchor is placed 1 cm above the first anchor site. This location is usually just below the talar dome and allows an adequate bone bridge between the anchors (Figure 10-4). The second set of sutures is then shuttled with the sharp-tipped suture passer again using either an "inside-out" or "outside-in" technique.

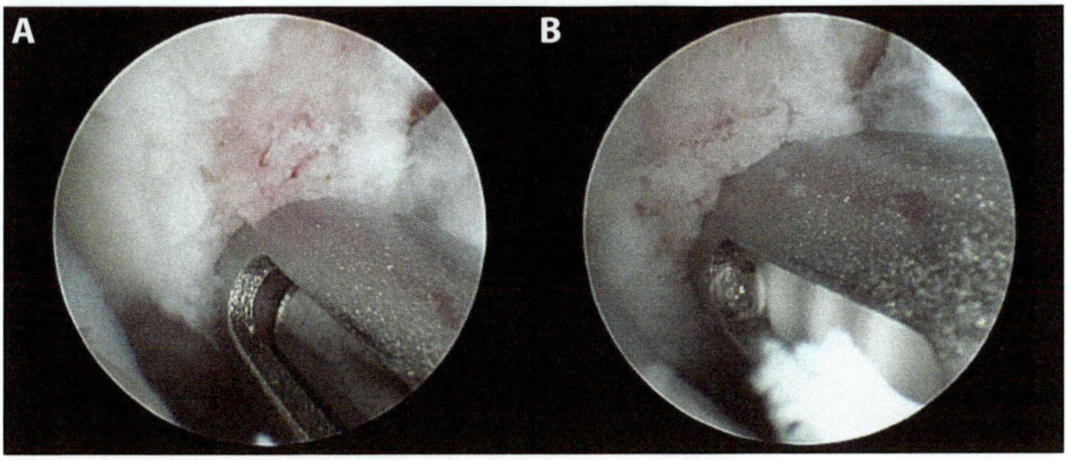

Figure 10-2. (A) Drilling of the first suture anchor through the arthroscopic cannula. (B) Insertion of the first suture anchor through the arthroscopic cannula.

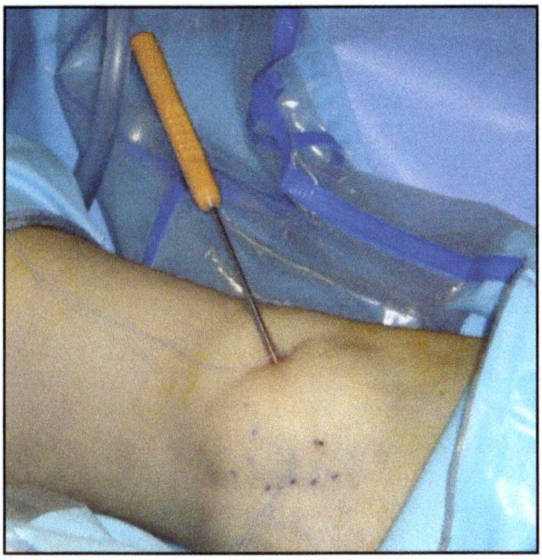

Figure 10-3. The suture passer shown in place for shuttling the second suture limb (inside-out technique). The first suture limb has already been passed and the suture passer is shown piercing the skin just above the peroneal tendon margin.

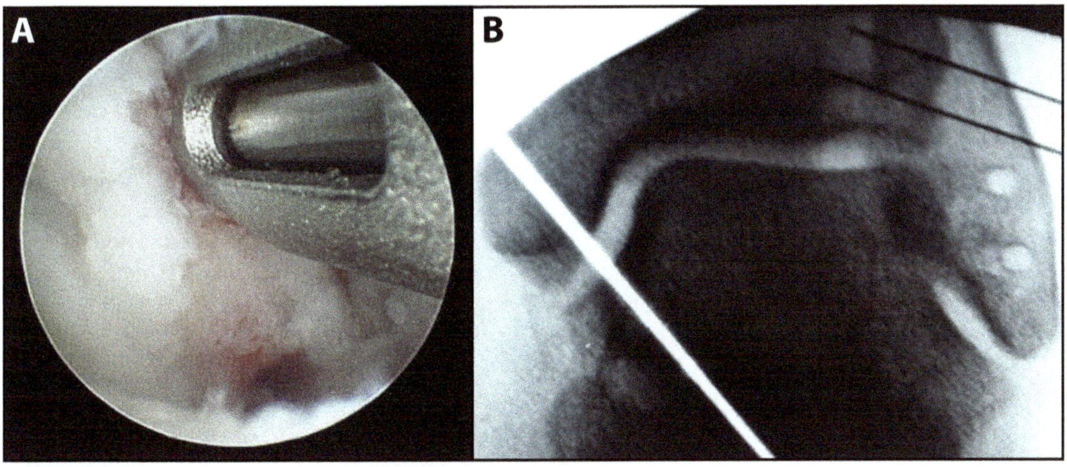

Figure 10-4. (A) Arthroscopic view of the second anchor placement relative to the first anchor location. (B) Fluoroscopic view of bone tunnel placement for anchors.

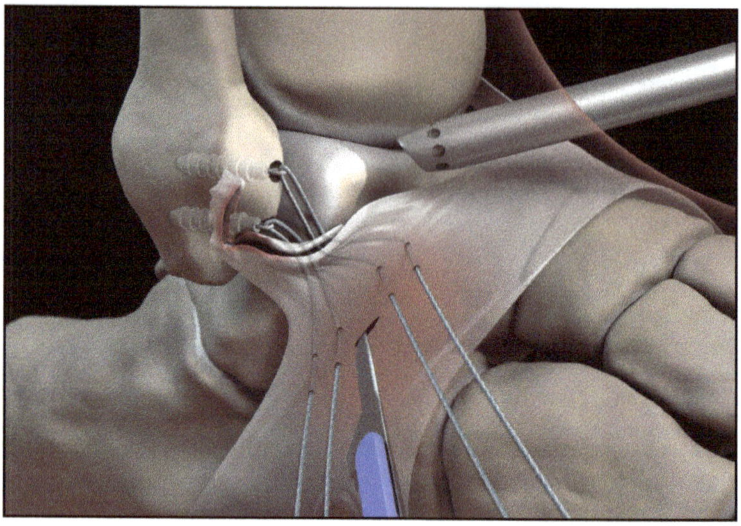

Figure 10-5. Diagrammatic representation of a central incision between the 2 sets of sutures once they have been shuttled through the lateral ligamentous complex.

The first suture limb (from the second anchor) is passed approximately 1 cm dorsal/anterior to the last suture (from the first anchor) along the arc of the IER. The second suture limb from the second anchor is then passed through the tissues 1 cm dorsal/anterior from the first suture limb (from the second anchor). This set of sutures is intended to capture the anterior capsule, ATFL, and part of the IER. However, it is important to stay inferior to the intermediate branch of the superficial peroneal nerve to avoid iatrogenic injury.

Subcutaneous passage of the 2 sets of sutures is next performed through a small (0.5-cm) incision between the suture sets (Figure 10-5). Using a small arthroscopic hook/probe, the 2 sets of sutures are delivered through this central incision. A small hemostat can facilitate subcutaneous dissection around the sutures. If there is concern with injuring the superficial peroneal nerve, retract the tissues anteriorly through the incision to make sure the more superior set of sutures has been passed deep to the nerve to prevent entrapment. The sutures are then tied down to the capsule/IER with the ankle held in neutral to slight eversion, at 90 degrees dorsiflexion, with a posterior drawer pressure applied. The sutures can be tied down with either a traditional knot-tying technique or an arthroscopic knot-tying technique. The use of an arthroscopic knot pusher can be helpful as well. If the arthroscope is inserted through the anteromedial portal during this process, the lateral ligamentous complex can be seen imbricating and drawing up to the anterior fibular surface.

Any residual laxity can be corrected by adding a second suture row (suture bridge) to the lateral fibula by passing the sutures in a percutaneous fashion. Should the surgeon decide that the arthroscopic technique has not adequately stabilized the lateral ligaments, the procedure can easily be converted to an open technique at any point during the procedure. All incisions are then closed with 4.0 nylon sutures and a simple horizontal mattress technique.

In cases where peroneal tendon pathology is concerned, a small ancillary incision is made directly over the peroneal tendon sheath. In the authors' experience, a 2-cm incision will suffice to address the majority of associated tendon pathology and limits the morbidity involved with more extensive approaches. Alternatively, the surgeon may also perform a peroneal tendoscopy if debridement and primary repair is all that is necessary.

"Inside-Out" Technique

Although the overview described previously does not change for the basic procedure, here the authors describe 2 methods of achieving the same outcome. When using the inside-out technique, the sharp-tipped suture passer is inserted through the anterolateral portal while viewing its entry with the scope in the anteromedial portal. When properly inserted, the suture passer will follow a trajectory between the lateral surface of the talus and the suture limbs, which initially exit the anterolateral portal. The suture passer will then pierce through the capsule, ATFL, and IER to exit at least 1.5 cm distal to the fibula and anterior/dorsal to the margin of the peroneal tendons (see Figure 10-3). If using the Micro SutureLasso (Arthrex), the looped wire is left in place and the SutureLasso is removed. The looped wire is then used to shuttle the first suture limb (first anchor) from the anterolateral portal out through the exit point as described previously. After passage of the first suture limb, the SutureLasso is then reinserted through the anterolateral portal for shuttling of the second suture limb (first anchor) following the same trajectory and exiting along the arc of the IER. A similar sequence of steps is used for shuttling the 2 suture limbs after placement of the second anchor.

"Outside-In" Technique

The outside-in technique follows the same course as the inside-out technique but differs in the entry point of the suture passer. Instead, the suture passer is inserted at the exit points on the skin of the inside-out technique. In other words, the sharp-tipped Micro SutureLasso is passed through the skin, subcutaneous tissue, IER, and ankle joint capsule and brought up into the joint under direct visualization of the arthroscope (viewing from the anteromedial portal). The looped wire is then advanced into the joint through the SutureLasso and an arthroscopic grasper is placed through the anterolateral portal to grab the wire and pull it out of the joint. The use of the blunt grasper device to pull the looped wire out of the portal decreases the chance of creating a tissue bridge that can occur more frequently if the surgeon tries to advance the SutureLasso device fully through the anterolateral portal. The looped wire is then used to shuttle each individual suture limb from the anterolateral portal and pulled back through the tissues and out of the skin. The remainder of the procedure was described previously in the overview.

Postoperative Protocol

Patients are discharged on the day of surgery in a short leg splint and then seen in the office for follow-up 10 days after surgery. Suture removal is usually performed at that time; however, this can be delayed 14 to 20 days after surgery if there are any concerns with wound healing. Patients remain in a walking boot until 3 to 4 weeks postoperatively and allowed 50% weightbearing during this time period. Transition is then made to a lace-up style gauntlet ankle brace and the patient progresses to full weightbearing as tolerated. Recently, the authors have started to use a brace as soon as the first postoperative visit in carefully selected, highly compliant patients. Protected active range of motion in the sagittal plane (dorsiflexion/plantarflexion) is started to help promote collagen alignment during healing. This has also helped to lessen lower leg atrophy during recovery. Formal physical therapy is initiated at 6 weeks after surgery, including a range of motion and TheraBand (The Hygenic Corporation) program with avoidance of passive inversion stretching. The ankle brace is continued for 6 to 9 months after surgery for athletic and higher impact activities. Return to competitive athletics will vary depending on the patient and the sport, but in most cases, this will be between 3 to 4 months after surgery.

Potential Complications

The authors have reviewed their latest follow-up of 93 patients who have undergone the ArthroBroström procedure since November 2007. Four patients were dissatisfied. Of the dissatisfied patients, 1 had recurrent instability and 3 had persistent pain symptoms postoperatively. Two of the 4 patients were receiving workers' compensation. Five patients developed postoperative neuritis, which was self-limited in all cases except for one patient whose symptoms resolved only after removal of the sutures that had entrapped the intermediate branch of the superficial peroneal nerve. In addition, there was one patient who developed a deep vein thrombosis and one who had stiffness, both of which resolved with appropriate nonoperative treatment.

Top Technical Pearls for the Procedure

1. Mark the "safe zone" before beginning arthroscopy—the superior margin of the peroneal tendons, distal fibular tip, intermediate branch of the superficial peroneal nerve, and proximal border of the IER.
2. Make sure to perform an extensive debridement of the lateral gutter to allow for visualization of the inferior tip of the fibula.
3. Place the first anchor 1 cm above the tip of the fibula, then pass the first set of sutures. Place the second anchor 1 cm above the first anchor (this should be below the level of the talar dome) and then pass the second set of sutures. This helps prevent crossing suture sets.
4. After placement of each suture anchor, use an arthroscopic ring grabber to identify the superior vs inferior limb of the suture. Pass the more inferior limb of the suture first to decrease the chance of crossing the sutures and inhibiting the ability to fully tie down the tissue on to the face of the fibula.
5. The distractor should be released and the ankle held in a neutral position with slight posterior drawer force prior to tying the sutures down.

References

1. Broström L. Sprained ankles. VI. Surgical treatment of "chronic" ligament ruptures. *Acta Chir Scand.* 1966;132(5):551-565.
2. Cannon LB, Slater HK. The role of ankle arthroscopy and surgical approach in lateral ankle ligament repair. *J Foot Ankle Surg.* 2005;11:1-4.
3. Hua Y. Modified Broström procedure plus ankle arthroscopy may be effective for ankle instability. *Arthroscopy.* 2010;26:524-528.
4. Karlsson J, Bergsten T, Lansinger O, Peterson L. Reconstruction of the lateral ligaments of the ankle for chronic lateral instability. *J Bone Joint Surg Am.* 1988;70(4):581-588.
5. Lee KT, Park YU, Kim JS, Kim JB, Kim KC, Kang SK. Long-term results after modified Broström procedure without calcaneofibular ligament reconstruction. *Foot Ankle Int.* 2011;32(2):153-157.
6. Clanton TO, Viens NA, Campbell KJ, Laprade RF, Wijdicks CA. Anterior talofibular ligament ruptures, part 2: biomechanical comparison of anterior talofibular ligament reconstruction using semitendinosus allografts with the intact ligament. *Am J Sports Med.* 2014;42(2):412-416.
7. Lee KT, Lee JI, Sung KS, et al. Biomechanical evaluation against calcaneofibular ligament repair in the Broström procedure: a cadaveric study. *Knee Surg Sports Traumatol Arthrosc.* 2008;16(8):781-786.
8. Viens NA, Wijdicks CA, Campbell KJ, Laprade RF, Clanton TO. Anterior talofibular ligament ruptures, part 1: biomechanical comparison of augmented Broström repair techniques with the intact anterior talofibular ligament. *Am J Sports Med.* 2014;42(2):405-411.

9. Waldrop NE 3rd, Wijdicks CA, Jansson KS, LaPrade RF, Clanton TO. Anatomic suture anchor versus the Broström technique for anterior talofibular ligament repair: a biomechanical comparison. *Am J Sports Med.* 2012;40(11):2590-2596.
10. Ferkel RD, Chams RN. Chronic lateral ankle instability: arthroscopic findings and long-term results. *Foot Ankle Int.* 2007;25:24-31.
11. Hintermann B, Boss A, Schäfer D. Arthroscopic findings in patients with chronic ankle instability. *Am J Sports Med.* 2002;30:402-409.
12. Komenda GA, Ferkel RD. Arthroscopic findings associated with the unstable ankle. *Foot Ankle Int.* 1999;20:708-713.
13. Acevedo JI, Mangone PG. Arthroscopic lateral ankle ligament reconstruction. *Tech Foot Ankle Surg.* 2011;10(3):111-116.
14. Corte-Real NM, Moreira RM. Arthroscopic repair of chronic lateral ankle instability. *Foot Ankle Int.* 2009;30:213-217.
15. Cottom JM, Rigby RB. The "all inside" arthroscopic Broström procedure: a prospective study of 40 consecutive patients. *J Foot Ankle Surg.* 2013;52(5):568-574.
16. Kim ES, Lee KT, Park JS, Lee YK. Arthroscopic anterior talofibular ligament repair for chronic ankle instability with a suture anchor technique. *Orthopedics.* 2011;34(4).
17. Mangone PG, Acevedo JI. Arthroscopically assisted lateral ligament reconstruction. Paper presented at: AOFAS 2010, Proceedings of the 26th Annual Meeting of the American Orthopaedic Foot and Ankle Society; July 7-9, 2010; Washington, DC.
18. Nery C, Raduan F, el Buono A, Asaumi ID, Cohen M, Maffulli N. Arthroscopic-assisted Broström-Gould for chronic ankle instability: a long-term follow-up. *Am J Sports Med.* 2011;39(11):2381-2388.
19. Vega J, Golanó P, Pellegrino A, Rabat E, Peña F. All-inside arthroscopic lateral collateral ligament repair for ankle instability with a knotless suture anchor technique. *Foot Ankle Int.* 2013;34(12):1701-1709.
20. Acevedo JI. ArthroBroström lateral ankle stabilization technique: an anatomical study. Paper presented at: AANA 2014, Proceedings of the 33rd Annual Meeting of the Arthroscopy Association of North America; May 1-3, 2014; Hollywood, FL.
21. Drakos M, Behrens SB, Mulcahey MK, Paller D, Hoffman E, Digiovanni CW. Proximity of arthroscopic ankle stabilization procedures to surrounding structures: an anatomic study. *Arthroscopy.* 2013;29(6):1089-1094.
22. Berlet GC, Saar WE, Ryan A, et al. Thermal-assisted capsular modification for functional ankle instability. *Foot Ankle Clin.* 2002;7:567-576.
23. de Vries JS, Krips R, Blankevoort L, Fievez AW, van Dijk CN. Arthroscopic capsular shrinkage for chronic ankle instability with thermal radiofrequency: prospective multicenter trial. *Orthopedics.* 2008;31(7):655.
24. Hawkins RB. Arthroscopic stapling repair for chronic lateral instability. *Clin Podiatr Med Surg.* 1987;4(4):875-883.
25. Drakos M, Behrens S, Hoffman E, et al. A biomechanical comparison of an open vs. arthroscopic approach for the treatment of lateral ankle instability (SS-57). *Arthroscopy.* 2011;27(5):e60–e61.
26. Giza E, Shin EC, Wong SE, et al. Arthroscopic suture anchor repair of the lateral ligament ankle complex: a cadaveric study. *Am J Sports Med.* 2013;41(11):2567-2572.

Please visit www.routledge.com/9781617119989
to access additional material.

11

Arthroscopic Anatomical Reconstruction of the Lateral Ankle Ligaments

Stephane Guillo, MD; Masato Takao, MD, PhD;
James W. Stone, MD; and Mark Glazebrook, MD

Introduction

Chronic ankle instability secondary to lateral ligament insufficiency is very common after sports injury.[1] When neglected, the recurrent "giving way" episodes may lead to articular cartilage injury and the subsequent development of degenerative arthritis of the tibiotalar joint. Many surgical techniques have been described for the treatment of the lateral ankle ligament complex. They can be classified by 2 definitions: repair or reconstruction and nonanatomical or anatomical.[2] Nonanatomical reconstructive techniques (so called *tenodesis*) (Evans, Watson-Jones, Chrisman-Snook) give very good results in the short term, but they may lead to restrictions in range of motion of the ankle or may result in persistent lateral instability after surgical intervension.[3-8] Accordingly, nonanatomical reconstructive techniques have gone out of favor because of the problems they generate in the long term.[9] Arthroscopy is commonly utilized as an adjunct to open ligament surgery, but it has traditionally been used to improve the diagnosis and management of any associated intra-articular lesions. A few authors have recently published innovative techniques for arthroscopic repair,[10-13] but only one was about the anatomical reconstruction.[14] The authors present here an all-arthroscopic technique for reconstruction of the anterior talofibular ligament (ATFL) and the calcaneofibular ligament (CFL) by means of anatomical placement of gracilis graft (auto or allograft). Although it is a new technique, it has been validated by an international expert group of surgeons specializing in ankle surgery (the Ankle Instability Group).

Indications

- Severe chronic ankle instability
- Revision case of chronic ankle instability
- High demand or high risk in chronic instability

Stone JW, Kennedy JG, Glazebrook M, eds. *The Foot and Ankle: AANA Advanced Arthroscopic Surgical Techniques* (pp 95-104).

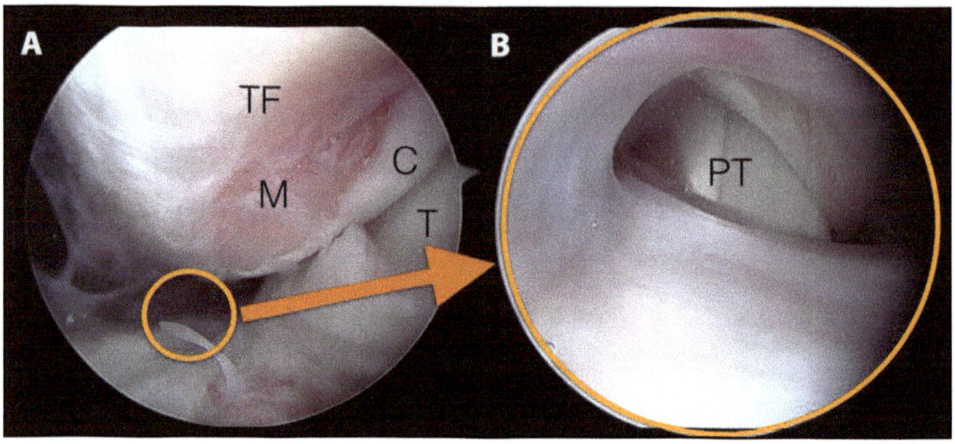

Figure 11-1. Lateral gutter of the ankle. (A) The ATFL has disappeared. (B) Inferior view with a view on the peroneal tendon (PT). C, cartilage side of the malleolus; M, malleolus; T, lateral side of the talus; TF, inferior part of the anterior tibiofibular ligament.

Surgery is indicated for patients with recurrent instability of the ankle secondary to injury to the lateral ligament complex after failure of nonoperative management, which may include physical therapy modalities, shoe modifications, and bracing. The Broström-Gould is a popular procedure to address chronic lateral instability. However, that procedure may not be adequate in cases where the patient's tissue is insufficient for repair, congenital ligament laxity, excessive body mass index, or failed previous repairs, and also if the time between injury and reconstruction is extremely long. In these difficult cases, reconstruction of the lateral ligament complex using autograft or allograft material is indicated (Figure 11-1). Several long-term studies have demonstrated a gradual deterioration of the joint, including postoperative loss of range of motion, recurrence of instability, ankle pain under conditions involving stress, a postoperative increase in radiographic arthritis changes, longer peroneal reaction time, and changes in both static and dynamic plantar pressure distribution.[15-18] According to these previous reports, it is supposed that the anatomical reconstruction should be performed to maintain long-term satisfactory clinical results.

Pertinent Physical Findings

It is important to obtain a detailed history of the patient's complaints to help differentiate between instability due to recurrent ligament injury and functional instability not related to increased ligament laxity. Physical examination must include the following:

- Overall assessment of lower extremity alignment
- Assessment for generalized ligament laxity
- Assessment for hindfoot varus malalignment, which may predispose to lateral ligament problems and which, if not addressed at the time of surgery, will result in a high likelihood of failure of surgical repair or reconstruction
- The range of motion (passive and active) of the ankle and subtalar joints is also noted.
- Gastrocnemius retraction is assessed with the lack of ankle dorsiflexion when the knee is in extension, comparing between the left and right sides.
- The ankle is assessed for lateral ligament laxity using both an anterior drawer test and an inversion test.
- ATFL is assessed in plantarflexion over 16.2 degrees,[19] so it is performed at neutral and at 30 degrees of plantarflexion, comparing the ankle to the opposite normal ankle.

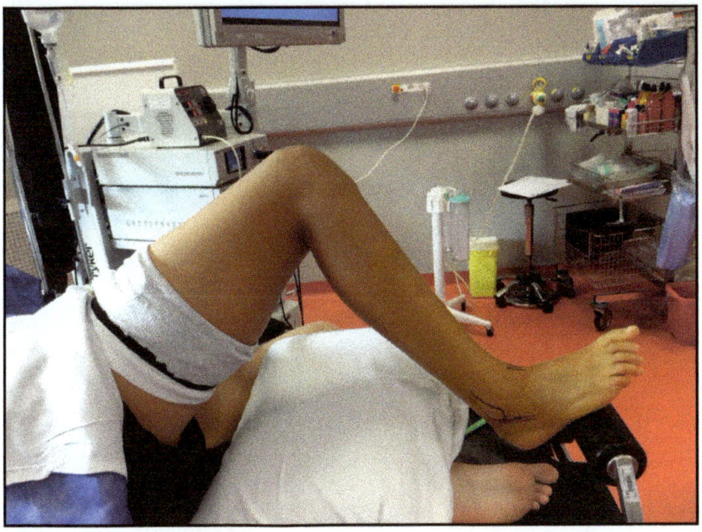

Figure 11-2. Position 1 for harvesting the graft.

Pertinent Imaging

- Ultrasound by hyper-specialist radiologist
- Standard plain radiographs: standing anteroposterior view, lateral and mortise views, and a comparative Saltzmann view, which is helpful to assess hindfoot alignment
- Magnetic resonance imaging may be helpful in the presence of deep pain to assess for osteochondral lesions and tendon injuries.

Equipment

The technique is carried out with a standard 4- or 2.7-mm diameter arthroscope, depending on surgeon preference. The 4.0-mm, 30-degree angle gives a better view and the laxity allows the use of this scope for the complete exploration of the joint. The surgical approaches are using, after the skin incision, a blunt dissection with a mosquito pean in order to not injure the nerves. Irrigation is provided by gravity pressure with a hanging saline serum by pockets of 3 L, or 50 to 60 mm Hg pressure using an irrigation system. The dissection is done arthroscopically with a shaver blade of 4-mm aggressive. The surgery is made in 5 steps: 3 steps for dissection and making tunnels, and 2 steps to introduce and fix the graft.

Achieving the tunnels requires a 2.4-mm Beath pin and 2 cannulated drills (4.5 and 6 mm). The fixation of the graft will use the following: for the malleolar fixation, a Toggle lock (Biomet); for the calcaneus, an interference screw of 7 x 25 mm; and for the talus, a 1.4-mm JuggerKnot bone anchor (Biomet) with an interference screw of 5x15 mm for the talus.

Positioning and Portals

The patient is placed in the lateral decubitus position with the pelvis slightly rotated 30 degrees posteriorly. For position 1, the hip is externally rotated and the knee is flexed (Figure 11-2) to harvest the gracilis tendon for the autograft. Position 2 is used for anterior arthroscopy with the knee extended and the hip externally rotated (Figure 11-3). Position 3 is utilized for lateral endoscopy with neutral rotation of the hip and the knee extended (Figure 11-4).

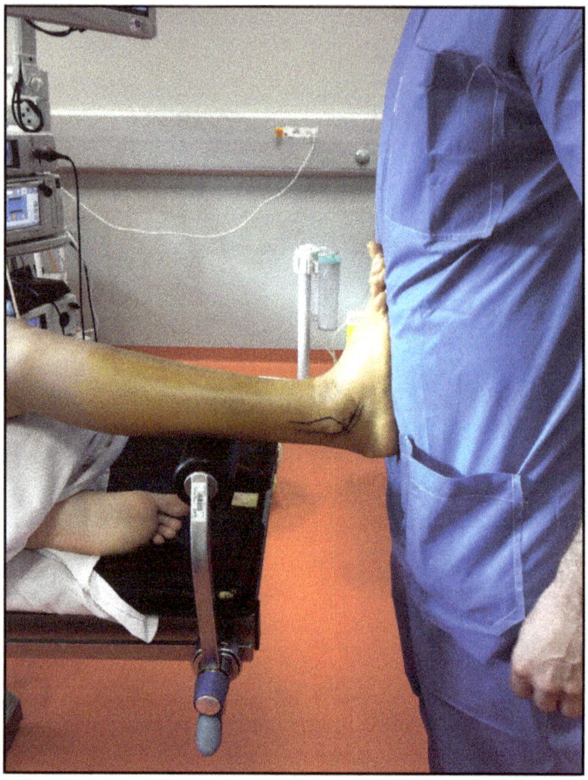

Figure 11-3. Position 2 for anterior arthroscopy.

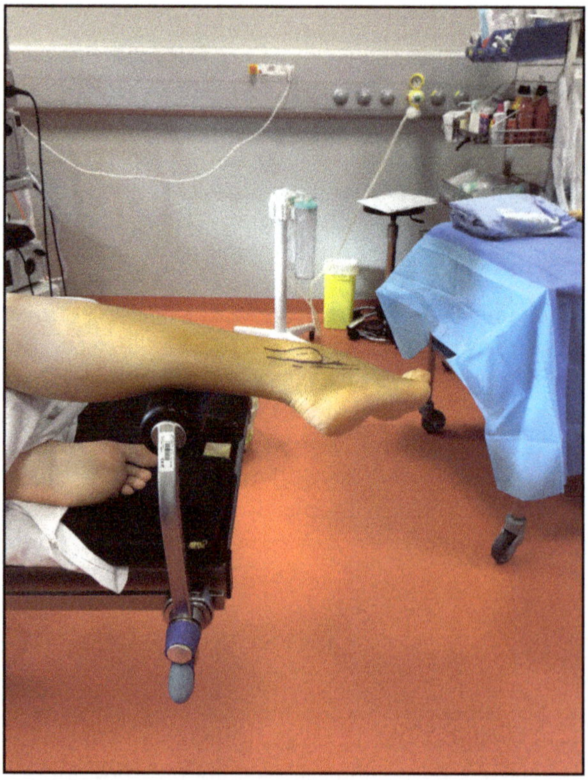

Figure 11-4. Position 3 for lateral hindfoot endoscopy.

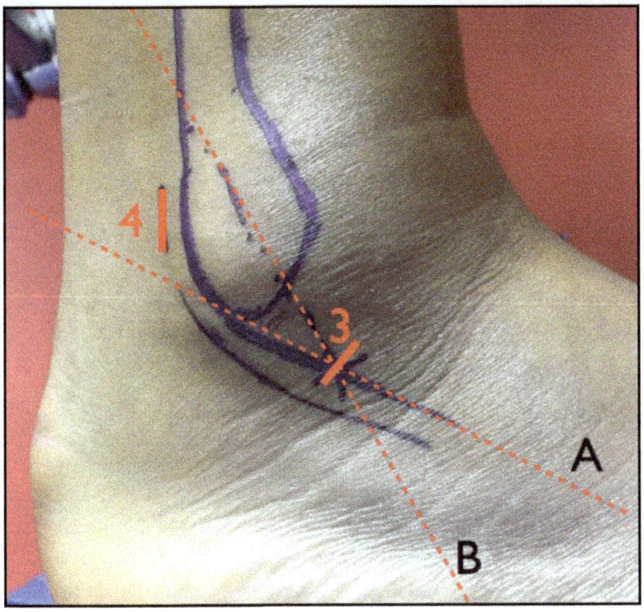

Figure 11-5. Landmark of portal 3.

Step-by-Step Description of the Procedure

Graft Harvesting

After harvesting, the graft is folded to create a 1-cm long doubled segment with 2 single strand limbs, one for the ATFL reconstruction and one for CFL. A whip-stitch is placed on the 1-cm doubled end (which will be placed into the fibular tunnel) attached to a malleolar fixation device, which is used for internal fixation. Whip-stitches are also placed on the CFL end, which should be approximately 5.5 cm in length, and the ATFL end, which should be approximately 4 cm in length. A similar preparation is used in the case of an allograft gracilis tendon.

Landmarks

The patient is placed into position 2. Three portals are created to perform the procedure. A fourth additional portal is possible to explore the peroneal tendon.

The anteromedial portal is the first portal (portal 1). The second portal is the accessory anterolateral portal (portal 2). This portal is not marked on the skin as it is made under transillumination guidance when the arthroscope is positioned in portal 1 and viewing the lateral gutter. Portal 3 is the sinus tarsi portal. This portal is very important to have a vision of the CFL and to make an endoscopic dissection of the ligaments and their footprint. Portal 3 is made at the cross section of 2 lines. To make the first line, follow the superior border of the peroneus brevis tendon. The second line follows the direction of the lateral malleolus tunnel. This axis of the malleolus tunnel is 10 degrees, rotating anteriorly to the axis of the fibula (Figure 11-5). The portal is made at the cross section of these lines.

Portal 4 is an accessory portal made for tendoscopy. For this portal, an incision is placed 1 cm proximal and 1 cm posterior to the tip/apex of the fibula.

Step 1

The arthroscope is placed in the anteromedial portal (portal 1). It is important to make the portal with the ankle positioned in dorsiflexion and very close to the tibialis anterior tendon in order to achieve a good vision of the lateral gutter. Proper positioning of this portal allows for viewing the anterolateral gutter, including the fibular origin of the ATFL, the ATFL itself, and the insertion of the ATFL on the talus. Transillumination is used to create the accessory anterolateral portal (the position of the anterolateral portal is determined using the transillumination technique; portal 2) and a shaver is introduced through this portal to debride the lateral gutter exposing the fibular origin of the ATFL, the ATFL itself, and the insertion of the ATFL on the talus. Once the ATFL footprint has been debrided, the position for the fibular tunnel guide pin insertion between the CFL and the ATFL is identified.

Step 2

The arthroscope is now placed in portal 2. Portal 3 is created at the sinus tarsi in the marked position as described previously. A shaver is then introduced through portal 3 to complete the preparation at the malleolar ligament insertion. A Beath pin is then inserted and drilled across the fibula, exiting the fibula posteriorly and proximally, with care taken to protect the peroneal tendons. The pin is overdrilled using a 4.5-mm cannulated drill, and then a 6-mm cannulated drill is used to make the tunnel to a depth of 1 cm. With the arthroscope in portal 2, the dissection is continuing along the lateral articular surface of the talus and then the anterior side of the posterior subtalar joint. This dissection is guided by the remaining CFL until the insertion on the calcaneus, between the lateral cortex of the calcaneus and the peroneal tendons. This step must be performed with great care in order to properly identify the fibers of the CFL insertion. A Beath pin is then placed in the footprint and drilled through the calcaneus. The direction is inferior, posterior, and medial. A cannulated 6-mm drill is then introduced through the 2 cortexes.

Step 3

The arthroscope is now inserted into portal 3. Using a shaver placed in portal 2, the talar insertion of the ATFL is completely exposed. A pin is then placed under direct visualization into the center of the talar insertion of the ATFL, and then the pin is overdrilled to a depth of 20 mm using a 6-mm cannulated drill. The direction of the tunnel is slightly upward, centered toward the middle of the talus. A JuggerKnot 1.4 anchor is then placed in the tunnel. It is used as a pulley to introduce the transplant.

Step 4

Step 4 corresponds to the placement of the ATFL transplant. One of the JuggerKnot sutures exiting portal 3 is tied to the suture of the talar ATFL limb. The transplant must have a final length of at least 4 cm. The Toggle lock is then introduced through portal 3, advanced through the lateral malleolus, and then hooked on the posterior and a bit lateral cortex of the malleolus. By pulling the free suture of the JuggerKnot, the talar transplant is now introduced into the tunnel by a pulley effect. The talar fixation is then completed with a 5x15-mm Bio-Interference screw (Arthrex). The final tension is achieved by closing the loop of the Toggle lock in the ankle. Tensioning transplants (ATFL and CFL) are made with the ankle in the neutral position.

Step 5

The arthroscope is now placed in portal 2. By pulling the traction suture on the opposite side, the CFL limb of the transplant will be introduced into the calcaneal tunnel. The final fixation

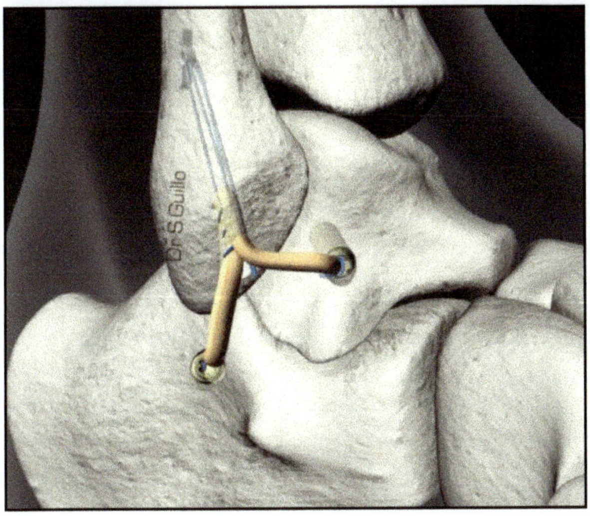

Figure 11-6. Final aspect of the transplant in position.

is achieved with a 7x25-mm interference screw introduced into the tunnel. Because of the poor quality of the calcaneal bone, the screw is oversized and a long screw is used. For a tunnel of 6 mm, it is recommended to use a 7x25-mm screw. It is important to use the arthroscope to control the complete introduction of the screw head to avoid impingement on the peroneal tendons (Figure 11-6).

Accessory Step: The Tendoscopy

A significant number of patients with chronic lateral ligament insufficiency also have pathology of the peroneal tendons, including tendinopathy and partial longitudinal ruptures. Tendoscopy allows visualization of the peroneal tendons and may be helpful as an adjunct. However, the deeper dissection of the peroneal bed in order to visualize the CFL can be technically demanding. Once familiar with the procedure, an experienced arthroscopic surgeon can perform peroneal tendoscopy in a few additional minutes.

Nevertheless, it seems important to some authors to check the status of the CFL and the peroneal tendon. It can be time well spent because a good exposure of the peroneals can help minimize the risk of trauma to peroneal tendons.

If the surgeon decides to do this portal, it has to be made after step 2. The arthroscope is inserted through portal 4. To make this portal, it is important after the skin incision to release and expose the upper peroneal retinaculum. A longitudinal incision of this retinaculum is made and a mosquito clamp is introduced into the tendon sheath from proximal to distal. The 4-mm arthroscope is then introduced. It is important to understand the anatomy of the peroneal tendons. From the tip of the malleolus, looking downward and forward, the 2 tendons are visualized. The beginning of proper tunnels is marked by a small but easily visible distal septum between the 2 tendons. In this position, moving to the top edge of the peroneus brevis, we are left at the entrance of the tarsal sinus. Normally, this gap is filled by a fat pad. It is in this space that dissection using the shaver is performed, between the entrance of the proper tunnel of the peroneus brevis and proximally to the CFL (Figure 11-7). Those landmarks will secure the step 3 dissection of the sinus tarsi. This dissection must end with a clear view of the front edge of the CFL and the subtalar joint. It is then important to search for a peroneal tendon tear and tear or degenerative changes of the CFL.

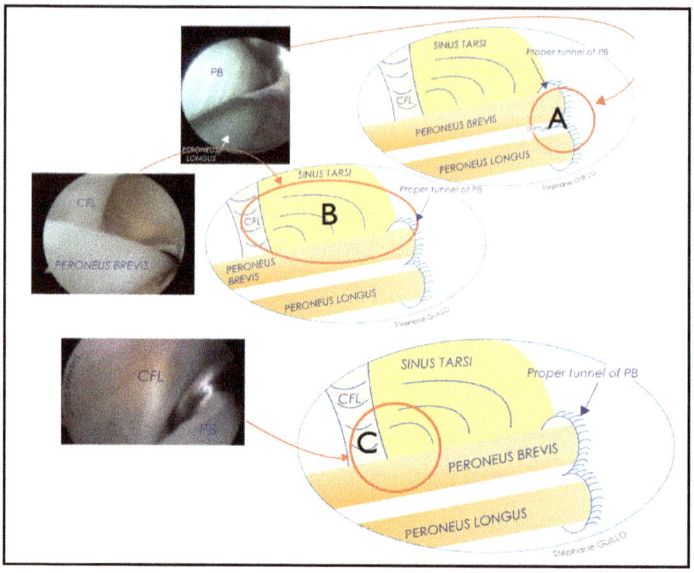

Figure 11-7. Endoscopic dissection around the peroneal tendon. Landmark A, septum between the tendons; B, sinus tarsi; C, CFL.

Postoperative Protocol

The patient is immobilized in a walker boot for 15 days. Although the authors allowed full weightbearing at 15 days after surgery, a previous paper showed there is a little effect of weightbearing during stance phase, maximally 11.3 Newton force on ATFL and 0 Newton force on CFL.[20]

The passive range of motion in dorsi- and plantarflexion is started at 15 days with full weightbearing. Inversion and eversion exercises are started at 6 weeks after surgery and full athletic activity at 12 weeks after surgery.

Potential Complications

Out of the known complications that are common for anterior arthroscopy, there is a risk of a bad placement of the tunnel if there is not perfect arthroscopic control of the entrance point and direction of the bone tunnel. This can end up with cartilage or tendon damage or nonanatomical reconstruction.

Conclusion

Following the now universally accepted principles of anterior cruciate ligament knee surgery, anatomical reconstruction with autograft could be a reliable surgical option because it leads to an anatomical repair using a sufficiently resistant transplant. However, the indication is still not clear today.

The concept of lateral hindfoot endoscopy makes possible the complete dissection of the CFL and ATFL. It allows an anatomical reconstruction of those 2 ligaments with probably more accuracy than with open technique. This description in 5 steps makes the procedure more simple and reproducible. However, cadaveric training is very important to perform this technique, which is technically demanding. To improve the technique, it will be necessary in the future to have specific implant and instrumentation. Further work needs to be done to confirm the superiority of the arthroscopic procedure vs open technique.

Top Technical Pearls for the Procedure

1. The anteromedial portal has to be made in dorsiflexion very close to the tibialis anterior in order to have the optimum view of the lateral gutter.
2. To do the malleolar tunnel, the scope is used in portal 2 and the instruments in portal 3 in order to have an anatomical placement of the tunnel.
3. The placement of the talar tunnel is halfway up the anterior border of the lateral facet of the talus.
4. The scope is placed in portal 3 and the instruments in portal 2 to find the calcaneal footprint of the CFL.
5. The placement of the transplant in the malleolar tunnel requires a tension with the foot at 90 degrees for the ATFL and a tension in plantarflexion for the CFL.

References

1. Lewis JE, Marymont JV. Ankle arthroscopy and sports-related injuries. Orthopaedic Knowledge Update. *Foot Ankle Int.* 1988;2:39-54.
2. Takao M, Oae K, Uchio Y, Ochi M, Yamamoto H. Anatomical reconstruction of the lateral ligaments of the ankle with a gracilis autograft: a new technique using an interference fit anchoring system. *Am J Sports Med.* 2005;33(6):814-823.
3. Bahr R, Pena F, Shine J, Lew WD, Tyrdal S, Engebretsen L. Biomechanics of ankle ligament reconstruction. An in vitro comparison of the Brostrom repair, Watson-Jones reconstruction, and a new anatomic reconstruction technique. *Am J Sports Med.* 1997;25(4):424-432.
4. Colville MR, Marder RA, Zarins B. Reconstruction of the lateral ankle ligaments. A biomechanical analysis. *Am J Sports Med.* 1992;20(5):594-600.
5. Hollis JM, Blasier RD, Flahiff CM, Hofmann OE. Biomechanical comparison of reconstruction techniques in simulated lateral ankle ligament injury. *Am J Sports Med.* 1995;23(6):678-682.
6. Rosenbaum D, Becker HP, Wilke HJ, Claes LE. Tenodeses destroy the kinematic coupling of the ankle joint complex. A three-dimensional in vitro analysis of joint movement. *J Bone Joint Surg Br.* 1998;80(1):162-168.
7. Sammarco GJ, Idusuyi OB. Reconstruction of the lateral ankle ligaments using a split peroneus brevis tendon graft. *Foot Ankle Int.* 1999;20(2):97-103.
8. Tohyama H, Beynnon BD, Pope MH, Haugh LD, Renstrom PA. Laxity and flexibility of the ankle following reconstruction with the Chrisman-Snook procedure. *J Orthop Res.* 1997;15(5):707-711.
9. Guillo S, Bauer T, Lee JW, et al. Consensus in chronic ankle instability: aetiology, assessment, surgical indications and place for arthroscopy. *Orthop Traumatol Surg Res.* 2013;99(8 Suppl):S411-S419.
10. Acevedo J, Mangone PG. Arthroscopic lateral ankle ligament reconstruction. *Tech Foot Ankle Surg.* 2011;10(3):111-116.
11. Nery C, Raduan F, Del Buono A, Asaumi ID, Cohen M, Maffulli N. Arthroscopic-assisted Brostrom-Gould for chronic ankle instability: a long-term follow-up. *Am J Sports Med.* 2011;39(11):2381-2388.
12. Corte-Real N, Moreira R. Arthroscopic repair of chronic lateral ankle instability. *Foot Ankle Int.* 2009;30(3):213-217.
13. Vega J, Golano P, Pellegrino A, Rabat E, Pena F. All-inside arthroscopic lateral collateral ligament repair for ankle instability with a knotless suture anchor technique. *Foot Ankle Int.* 2013;34(12):1701-1709.
14. Guillo S, Archold P, perera A, Bauer T, Sonnery-Cottet B. Arthroscopic anatomic reconstruction of the lateral ligaments of the ankle with gracilis autograft. *Arthroscopy.* 2014;3(5):e593-e598.

15. Becker HP, Ebner S, Ebner D, et al. 12-year outcome after modified Watson-Jones tenodesis for ankle instability. *Clin Orthop Rel Res.* 1999;(358):194-204.
16. Rosenbaum D, Becker HP, Sterk J, Gerngross H, Claes L. Functional evaluation of the 10-year outcome after modified Evans repair for chronic ankle instability. *Foot Ankle Int.* 1997;18(12):765-771.
17. Snook GA, Chrisman OD, Wilson TC. Long-term results of the Chrisman-Snook operation for reconstruction of the lateral ligaments of the ankle. *J Bone Joint Surg Am.* 1985;67(1):1-7.
18. Vienne P, Schoniger R, Helmy N, Espinosa N. Hindfoot instability in cavovarus deformity: static and dynamic balancing. *Foot Ankle Int.* 2007;28(1):96-102.
19. Ozeki S, Yasuda K, Kaneda K, Yamakoshi K, Yamanoi T. Simultaneous strain measurement with determination of a zero strain reference for the medial and lateral ligaments of the ankle. *Foot Ankle Int.* 2002;23(9):825-832.
20. Haraguchi N, Armiger RS, Myerson MS, Campbell JT, Chao EY. Prediction of three-dimensional contact stress and ligament tension in the ankle during stance determined from computational modeling. *Foot Ankle Int.* 2009;30:177-185.

Please visit www.routledge.com/9781617119989 to access additional material.

12

Medial Ankle Stabilization

Beat Hintermann, MD

Introduction

There is evidence that the medial ankle ligaments are injured more often than generally believed.[1,2] They may be involved in injuries obtained while running down stairs, landing on uneven surfaces, or dancing while the body simultaneously rotates in the opposite direction. In practice, however, it is not so easy to elicit the injury mechanism because patients often report having had multiple ankle sprains and are therefore not able to clearly indicate their specific injury mechanism. In all patients, a key feature of the patients' histories is that they have sustained a pronation (eversion) trauma (eg, an outward rotation of the foot during simultaneous inward rotation of the tibia).[3] In cases with extreme rotational forces, such as in excessive lateral rotation, the tibiofibular and interosseous ligaments at the syndesmosis may be injured and, furthermore, the anterior fibers of the deltoid ligament may be involved.

Complete deltoid ligament ruptures are sometimes seen in association with lateral malleolar fractures[4] or in specific bimalleolar fractures.[5] Chronic deltoid ligament insufficiency can be found in a number of conditions, including posterior tibial tendon disorder, trauma, and sports-related deltoid disruptions, as well as valgus talar tilting in patients with previous triple arthrodesis or total ankle arthroplasty.

One concern may be the question of whether posterior tibial dysfunction and medial ankle instability are distinct conditions. Although possible, it is not yet clear whether, or to which extent, a medial ankle instability may cause a secondary posterior tibial dysfunction over time as the tendon may become elongated and/or ruptured.[6]

Indications

- Failed conservative treatment
- Symptomatic medial ankle instability following pronation injuries of the ankle joint complex that have resulted in a partial or complete disruption of the superficial anterior bundles of the deltoid ligament

Stone JW, Kennedy JG, Glazebrook M, eds. *The Foot and Ankle: AANA Advanced Arthroscopic Surgical Techniques* (pp 105-118).

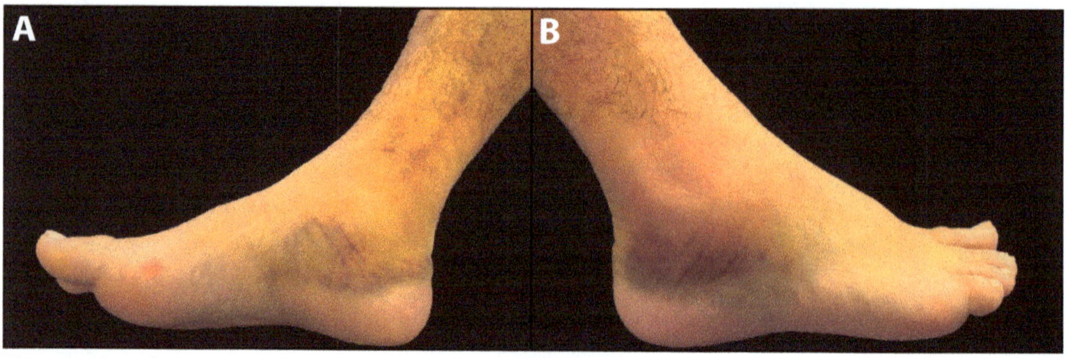

Figure 12-1. After an acute injury, a tenderness and hematoma can be found (A) medially and (B) laterally.

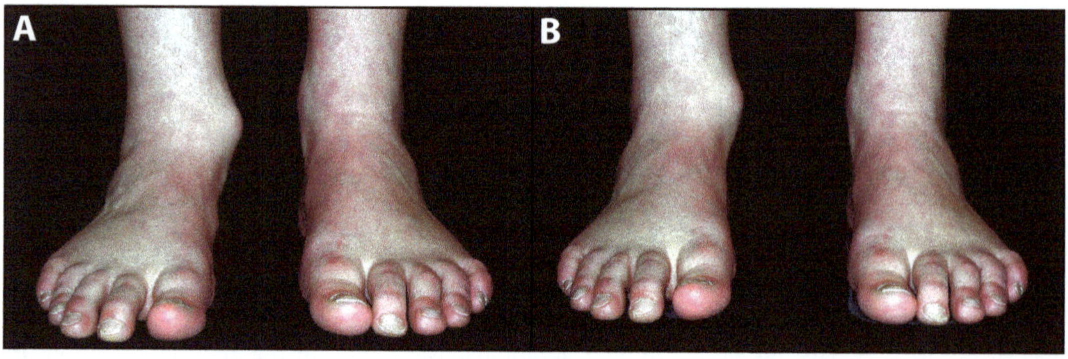

Figure 12-2. A 24-year-old female sports teacher with a symptomatic medial instability of her right foot after a severe pronation trauma 18 months earlier. (A) Frontal view, showing the excessive valgus and pronation of the right foot, with a prominent medial malleolus. (B) When the patient is asked to activate the posterior tibial muscle to correct the valgus position, the deformity is partially but not completely corrected. *(continued)*

- Symptomatic chronic medial ankle instability that has caused a secondary posterior tibial dysfunction over time as the tendon has became elongated and/or ruptured

Pertinent Physical Findings

- Acute injuries may evidence tenderness and hematoma in the region of the deltoid ligament (Figure 12-1A), and often in the region of the lateral ankle ligaments as well (Figure 12-1B).
- For patients with chronic injuries of the deltoid ligament, a key finding is pain in the medial gutter, as typically provoked by palpation of the anterior border of medial malleolus.[1,3]
- With the patient bearing weight, asymmetrical planus and pronation deformity of the affected foot has been found to indicate medial ankle instability.[1,3,6]
- Typically, the excessive valgus of the hindfoot and pronation of the foot (Figure 12-2A) disappears when the patient is asked to correct the hindfoot pronation and thereby activates the posterior tibial muscle (Figure 12-2B). Analogously, as seen from posteriorly, the excessive valgus of the hindfoot and pronation of the foot (Figure 12-2C) disappears when the patient is asked to stand on the tip of his or her toes (Figure 12-2D).
- Posterior tibial dysfunction can be excluded when flattening of the medial longitudinal arch, hindfoot valgus, and forefoot abduction are corrected after the patient is asked to perform the single-heel rise.

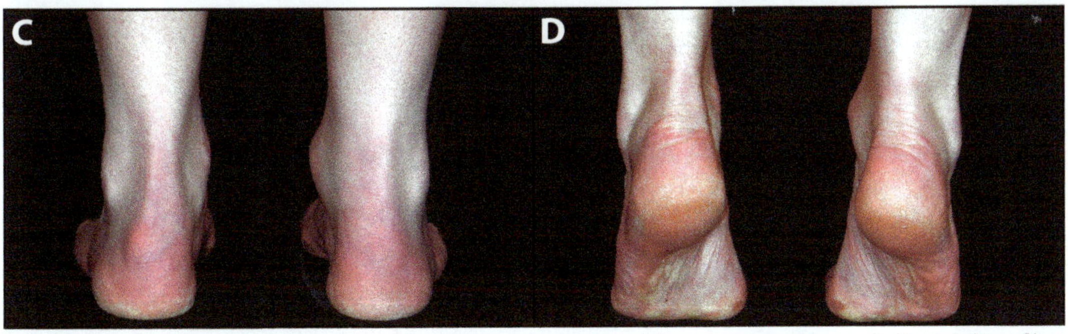

Figure 12-2 (continued). A 24-year-old female sports teacher with a symptomatic medial instability of her right foot after a severe pronation trauma 18 months earlier. (C) The asymmetrical position of the medial malleolus can also be seen from posterior. In contrast to an acquired flatfoot due to a posterior tibial dysfunction, no abduction of the forefoot is seen here. (D) The posterior tibial muscle is intact and can produce power, which can be seen when the patient is asked to go in a tip-toe position.

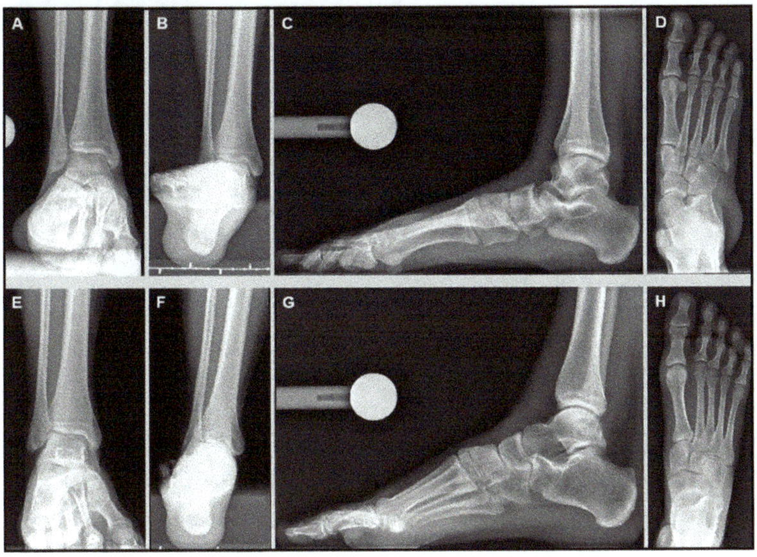

Figure 12-3. In this 16-year-old female patient with an acute type III injury of the deltoid-spring ligament complex after a pronation trauma, the destabilization of the peritalar joints can nicely be seen on the radiographs taken in a relaxed position (A through D); whereas, the deformity is completely corrected when the patient is asked to activate her posterior tibial muscle as seen in E through H. (A and E) Anterior ankle view. (B and F) Saltzman view. (C and G) Lateral view of the foot. (D and H) Dorsoplantar view of the foot.

- Clinical stress investigation has been found to be the most reliable when the patient is seated on the table with hanging feet.[3] The heel is held in one hand and the tibia is held in the other hand. First, a varus and then a valgus tilt stress are applied to the heel, and the resulting range of motion is compared with the contralateral side. Second, an anterior drawer stress is applied and, again, the resulting motion is compared with the contralateral side.

Pertinent Imaging

- Plain standard x-rays are used to exclude a fracture and/or bony pathologies.
- Weightbearing x-rays should be obtained to assess the presence and extent of a deformity in chronic conditions. This is particularly true for a valgus deformity of the hindfoot because of a severe incompetence of the medial ankle ligaments (Figures 12-3A through D). Typically, a correction of the deformity can be seen when the patient is asked to activate his or her posterior tibial muscle (Figures 12-3E through H).

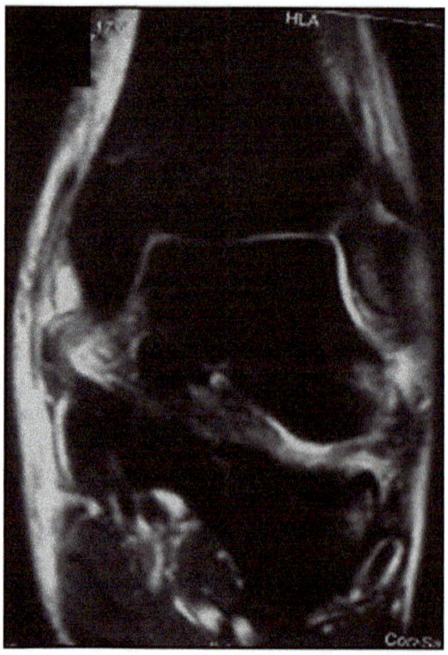

Figure 12-4. MRI (frontal view) of the left ankle joint of a 32-year-old male volleyball player after a pronation trauma, showing a major lesion of the superficial part of the deltoid ligament.

- Stress x-rays have been found to be helpful to discern an incompetence of the deltoid ligaments in the treatment of acute ankle fractures[5]; however, this has not been the case in chronic conditions.[3]
- Computed tomography may be additionally initiated if a talocalcaneal coalition or a bony fragmentation that involves the articular surfaces is suspected.
- Although magnetic resonance imaging (MRI) may evidence an injury to the deltoid ligament, particularly in acute conditions (Figure 12-4), there is no need for MRI investigation on a regular basis.
- Ankle arthroscopy may be a further helpful diagnostic tool to confirm clinically suspected instability of the medial and lateral ankle and to detect additional structural changes.[3,7]

Equipment

- Equipment for arthroscopy with 4.5- or 2.7-mm optic
- Standard instruments for foot and ankle surgery
- For soft tissue reconstruction:
  - Bony anchor
  - Suture material
- In the case of additional calcaneal lengthening osteotomy:
  - Saw
  - Hintermann distractor
  - Allograft

Positioning and Portals

- The patient is in a supine position with the feet at the edge of the table.

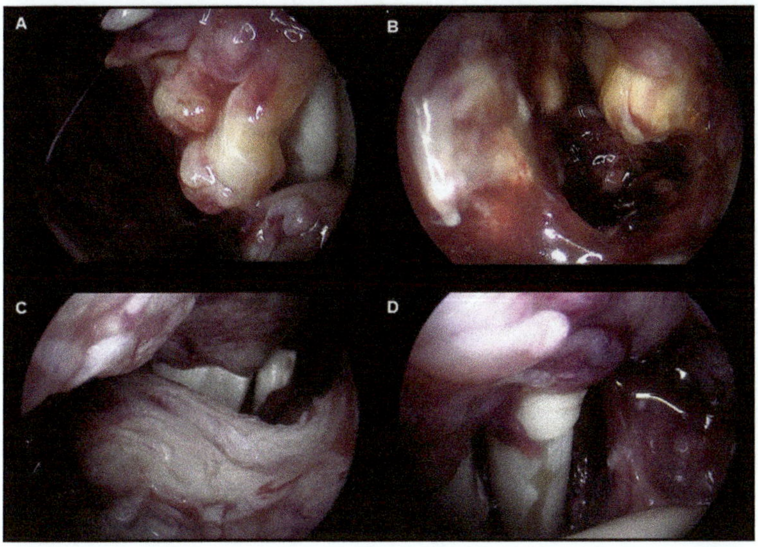

Figure 12-5. Arthroscopic assessment of the ankle in a 28-year-old male police officer after an acute pronation trauma of his left ankle (same patient as in Figure 12-1). (A) The anterior superficial layers of the deltoid are completely torn. (B) The deep tibiotalar layers of the deltoid ligament are also ruptured. (C) The posterior tibial and flexor digitorum tendon can be seen behind the ruptured tibiotalar layers. (D) More posteriorly, both tendons can be seen even more extensively.

- A commercially available knee holder is used to support the distal femur and to place the foot into a hanging position.
- This allows the surgeon to move the foot freely while arthroscopy is done prior to open reconstruction.
- After arthroscopy, the knee holder is removed, leaving the foot on the table.

Step-by-Step Description of the Procedure

Surgical Approach

- An anteromedial approach is used for ankle arthroscopy[7]
- A gently curved incision of 3 to 5 cm is made, starting 1 cm cranially to the tip of the medial malleolus and running toward the medial aspect of the navicular bone.
- If additional instability of the lateral ankle ligaments is suspected due to the preoperative clinical examination and confirmed by arthroscopy, a lateral approach to the ankle is also performed to explore the anterior talofibular and calcaneofibular ligaments.

Ankle Arthroscopy

- After visual evaluation of the ligaments (Figures 12-5 and 12-6), lateral and medial ligament stability is tested by applying gentle varus, valgus, and anterior pull stress to the ankle joint under arthroscopic control.
- Ligament lesions are graded as "distended" if the ligament is thinned or elongated and as "ruptured" if continuity is lost. Most ligament tears are located on the proximal insertion; this is best seen by a completely free insertion area of the ligament on the malleoli (see Figure 12-5C).
- As the foot is everted and pronated, the deltoid ligament is tensioned. It is considered incompetent when, despite the tension applied, no strong medial buttress is created. A further indicator for an overstretched deltoid ligament is an excessive lifting away of the talus from the medial malleolus when pulling the foot anteriorly.

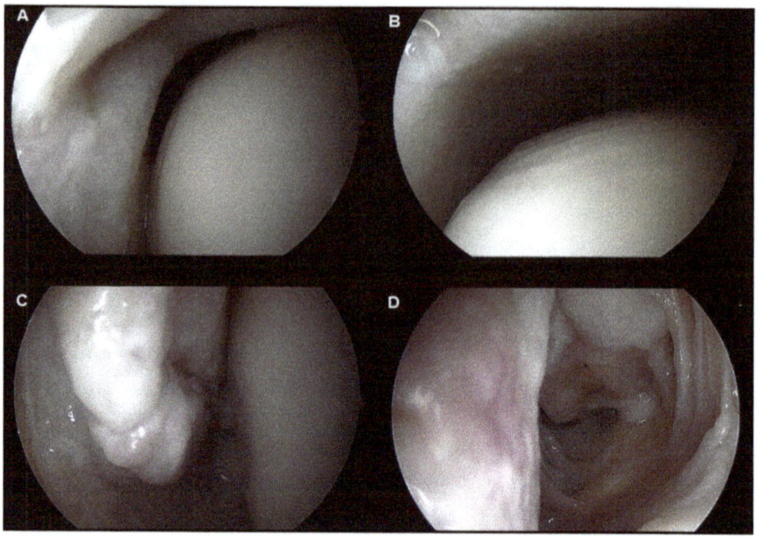

Figure 12-6. Arthroscopic assessment of the ankle in a 36-year-old male runner who is suffering from chronic medial ankle instability of his right ankle after a bad sprain 3.5 years earlier. He complains of having a feeling of severe instability. (A) The anteromedial corner of the tibia shows bony apposition as a result of the chronic battement of the talus against the medial malleolus. (B) As a result of incompetence of the superficial anterior layers of the deltoid ligament, the medial malleolus moves easily out of the mortise when applying slight pull on the foot. (C) The tip of the medial malleolus is free of ligaments. (D) The lateral ligaments are also detached from the fibula, which allows for full exposure of the tip of fibula and to see the posterior tibiofibular ligament.

- Lateral instability is considered to be present when talar tilting occurs during supination stress of the foot.
- Evaluated for both the medial and lateral side, the ankle joint is graded as follows:
  - Stable when there is some translocation of the talus but not enough to open the tibiotalar joint by more than 2 mm (as measured by the 2-mm hook) and not enough to introduce the 5-mm arthroscope into the tibiotalar space
  - Moderately unstable when the talus moves to some extent out of the ankle mortise, allowing introduction of the 5-mm arthroscope into the tibiotalar space but not enough to open the tibiotalar joint by more than 5 mm
  - Severely unstable when the talus moves easily out of the ankle mortise, typically allowing free insight into the posterior aspect of the ankle joint without applying significant pulling stress on the heel[7]

Reconstruction of the Medial Ankle Ligaments

- Complete acute rupture: Since the rupture is mostly situated at the proximal end of the deltoid ligament (Figure 12-7A), reattachment to the medial malleolus is achieved by interosseous sutures; a bony anchor can also be used to refix the ligament to the bone (Figures 12-7B through D).
- Chronic rupture of the superficial deltoid ligament: Classification of these injuries is shown in Table 12-1.
  - Type I lesion
    - Exposure of the anterior border of the medial malleolus by making a short longitudinal incision between the tibionavicular and tibiospring ligaments, where there is usually a small fibrous septum without adherent connective fibers between the 2 ligaments (Figure 12-8A).

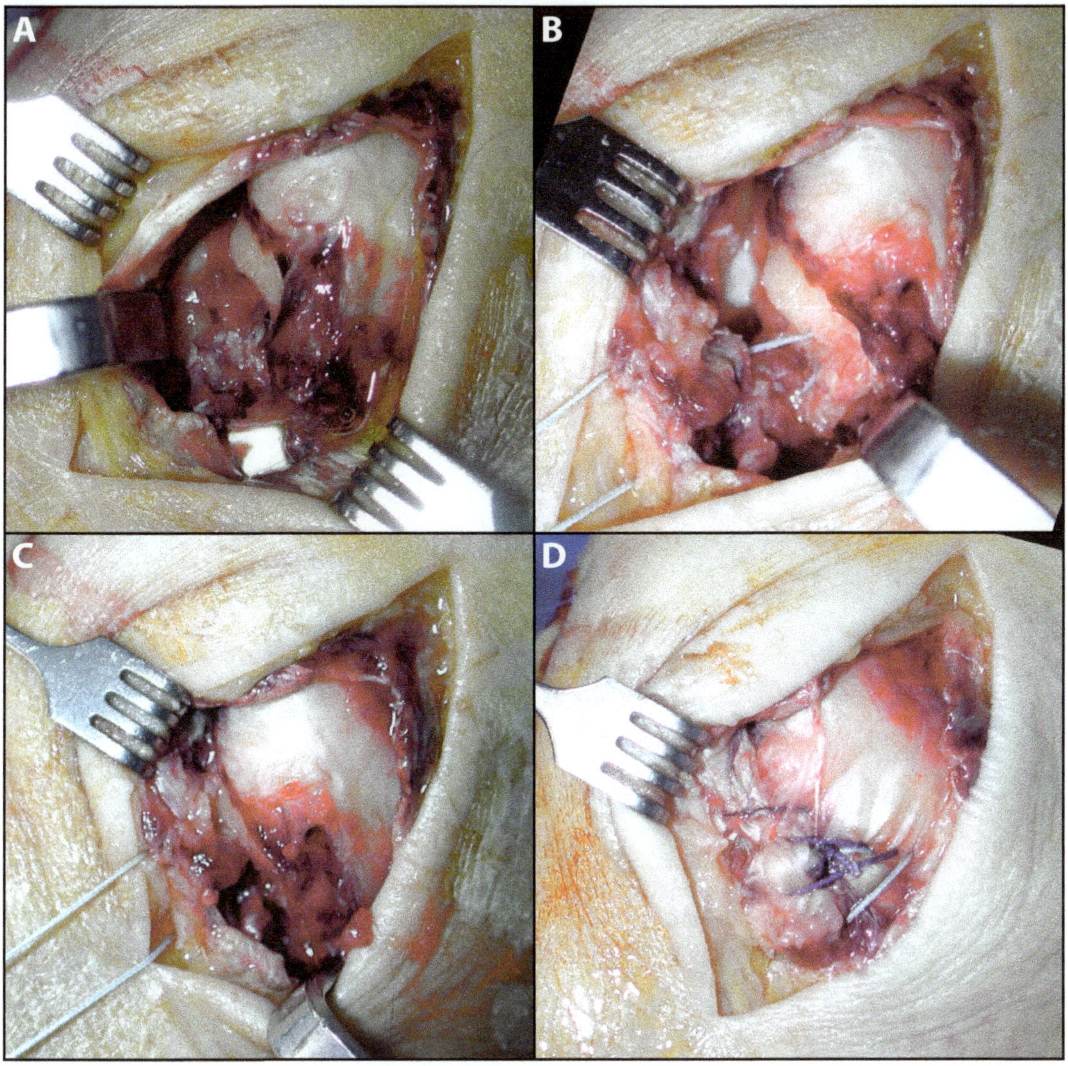

Figure 12-7. Reconstruction of the deltoid ligament (same patient as in Figures 12-1 and 12-5). (A) The deltoid ligament is completely detached from the medial malleolus; the lesion also involves the sheath of the posterior tibial tendon. (B) An anchor is placed on the anterior aspect of the tip of the medial malleolus. (C) The deltoid ligament is reattached with a suture. (D) Final reconstruction.

Table 12-1. Classification of Chronic Superficial Lesions of the Deltoid Ligament

Lesion	Location of Tear
Type I	Proximal tear/avulsion of the deltoid ligament
Type II	Intermediate tear of the deltoid ligament
Type III	Distal tear/avulsion of the deltoid and the spring ligaments

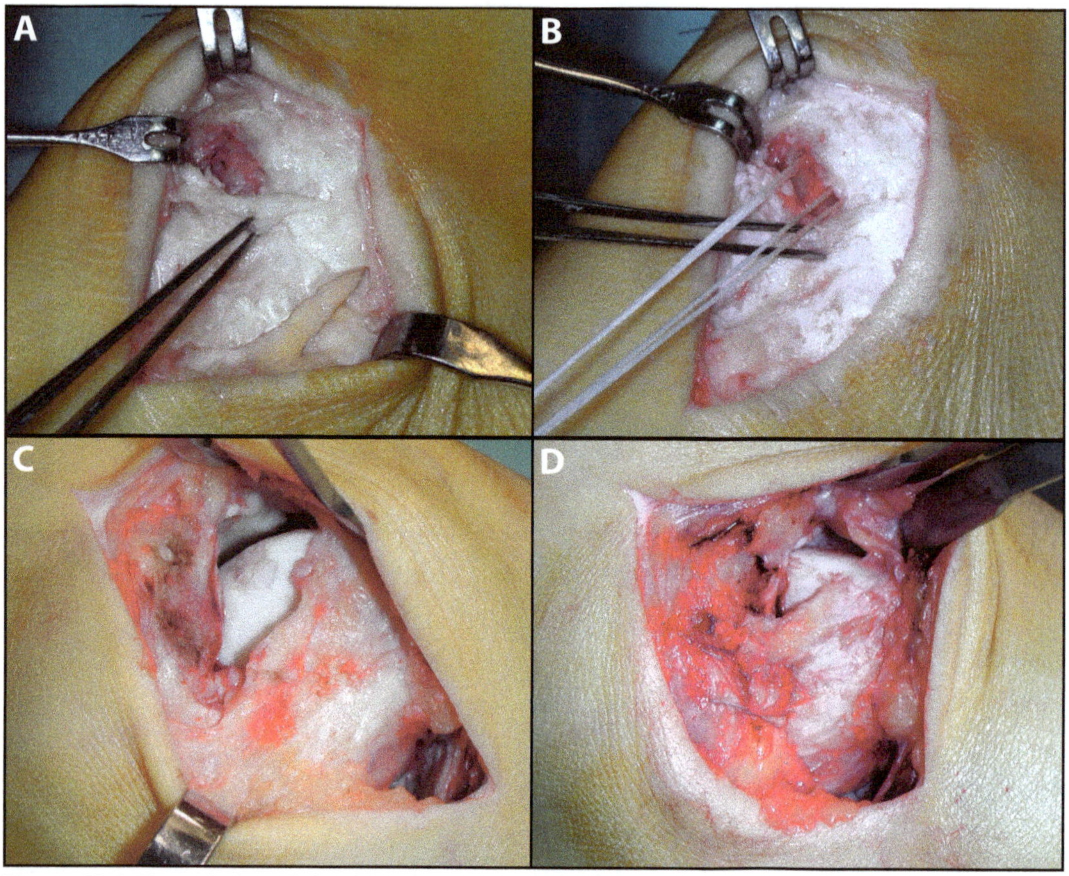

Figure 12-8. Type I lesion of the deltoid ligament in a 34-year-old male soccer player. (A) The lesion is located in the interval between the tibiospring and tibiocalcaneal ligament (superficial deltoid ligament). (B) After roughening the anterior surface of the medial malleolus, a bony anchor is used to reattach the deltoid ligament and to close the interval. (C) The lateral ankle ligaments are typically detached from the fibula, thus allowing the talus to move anteriorly, out of the mortise. The cartilage lesion seen here may be a result of this shifting movement. (D) The lateral ligaments are reattached to the anterior aspect of the fibula by a bony anchor or by intraosseous sutures, which results in a stable reduction of the talus in the ankle mortise.

- After roughening the medial aspect of the medial malleolus, an anchor is placed 6 mm above the tip of the malleolus (Figure 12-8B). The anchor is used to shorten the tibionavicular and tibiospring ligaments and, at the same time, refix them to the medial malleolus.
- The lateral ankle ligaments are exposed (Figure 12-8C) and reattached to the anterior aspect of the fibula with the use of an anchor or intraosseous sutures (Figure 12-8D).
- #0 resorbable sutures are used to refix the tibionavicular and tibiospring ligaments.

▹ Type II lesion

- The scarred insufficient ligament is carefully exposed (Figures 12-9A and B). If possible, it is divided into 2 flaps: the deep flap remains reattached distally and the superficial flap remains reattached to the medial malleolus.
- Two anchors are placed 6 mm above the tip of the malleolus, and another anchor is placed at the superior edge of the navicular tuberosity. The 2 anchors are used to refix

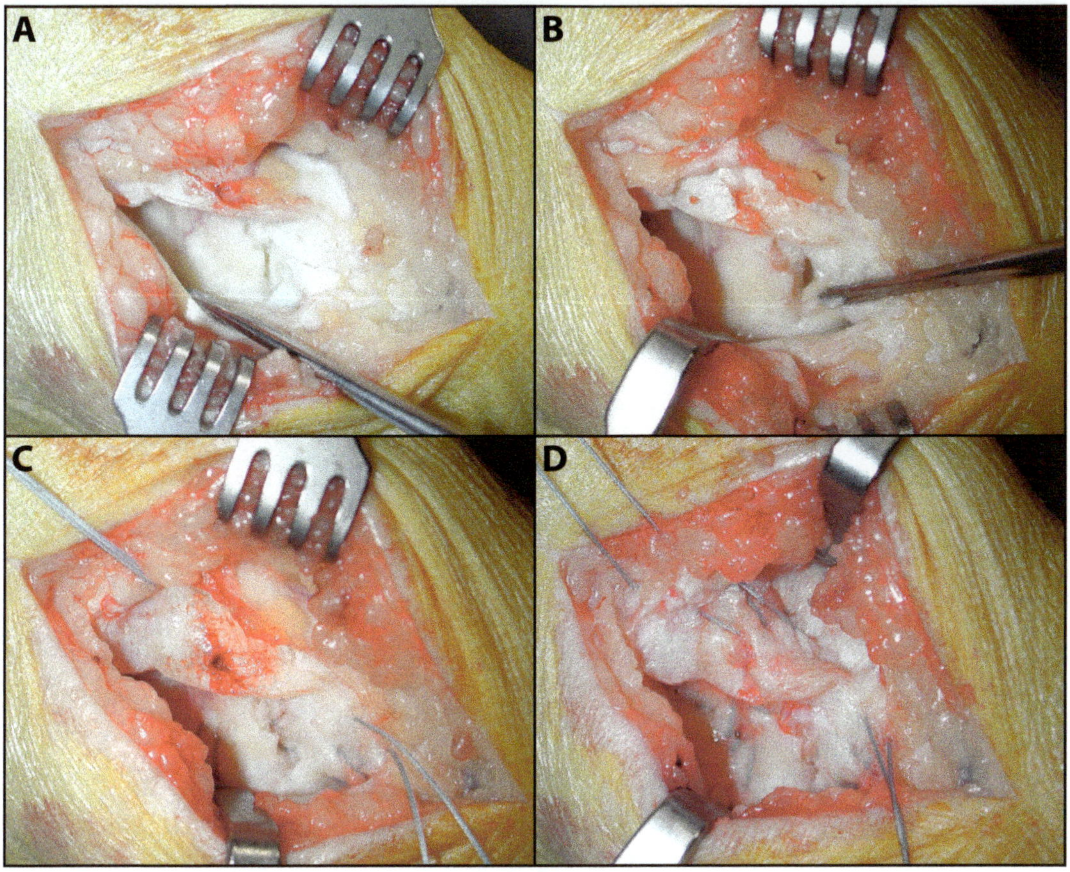

Figure 12-9. A type II lesion of the deltoid ligament in a 42-year-old female tennis player with a persisting feeling of instability and medial ankle pain since a complex ankle sprain 8 months earlier. (A) Surgical exploration of the deltoid ligament evidences a lesion of the intermediate portion of the anterior superficial deltoid. (B) A complete rupture of parts of the tibiospring ligament can be found. (C) One anchor is placed in the medial malleolus and another one in the tuberosity of navicular; the distal part of the ligament is reconstructed first. (D) Then, the proximal part of the ligament is reconstructed. Additional sutures are then used to complete the reconstruction.

the distal flap to the navicular tuberosity (Figure 12-9C) and the proximal flap to the medial malleolus (Figure 12-9D), thereby reconstructing a strong and well-tightened ligament.

- Additional #0 resorbable sutures are used to further stabilize the reconstructed tibionavicular and tibiospring ligaments.

▹ Type III lesion

- The distal insertion of the deltoid ligament and spring ligament are carefully inspected (Figure 12-10A) and manually tested (Figure 12-10B). If necessary, the tear is debrided.
- Two nonresorbable sutures are placed in the spring ligament (Figure 12-10C).
- If the tibionavicular ligament is completely detached from its insertion, an anchor is placed at the superior edge of the navicular tuberosity.
- After tightening the sutures (Figure 12-10D), additional #0 resorbable sutures are used to further stabilize the reconstructed tibionavicular and spring ligaments.

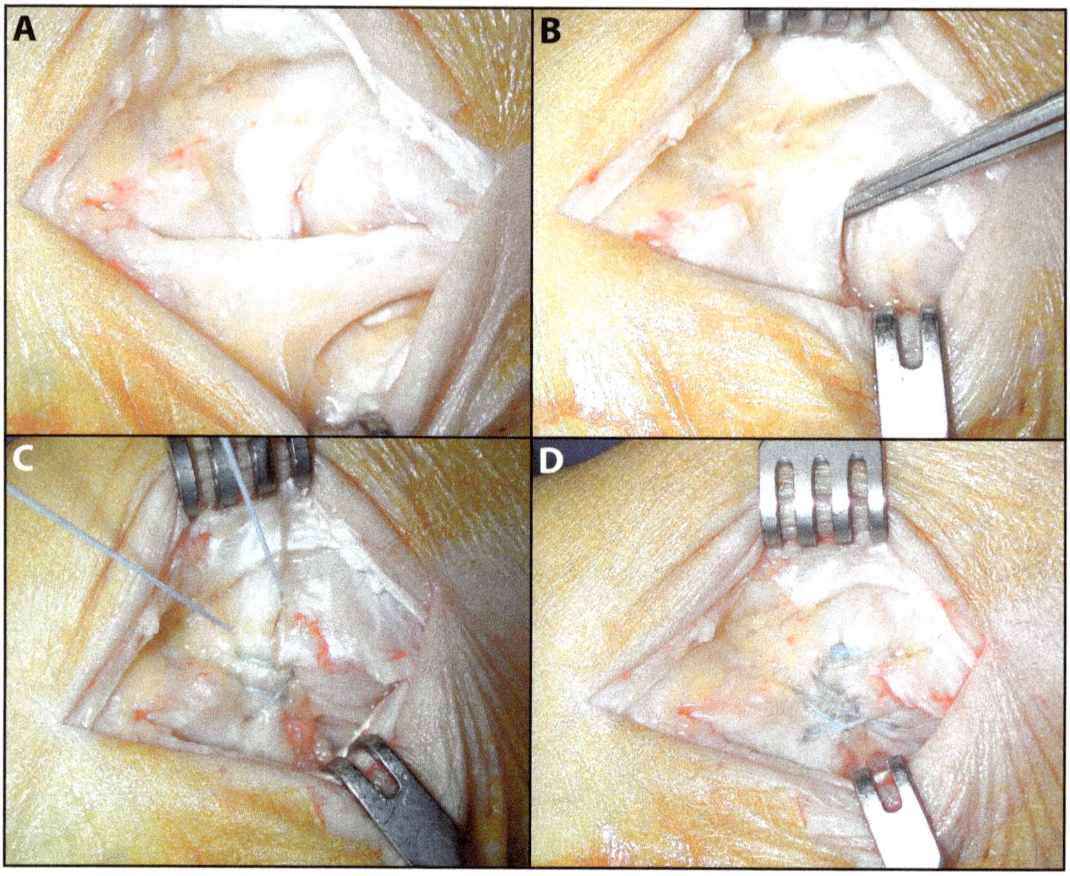

Figure 12-10. A type III lesion of the deltoid ligament in a 40-year-old female patient with a progressive pronation deformity since a pronation trauma 11 months earlier, not allowing her to engage in any sports activity since. In the last weeks, she experienced some tenderness along the posterior tibial tendon, but there was clinically no evidence of a posterior tibial dysfunction. (A) Surgical exploration reveals an intact distal posterior tibial tendon and a vertical tear of the distal deltoid and spring ligament. (B) The ligament lesion can be seen better when manually explored. (C) After having fixed a bony anchor to the tuberosity of navicular, the lesion is reconstructed by a suture with nonresorbable material. (D) Final result with a strong ligament repair.

- Chronic rupture of the deep deltoid ligament
  - Since this condition usually includes an extended tear of the superficial anterior bundles of the deltoid ligament, every reconstructive surgery should attempt to address the whole deltoid ligament.
  - The posterior tibial tendon can be used as a graft to augment the reconstructed deltoid ligament by passing it through a drill hole from the tip of the medial malleolus to the medial aspect of the distal tibia.
  - However, this technique has been found to be disappointing as it does not sufficiently reinforce the deep tibiotalar ligaments (Hintermann, unpublished data). The use of a bone-tendon-bone transplant has also been proposed for reconstruction of the deltoid ligament.[8] In this in vitro study, 2 limbs were created on a distal transplant, of which one was fixed to the medial aspect of the talus and the other to the sustentaculum tali, whereas the proximal end was fixed either to the distal tibia, medial malleolus, or lateral tibia.

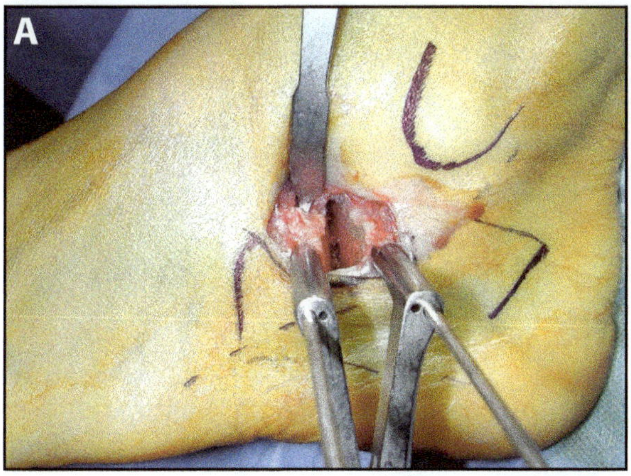

Figure 12-11. In this 36-year-old female patient with a long-standing pronation deformity 4 years after a pronation trauma, a lateral column lengthening osteotomy is done to correct the deformity (see text). (A) After exposure of the calcaneus at the level of the sinus tarsi, the osteotomy is carried out and then widened with the use of a distractor mounted over 2 Kirschner wires (Hintermann distractor). *(continued)*

Reconstruction of the Lateral Ankle Ligaments

- Approximately 75% of all patients with chronic medial ankle instability were found to evidence an associated avulsion of the anterior talofibular ligament that resulted in a complex rotational instability of the talus within the ankle mortise (see Figure 12-6D).[7]
- If the condition of the anterior talofibular ligament and calcaneofibular ligament allows an adequate primary repair, these ligaments are reconstructed by shortening and reinsertion (see Figures 12-8C and D).
- When no substantial ligamentous material is present, augmentation with a free plantaris tendon graft is performed.

Debridement/Reconstruction of the Posterior Tibial Tendon

- The posterior tibial tendon is meticulously inspected during surgery, especially in the case of a type II and type III lesion of the anterior deltoid ligament.
- If there is some degeneration of the tendon, debridement of the tendon is performed.
- If there is an elongation of the tendon, shortening of the tendon is considered.
- If there is an accessory bone (os tibiale externum), reattachment of the bone with the tendon insertion is considered. The posterior tibial tendon can additionally be tightened if the bone is reattached more distally to the navicular bone.
- A transfer of the flexor digitorum tendon might be considered in the case of a diseased or ruptured tendon. This is, however, seldom the case.

Lateral Lengthening Calcaneal Osteotomy

- This procedure is considered in the case of a pre-existing valgus and pronation deformity of the foot (eg, when a valgus and pronation deformity is also present on the contralateral, asymptomatic foot) or in the case of a severe attenuation or defect of the tibionavicular, tibiospring, or spring ligaments (see Figure 12-3).
- A calcaneal osteotomy is performed along and parallel to the posterior facet of the subtalar joint, from lateral to medial, preserving the medial cortex intact (Figure 12-11A).
- As the osteotomy is widened, the pronation deformity of the foot disappears (Figures 12-11B and C).

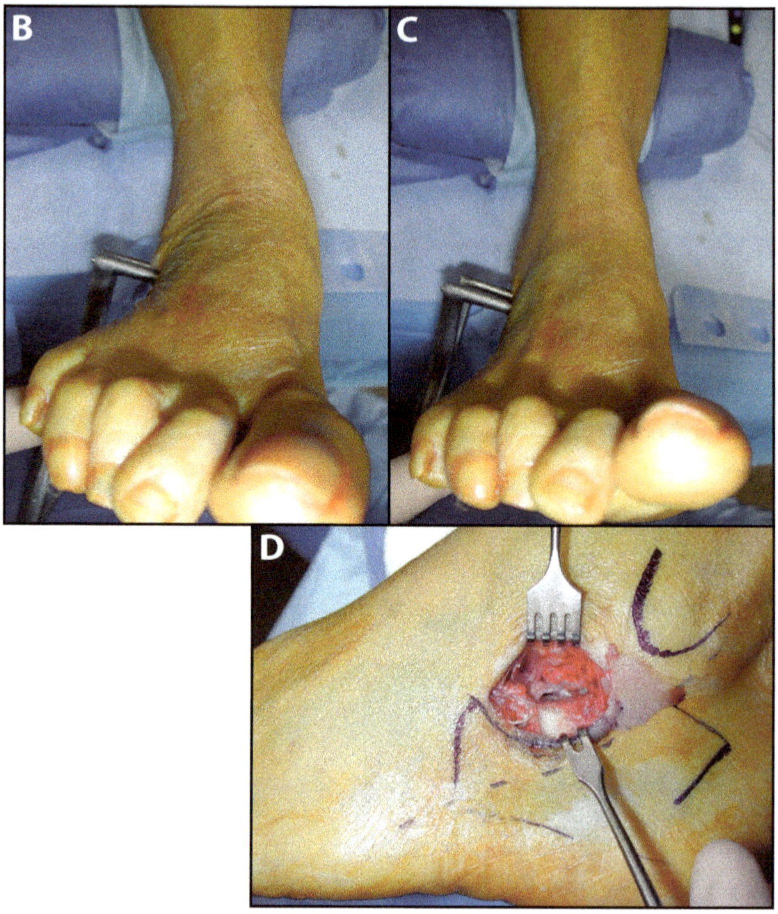

Figure 12-11 (continued). In this 36-year-old female patient with a long-standing pronation deformity 4 years after a pronation trauma, a lateral column lengthening osteotomy is done to correct the deformity (see text). A picture of the pronation of the foot (B) before and (C) after the osteotomy is widened. The osteotomy is widened until a normal foot position is obtained (usually 6 to 8 mm of widening is needed). (D) A bone graft is shaped according to the size of the defect and then inserted into the osteotomy site.

- A tricortical graft is fashioned from the iliac crest to the length required and placed into the osteotomy site; alternatively, an allograft (Figure 12-11D) or metal edge can be used.

Wound Closure

- The wounds are closed in layers.
- The subcutaneous tissue and skin are closed in a standard fashion.

Postoperative Protocol

- The foot is protected by a plaster cast for 6 weeks, and full weightbearing is allowed as soon as pain-free loading is possible.
- The rehabilitation program starts after cast removal. It includes passive and active mobilization of the ankle joint, training of the muscular strength, and protection with a walker or stabilizing shoe when walking.
- A walker or stabilizing shoe can be used for 4 to 6 weeks after cast removal, depending on the regained muscular balance of the hindfoot.
- The author recommends continued use for walks on uneven ground, high-risk sports activities, and professional outdoor work.

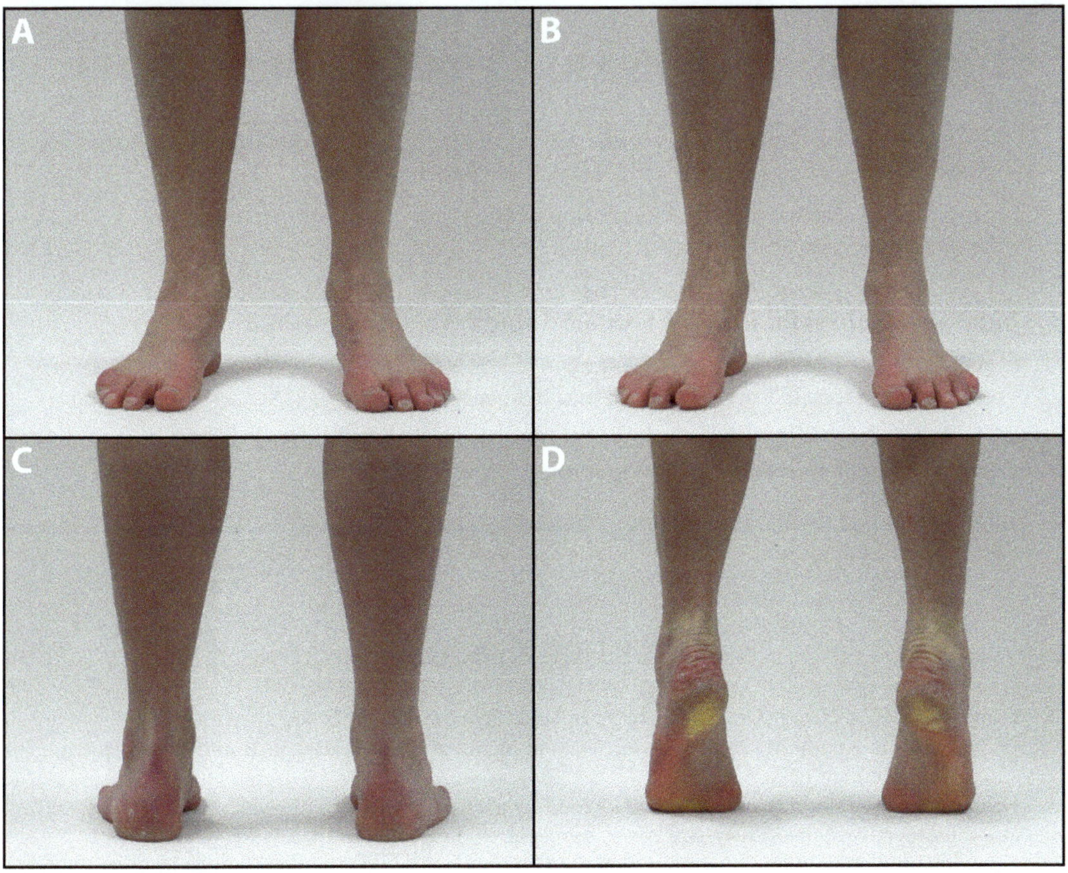

Figure 12-12. A sports teacher after reconstruction of the medial and lateral ligaments as well as an additional calcaneal lengthening osteotomy done 12 years earlier (same patient as in Figure 12-2). The patient is very pleased with the obtained results, allowing her to engage in unlimited sports activities. (A) A distinct pronation deformity of the right foot is left when standing in a relaxed position. (B) It completely disappears when activating the posterior tibial muscle. (C) Symmetric position of the heel as seen from posteriorly. (D) Symmetric varization of the heel in a tip-toe position.

- The overall rehabilitation time to get back to high-demanding sports activities is approximately 9 months (Figure 12-12).

Potential Complications

- Deficient stability due to inappropriate ligament reconstruction
- Recurrent instability due to an unaddressed valgus deformity
- Suture granuloma at the anterior margin of the medial malleolus when using nonresorbable sutures and placing the suture knot on a bony surface
- Deep venous thrombosis
- Infection
- Scarring of the anteromedial ankle causing soft tissue impingement

Top Technical Pearls for the Procedure

1. Arthroscopic assessment: This is the key to confirm the diagnosis of ankle instability and to detect associated intra-articular pathologies.
2. Surgical exploration: Careful exploration of the injured or incompetent ligament should be done routinely.
3. Ligament reconstruction: Strictly anatomical reconstruction of ankle ligaments will be the key of success for obtained functional outcome and ankle stability.
4. Associated problems: Careful assessment of the foot while weightbearing is mandatory to identify associated malalignment and deformity problems.
5. Overall reconstruction: All associated problems should be addressed to achieve an excellent functional outcome in the long term.

References

1. Hintermann B. Medial ankle instability. *Foot Ankle Clin.* 2003;8(4):723-738.
2. Hintermann B, Knupp M, Pagenstert GI. Deltoid ligament injuries: diagnosis and management. *Foot Ankle Clin.* 2006;11(3):625-637.
3. Hintermann B, Valderrabano V, Boss A, Trouillier HH, Dick W. Medial ankle instability: an exploratory, prospective study of fifty-two cases. *Am J Sports Med.* 2004;32(1):183-190.
4. Hintermann B, Regazzoni P, Lampert C, Stutz G, Gachter A. Arthroscopic findings in acute fractures of the ankle. *J Bone Joint Surg Br.* 2000;82(3):345-351.
5. Tornetta P, 3rd. Competence of the deltoid ligament in bimalleolar ankle fractures after medial malleolar fixation. *J Bone Joint Surg Am.* 2000;82(6):843-848.
6. Nelson DR, Younger A. Acute posttraumatic planovalgus foot deformity involving hindfoot ligamentous pathology. *Foot Ankle Clin.* 2003;8(3):521-537.
7. Hintermann B, Boss A, Schafer D. Arthroscopic findings in patients with chronic ankle instability. *Am J Sports Med.* 2002;30(3):402-409.
8. Buman EM KG, Haraguchi N, Myerson MS. Minimally invasive deltoid ligament reconstruction: a comparison of three techniques. Paper presented at: Proceedings of the 36th Annual Winter Meeting, Speciality Day AOFAS; March 25, 2006; Chicago, IL.

Please visit www.routledge.com/9781617119989
to access additional material.

Section III

Diagnostic Subtalar Arthroscopy

13

Subtalar Arthroscopy
Lateral Approach

Christopher E. Gross, MD and Mark E. Easley, MD

Introduction

Lateral approach subtalar arthroscopy confers diagnostic and potentially therapeutic value in treating subtalar trauma, arthrofibrosis, impingement, and cartilage pathology.[1] The orthopedic literature suggests that establishing a definitive diagnosis of subtalar pathology, based on physical exam and detailed imaging studies, improves the likelihood of successful outcome with subtalar arthroscopy.[2-4] Lateral approach subtalar arthroscopy affords satisfactory access to the majority of the talocalcaneal mechanism, including the major articular surfaces, the lateral (talocalcaneal-fibular) gutter, the anterior structures within the sinus tarsi, and the posterior subtalar structures.[1,5] Subtalar access is optimized and complications minimized with careful placement of the 3 standard portals used in lateral approach subtalar arthroscopy[4]: the anterior portal at the distal sinus tarsi, the middle portal immediately anterior to the tip of the fibula and centered over the sinus tarsi, and the posterior portal slightly proximal and posterior to the fibular tip. The authors recommend using small joint arthroscopy equipment. By switching the small joint arthroscope and instruments among the 3 portals, arthrofibrosis and impingement may be comprehensively debrided and all current arthroscopy cartilage repair procedures may be performed. Provided that subtalar arthroscopy confirms definitive diagnosis and pathology is treated appropriately using an arthroscopic technique, a postoperative protocol that includes physical therapy typically leads to a relatively rapid return to satisfactory function.

Indications

- Objective findings
  - Exploratory subtalar arthroscopy is discouraged
- Anterior and lateral subtalar pathology favored via a lateral approach
  - Posterior subtalar arthroscopy may be better accessed via a posterior approach
- Chronic subtalar and sinus tarsi synovitis and/or scarring

Stone JW, Kennedy JG, Glazebrook M, eds. *The Foot and Ankle: AANA Advanced Arthroscopic Surgical Techniques* (pp 121-130).

- Chondral and osteochondral lesions
- Adhesions, arthrofibrosis
- Loose bodies
- Mild arthritis
- Impingement (os trigonum)

Controversial Indications

- Diagnostic arthroscopy: Ideally, an objective finding on preoperative workup is recommended.
- Sinus tarsi syndrome: Nonspecific/nonobjective sinus tarsi pain
- Subtalar instability: Current subtalar arthroscopy techniques offer little in the way of stabilization procedures.
- Posterior subtalar pathology: May be better accessed via a posterior approach

Pertinent Physical Findings

- While some patients may complain of nonspecific hindfoot aching, most patients note pain in the sinus tarsi, particularly with walking on uneven surfaces.
- Sinus tarsi and subfibular tenderness: Occasionally, medial hindfoot tenderness
- Best tests
  - Hindfoot pain +/– stiffness with inversion and eversion
    - Inversion and eversion are tested by stabilizing the talus with one hand (thumb placed on the medial neck of the talus) and using the other hand to grasp and stress the heel into eversion and inversion.
    - Impingement with forced eversion is suggestive of lateral subtalar gutter impingement.
    - To assess stiffness, compare to the contralateral side.
  - Diagnostic subtalar injection with an anesthetic
    - With relief of the patient's pain, subtalar pathology is generally confirmed.
- Instability may also be suggested with the inversion/eversion examination maneuvers.
  - Isolated subtalar instability is often difficult to distinguish from ankle instability.
    - Making the diagnosis may be improved by performing stress testing under fluoroscopy.
    - However, current subtalar arthroscopy techniques need further development to reestablish subtalar stability.
- Pain with forced ankle/hindfoot plantarflexion
  - May be indicative of posterior subtalar pathology
  - Nonspecific as it may also be indicative of posterior ankle pathology

Pertinent Imaging

- Radiographs
  - Routine weightbearing 3-view foot series
    - Two-dimensional views of the complex subtalar joint are important but fail to provide comprehensive evaluation.

    - The lateral foot view provides the best view of the 3.
    - A 45-degree oblique view may provide more, but it is still a limited view of the anterior portion of the subtalar joint.
    - An anteroposterior foot radiograph offers little useful information but may reveal associated pathology and should be included for completeness.
  - Broden's view: posterior facet
    - With the ankle placed in a neutral sagittal plane position and the leg internally rotated 30 to 40 degrees, the x-ray beam is centered over the lateral malleolus and 4 x-rays are made with the tube angled at a 40-, 30-, 20-, and 10-degree cephalic tilt. In a graduated sequence, imaging of the subtalar posterior facet is optimized from anterior to posterior changing from 40 to 10 degrees.
  - Mortise ankle view also demonstrates some of the perspective provided by Broden's view.
  - Lateral oblique: posterior facet
    - The ankle is dorsiflexed, the foot is everted, and the leg is externally rotated 60 degrees.
    - The beam is centered 2 cm below the medial malleolus with a 10-degree cephalic tilt.
- Computed tomography
  - Provides important 3-dimensional analysis of the entire complex subtalar joint
  - Cystic component(s) of osteochondral lesions
  - Subtalar arthritis: Subchondral sclerosis, cystic changes
  - Bony loose bodies
- Magnetic resonance imaging
  - Osteochondral lesions
  - Subtalar chondral wear
  - Stress reactions: Bone marrow edema associated with osteochondral lesions
  - Fibrosis within subtalar joint, sinus tarsi, lateral subtalar gutter
  - Fibrous/cartilaginous loose bodies

Equipment

- Small joint arthroscopy equipment
- 2.3- or 2.7-mm arthroscope (25 vs 30 and 70 degrees)
- Camera
- Standard light source
- 2.9-mm aggressive shaver
- Small joint baskets and graspers
- Pump: To be used with caution as too much pressure may create considerable extravasation from the joint into the adjacent soft tissues

Positioning and Portals

- Two options: Full lateral decubitus position and semi-lateral decubitus (semi-lateral) position +/– noninvasive distraction

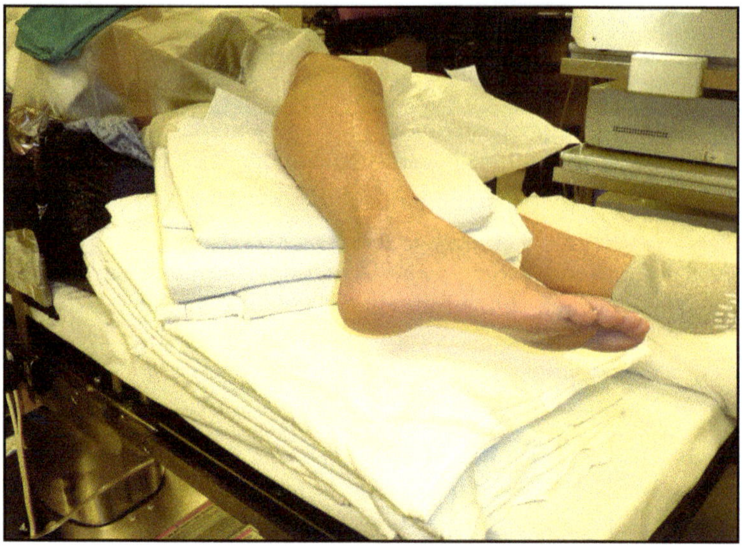

Figure 13-1. Lateral decubitus positioning. Lateral subtalar arthroscopy is facilitated with the patient in the lateral decubitus position and the operated ankle suspended from a support under the lower leg to open the subtalar joint.

- Thigh tourniquet
- Routine draping
- Full lateral decubitus position
  - Patient placed in full lateral decubitus position
  - Opposite (dependent) shoulder, greater trochanter, and fibular neck are well padded
  - Axillary roll to protect the brachial plexus
  - Operated ankle suspended from a firm support ending at the medial malleolus (Figure 13-1): Opens the lateral access to the subtalar joint facilitating arthroscopic instrument access
- Semi-lateral decubitus position
  - A support is placed under the ipsilateral hip
    - Allows for internal rotation to the operated extremity
  - A noninvasive distraction device may be used
    - The thigh may be placed in a thigh holder with the popliteal fossa protected
    - Noninvasive distraction device (Figure 13-2)
- Generally used for ankle arthroscopy
- May also provide distraction at the subtalar joint

Step-by-Step Description of the Procedure

Three Portals

- Anterior portal (Figure 13-3A)
  - 2-cm anterior and 1-cm distal lateral malleolus tip (distal portion of the sinus tarsi)
  - Typically immediately dorsal to the anterior calcaneus at the distal aspect of the angle of Gissane
  - Used primarily as a viewing portal

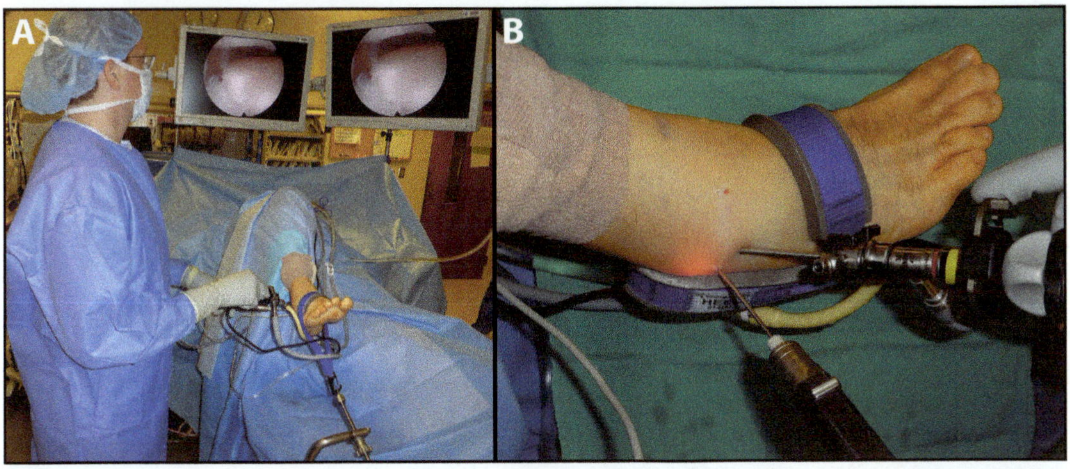

Figure 13-2. Modified lateral decubitus positioning with distraction. (A) Lateral subtalar arthroscopy with noninvasive ankle/hindfoot distraction. (B) Lateral access possible with noninvasive ankle/hindfoot straps in place.

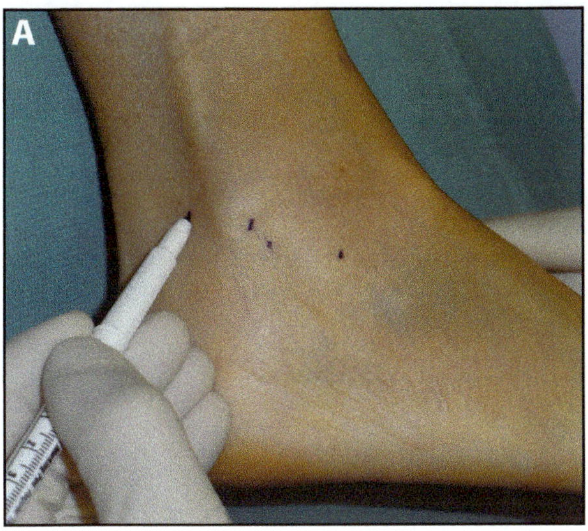

Figure 13-3. Lateral subtalar joint arthroscopy portals. (A) Tip of fibula marked. Middle portal immediately distal and inferior to the tip of the fibula. Anterior portal 1 cm inferior and 2 cm anterior to the tip of the fibula. The posterior portal is just proximal to the tip of the fibula and immediately posterior to the peroneal tendons. *(continued)*

- Middle portal (see Figure 13-3A)
  - Just distal and inferior to the tip of the lateral malleolar tip
  - Typically immediately dorsal to the anterior calcaneus at the proximal aspect of the angle of Gissane
  - Used primarily as an instrument portal
- Posterior portal (see Figure 13-3A)
  - 1-cm proximal to the lateral malleolus tip and anterior to Achilles tendon
  - Viewing and instrument portal
    - As an instrument portal, one may debride posterior and posterolateral subtalar pathology
- Including hypertrophic or inflamed synovium particularly in the lateral subtalar gutter
- Remove impinging structures, even an os trigonum (although best removed via posterior hindfoot arthroscopy)

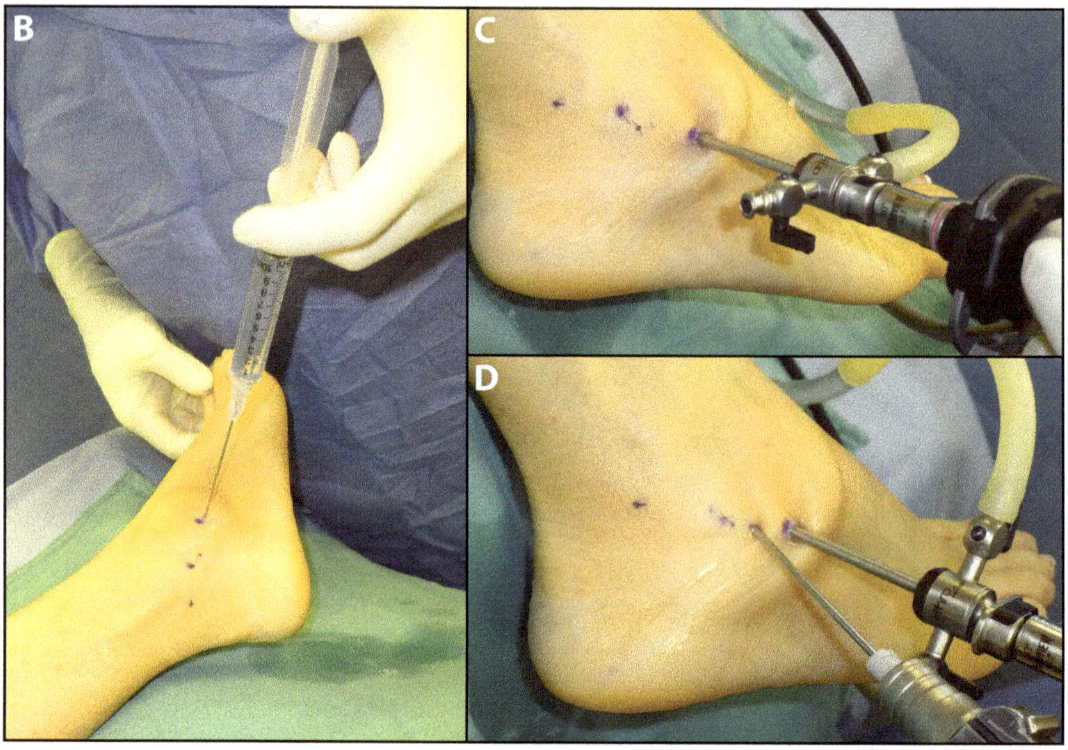

Figure 13-3 (continued). Lateral subtalar joint arthroscopy portals. (B) Anterior portal: spinal needle into sinus tarsi immediately superior to anterior calcaneus at the angle of Gissane with sterile saline introduced into expand anterior subtalar joint. (C) Introduction of the arthroscope. Note skin tension due to the anterior portal made too proximally; ideally, the portal should be created at the proper location without tensioning the skin. Initial visualization may be obscured by inflammatory and/or scar tissue. (D) The shaver introduced in trajectory determined with a spinal needle.

- Establishing the portals
  - Anterior portal
    - Identified first with palpation and an 18-gauge spinal needle
    - The anterior subtalar joint is insufflated with 10 cc of sterile saline through the spinal needle (Figure 13-3B).
    - A small skin incision is made with a #15 blade.
    - The subcutaneous tissue is spread with a hemostat clamp and the joint is entered with a hemostat clamp to avoid injury to the sural and lateral branches of the superficial peroneal nerve.
    - The trocar, followed by the arthroscope and camera with a fluid inflow source, is inserted (Figure 13-3C).
  - Middle portal
    - A spinal needle is inserted to determine the optimal trajectory based on direct visualization within the joint from the anterior portal arthroscope.
    - The middle portal is created through a small superficial incision, and subcutaneous tissue is spread with a hemostat clamp to avoid injury to the sural and lateral branches of the superficial peroneal nerve.
    - The shaver is introduced into the joint via the middle portal also under direct visualization (Figure 13-3D).

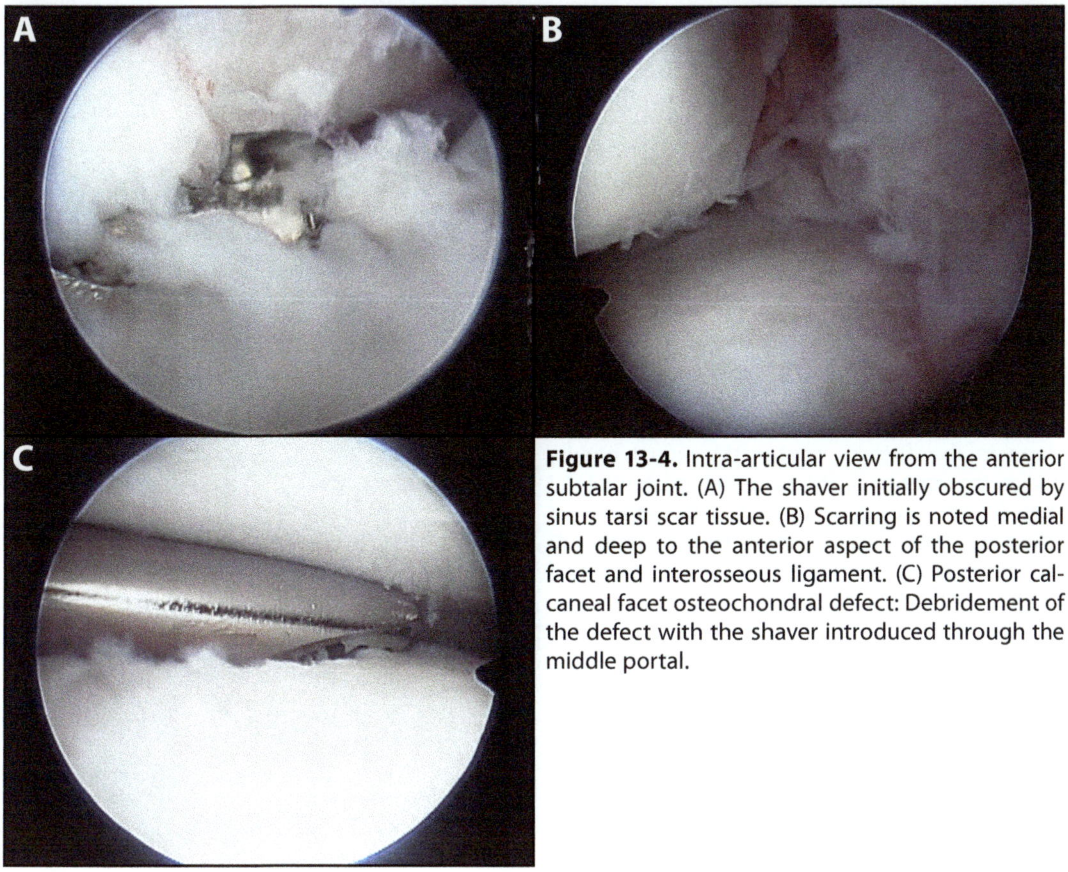

Figure 13-4. Intra-articular view from the anterior subtalar joint. (A) The shaver initially obscured by sinus tarsi scar tissue. (B) Scarring is noted medial and deep to the anterior aspect of the posterior facet and interosseous ligament. (C) Posterior calcaneal facet osteochondral defect: Debridement of the defect with the shaver introduced through the middle portal.

- ▹ Posterior portal
  - A spinal needle is inserted at the previously discussed posterior portal site.
  - Optimal trajectory is based on direct visualization from the subtalar lateral gutter from the anterior portal arthroscope; the subtalar lateral gutter may need to first be cleared of impinging fibrous tissue/scar and synovium.
  - The posterior portal is created through a small superficial incision and subcutaneous tissue is spread with a hemostat clamp to avoid injury to the sural nerve.
  - The shaver is introduced into the posterior lateral gutter and posterior subtalar joint also under direct visualization.

Viewing From the Anterior Portal and Working From the Middle Portal

- Viewing from the anterior portal, inspect the floor of the sinus tarsi.
  - ▹ Approximately 75% of the posterior facet may be visualized from this position.
    - The initial view may be obscured by the sinus tarsi scar or inflammatory tissue (Figure 13-4A).
    - With an arthroscopic shaver introduced through the middle portal, the reactive synovium and scar may be debrided to expose the anterior aspect of the posterior subtalar joint (Figure 13-4B).

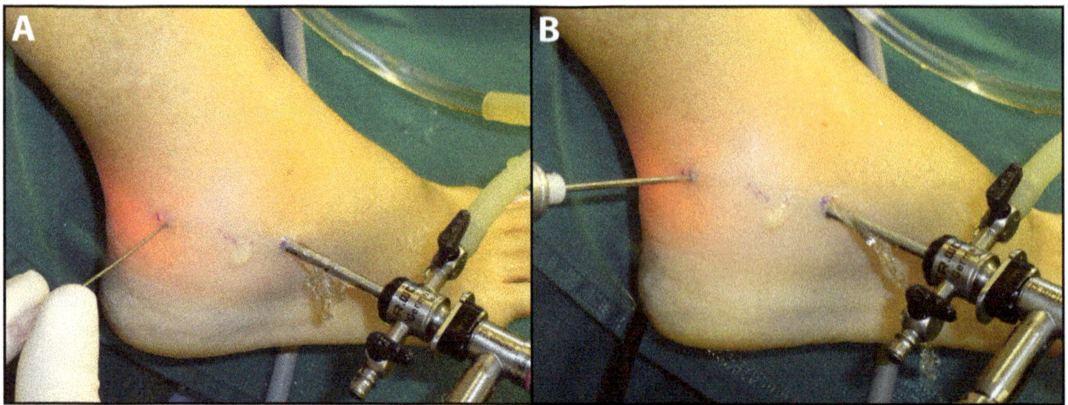

Figure 13-5. Posterior portal. (A) With the arthroscope in the anterior portal, the spinal needle is directly visualized entering the posterolateral joint. (B) The shaver is introduced posteriorly. (C) Visualization from the anterior arthroscope of lateral gutter debridement with the shaver introduced into the posterolateral portal.

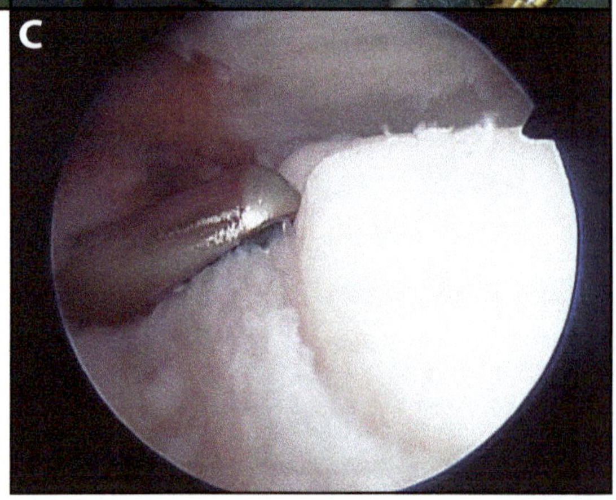

- Medially, the talocalcaneal interosseous ligament fills the tarsal canal.
  - Medial scar tissue may be visualized medial to the ligament and debrided under direct visualization.
  - The lens is rotated to visualize the middle facet medially and anterior calcaneal process laterally.
  - Occasionally, more anterior debridement may be facilitated by placing the arthroscope in the middle portal and the shaver in the anterior portal.
- After anterior debridement, the camera is rotated to inspect the posterior subtalar joint and the posterior calcaneal facet.
  - Pathology of anterior and central posterior calcaneal facet may be visible and accessed.
  - With the camera in the anterior portal and a shaver in the middle portal, intra-articular pathology such as an osteochondral defect of the posterior calcaneal facet may be effectively debrided (Figure 13-4C).
- With the camera still in the anterior portal, a posterior portal may be created by directing the arthroscope into the lateral subtalar gutter and directly visualizing the spinal needle inserted from the intended posterior portal (Figure 13-5A).
- To protect the sural nerve, the posterior portal should be created with a superficial stab incision in the skin and blunt dissection through the posterolateral subtalar capsule.
- The shaver is then introduced through the posterior portal (Figure 13-5B).
- Scar tissue in the lateral gutter may be readily debrided (Figure 13-5C).

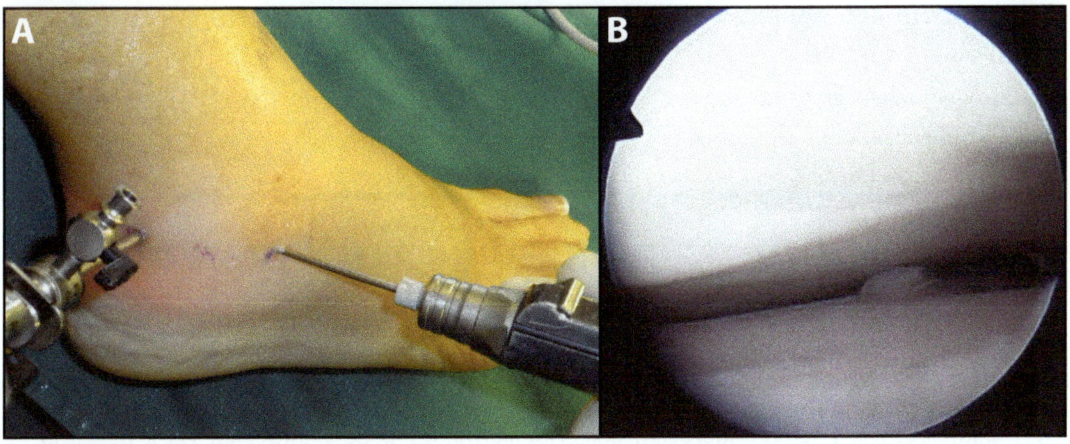

Figure 13-6. Visualization from the posterior portal. (A) Arthroscope introduced from the posterior portal with the shaver in the anterior portal. (B) Visualization of the subtalar joint and debrided osteochondral defect from the posterior portal.

Viewing From the Posterior Portal and Working From the Anterior or Middle Portal

- The arthroscope is removed from the anterior portal and the trocar and camera are introduced into the posterior portal (Figure 13-6A).
- The subtalar joint may be visualized, including findings such as a lateral osteochondral defect (Figure 13-6B).
- The lateral gutter may also be viewed from the posterior portal, and further debridement is possible by introducing the shaver from the middle or anterior portal.

Postoperative Protocol

- Early range of motion is possible, but if an osteochondral defect was managed surgically, consideration may want to be given to protected weightbearing for 3 to 4 weeks.
- An initial cam boot is recommended to protect the foot while the portal sites are healing.
- Partial weightbearing is allowed immediately and continued for 3 to 4 weeks if a microfracture was performed.
- Consideration may be given to physical therapy to be started after the portal sites are healed.
- Initial follow-up is at approximately 7 to 10 days for wound inspection and possible suture removal.
- Return to full activity may take 3 months or more.
- With an osteochondral defect, low-impact exercise is recommended.

Potential Complications

Potential complications are as follows[2]:

- Sural or superficial peroneal nerve injury

- Lack of relief of symptoms
- Infection
- Iatrogenic damage to cartilage
- Instrument failure

Top Technical Pearls for the Procedure

1. Avoid nerve injury at the portal sites by making a superficial sharp incision and access the joint with blunt dissection.
2. Maintain appropriate indications: anterior and lateral subtalar pathology is best addressed via a lateral approach; posterior pathology is best addressed via a posterior hindfoot arthroscopy.
3. To address anterior subtalar joint and sinus tarsi pathology, use the anterior portal for visualization and the middle portal as the working access.
4. Comprehensive lateral subtalar gutter debridement requires a variety of portal combinations: anterior visualization and middle portal instrumentation, anterior portal visualization and posterior portal instrumentation, and posterior portal visualization and middle vs anterior portal instrumentation.
5. A 70-degree arthroscope may improve visualization, particularly when viewing the lateral gutter or visualizing the posterior subtalar joint.

References

1. Hsu AR, Gross CE, Lee S, Carreira DS. Extended indications for foot and ankle arthroscopy. *J Am Acad Orthop Surg.* 2014;22:10-19.
2. Frey C, Feder KS, DiGiovanni C. Arthroscopic evaluation of the subtalar joint: does sinus tarsi syndrome exist? *Foot Ankle Int.* 1999;20:185-191.
3. Goldberger MI, Conti SF. Clinical outcome after subtalar arthroscopy. *Foot Ankle Int.* 1998;19:462-465.
4. Tuijthof GJ, Beimers L, Kerkhoffs GM, Dankelman J, Dijk CN. Overview of subtalar arthrodesis techniques: options, pitfalls and solutions. *Foot Ankle Surg.* 2010;16:107-116.
5. Beimers L, Frey C, van Dijk CN. Arthroscopy of the posterior subtalar joint. *Foot Ankle Clin.* 2006;11:369-990, vii.

Please visit www.routledge.com/9781617119989 to access additional material.

14

Diagnostic Subtalar Arthroscopy
Posterior Approach

Annunziato Amendola, MD and Jason A. Patterson, MD

Introduction

Since it was first published by Van Dijk et al in 2000, the posterior subtalar (ST) approach has gained in popularity for the management of the posterior ST joint and surrounding structures.[1-9] Current literature supports a posterior arthroscopic approach to the ST joint with regard to its increased visualization area,[10] low surgical morbidity and risk of complications, and, as a result, quicker recovery time.[11,12] Although the ST joint can be entered from a lateral approach and there are circumstances when such an approach may be advantageous, this chapter will focus on the diagnostic posterior ST arthroscopy in the prone position. Although posterior ST arthroscopy is still a relatively new procedure, recent literature has shown that it can be an important and valuable tool in the surgeon's armamentarium to safely and effectively treat debilitating and common problems of the hindfoot. This chapter will discuss the indications, describe the senior author's preferred method of the procedure and protocols, and discuss how to minimize any potential complications.

Indications

- ST joint arthritis/ST fusion
- Ankle and ST joint arthritis for tibiotalocalcaneal fusion
- Posterior impingement/os trigonum syndrome
- Flexor hallucis longus (FHL) tenosynovitis and impingement
- Pigmented villonodular synovitis
- Tarsal coalition
- Evaluation of talar/calcaneus fractures
- Lysis of adhesions (arthrofibrosis)
- Posterior ST synovitis

Stone JW, Kennedy JG, Glazebrook M, eds. *The Foot and Ankle: AANA Advanced Arthroscopic Surgical Techniques* (pp 131-139).

- Removal of loose bodies/avulsion fractures involving posterior ligaments
- Chondromalacia
- Osteochondral lesions of the ankle and ST joint

Controversial Indications

- Inadequate nonsurgical management
- Previous open surgery with excessive scar
- Posterior skin/soft tissue infection
- Severe trauma with posterior soft tissue damage
- Poor vascularity, diabetes

Pertinent Physical Findings

- Examination of the skin, sensation, and palpation for pulses
- Test of the muscle strength: extrinsic muscles that move the ankle, hindfoot, and toes
- Evaluation of the passive and active range of motion of the ankle and ST joint
- Tenderness over the anterior aspect of the posterior facet (sinus tarsi) or lateral aspect
- Performing the impingement test: ankle plantarflexion and hindfoot inversion first with palpation over sinus tarsi, followed by hindfoot eversion and ankle dorsiflexion
- Diagnostic injection of local anesthetic into the ST joint vs ankle joint vs tendon sheath to confirm the diagnosis (recommended "best" test)

Pertinent Imaging

- Weightbearing anteroposterior, mortise, and lateral views of the foot and ankle
- Consider hindfoot alignment view and standing bilateral long leg view
- Plantarflexed standing view if posterior impingement is a concern (Figure 14-1)
- Magnetic resonance imaging: cartilage, soft tissue evaluation, and effusion of the ST joint (Figure 14-2)
- Computed tomography scan (also with 3-dimensional reconstruction): bony irregularities such as osteochondral lesions, occult fractures, and joint trauma
- Dynamic ultrasound (with possible guided diagnostic injections): tendon and soft tissue pathology during active and passive joint motion
- Bone scan may be useful in conditions with multiple areas of pain

Equipment

- Sterile bump
- 18-gauge spinal needle
- 4.0-mm, 30-degree angled arthroscope for extra-articular procedures and 2.7-mm, 30-degree scope for intra-articular work

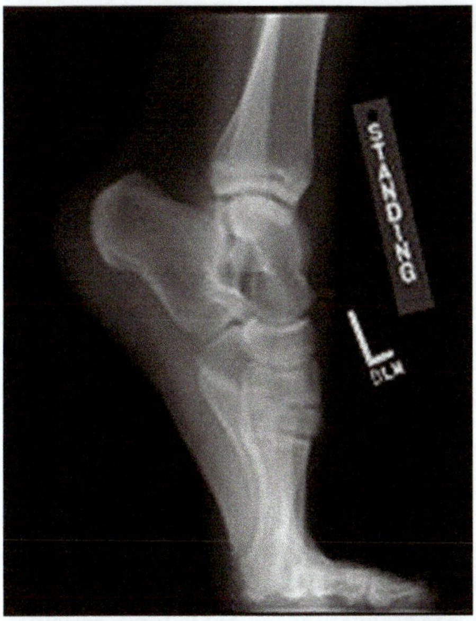

Figure 14-1. Standing plantarflexed view.

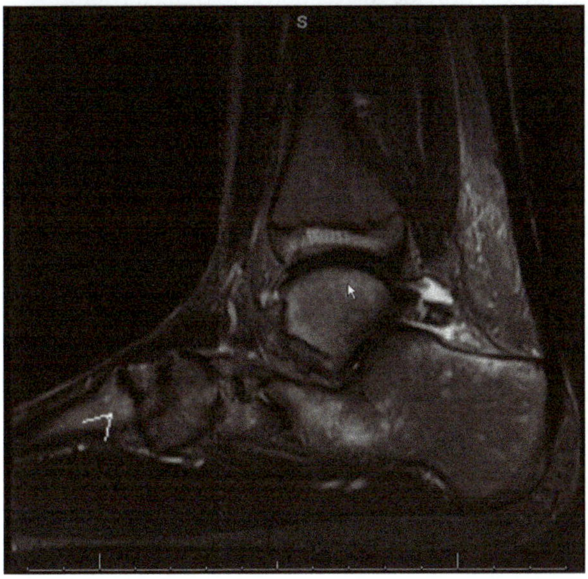

Figure 14-2. Magnetic resonance image showing os trigonum, posterior impingement.

- 3.5-mm full radius shaver
- 4.0-mm burr
- Arthroscopic instruments, including probe and pick set (Figure 14-3)

Positioning and Portals

Prior to positioning the patient prone, place a thigh tourniquet on the marked operative side. Make sure that the tourniquet tubing is lateral or posterior so that it does not cause pressure when the patient is flipped prone. Position the patient prone with use of longitudinal gel rolls on the chest and abdomen. Line up the end of the bed with the ankle joint so that the foot is just off the

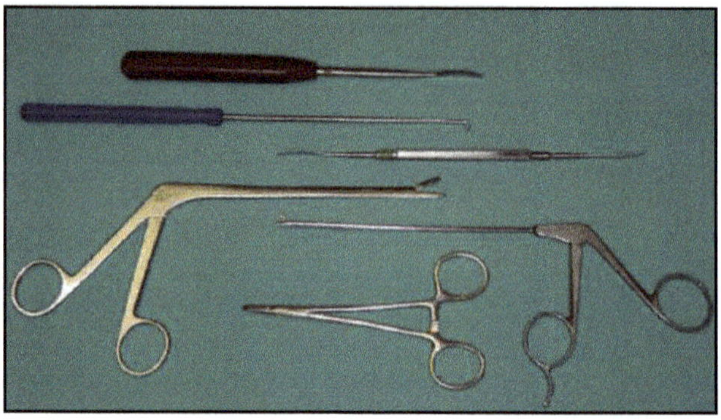

Figure 14-3. Instruments used in posterior diagnostic and basic scope.

table. Make sure both legs are well padded. Strap the patient to the bed securely in case the bed will be planed or traction will be used. A Trendelenburg tilt of the bed can also be used with traction to prevent the patient from sliding. The contralateral limb can be taped to the well-padded bed or can be bent at the knee and secured to a limb holder if fluoroscopy is anticipated to be used. Prep the patient and drape with U-drapes or an extremity drape.

As mentioned previously, traction can be used to improve visualization and aid in intra-articular procedures. There are a variety of different methods to provide distraction across the ST joint.[13,14] The authors prefer invasive distraction using a 1.6- or 2.0-mm wire through the calcaneus[13] for significant surgery (ie, arthrodesis) vs a noninvasive harness for debridement only.

Step-by-Step Description of the Procedure

As with any arthroscopic procedure, portal placement is crucial and depends on the anticipated procedure. Preoperative planning can greatly reduce intraoperative frustration. Review the images obtained to assess the angle of the posterior facet of the ST joint and the presence of osteophytes that may obstruct the view. In addition, placing the portals under fluoroscopic guidance with a C-arm or mini C-arm may be beneficial to confirm the correct placement.

The standard working portals for posterior ST arthroscopy are the posterolateral and posteromedial portals. Typically, the portals are placed 1.5 to 2.0 cm proximal to the superior border of the calcaneal tuberosity and are just on either side of the Achilles tendon near the midline while avoiding the tendon sheath (Figure 14-4).[10] The posterolateral portal will typically be slightly above a line connecting the tip of the lateral malleolus to the Achilles tendon. Establish either the posterolateral or posteromedial portal first by injecting 10 cc of saline centrally into the ST joint using an 18-gauge needle (Figure 14-5). The authors' preference is to go from medial to enter the joint initially to move away from the posteromedial neurovascular bundle, minimizing the risk. Make a vertical incision through the skin. Use a straight hemostat to bluntly dissect anteriorly through fat toward the center of the ST joint. Stay near the Achilles tendon border with the hemostat to minimize the risk to the sural nerve. A blunt 4.0-mm trocar can then be inserted with the 30-degree scope. Typically, water pressure of 30 to 40 mm Hg is usually sufficient in the hindfoot. A 2.7-mm scope with a 3-mm sheath is commonly used as well. The posterolateral portal is created in a similar fashion. After making the skin incision at the same level as the posteromedial portal, use the hemostat and slide down the trocar toward the ST joint. Stay central and to the lateral side of the ST joint to minimize the risk to the FHL tendon and neurovascular structures just medial to that tendon (Figure 14-6).[15] Spread gently to create space for the working instruments. Start with a 3.5-mm full radius shaver in the posteromedial portal to gently resect fat and synovium over the ST joint. Once again, start on the posterolateral aspect of the ST joint and work medially with the shaver pointed laterally. This is to prevent injury to the FHL tendon (see Figure 14-6).

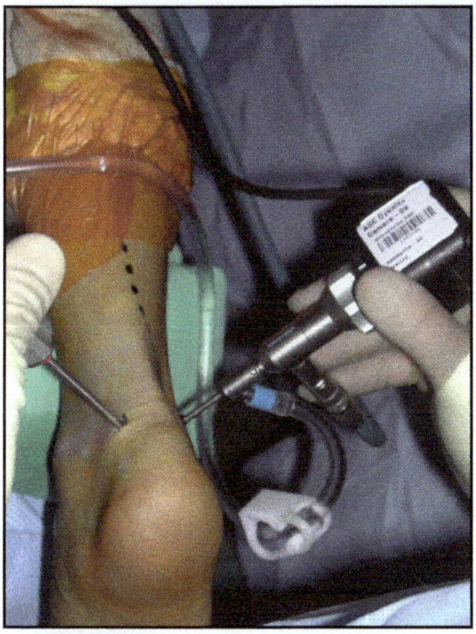

Figure 14-4. Posterior scope portals. The sural nerve (dotted line) is drawn out.

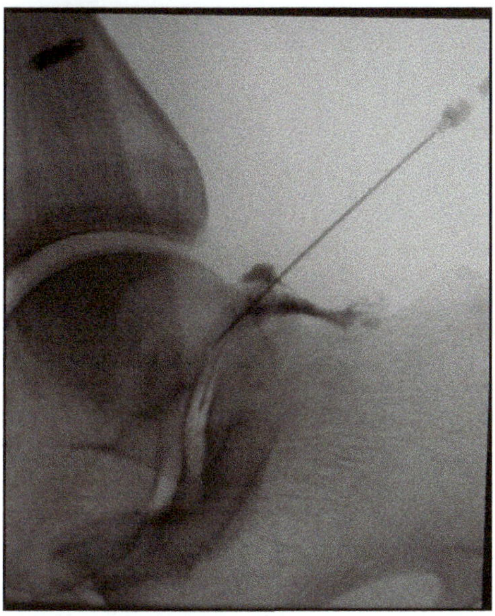

Figure 14-5. Fluoroscopy-guided injection of the ST joint to aid in portal position and instrumentation insertion.

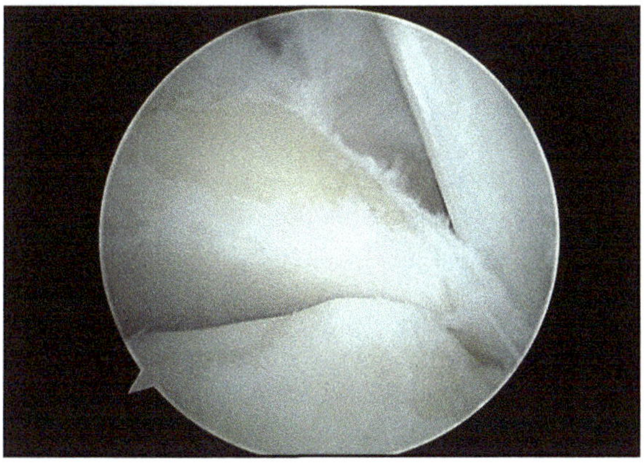

Figure 14-6. Medial aspect of ST joint just lateral to FHL.

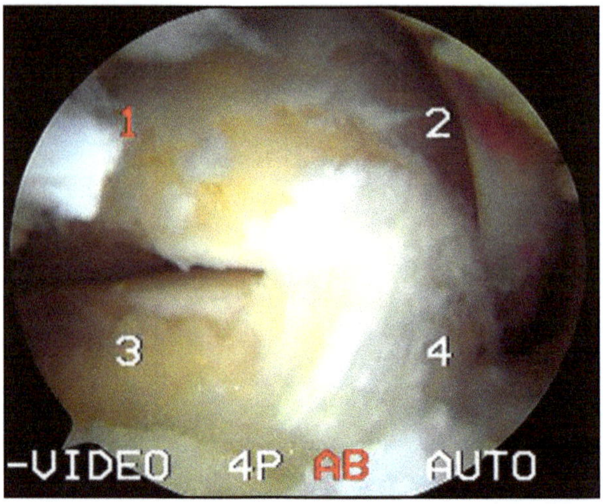

Figure 14-7. FHL tendon shown.

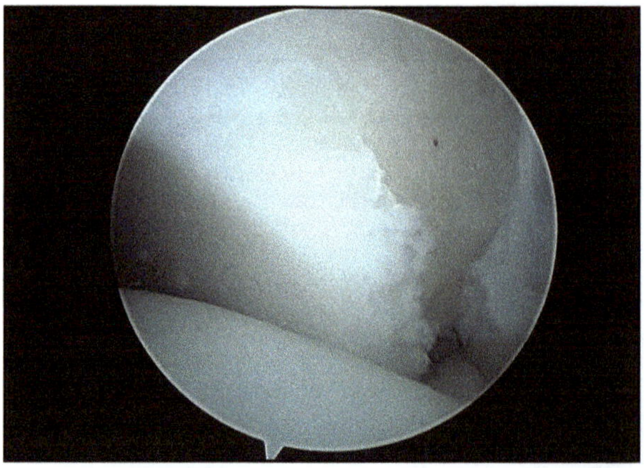

Figure 14-8. ST joint.

Soon, the FHL tendon will come into view as you work toward the posteromedial aspect (Figure 14-7). Once the tendon is identified, you can be slightly more aggressive resecting lateral to this important landmark as the neurovascular bundle lies just medial.[16,17] Usually the os trigonum, if present, and the posterior talofibular ligament will need to be resected to gain access to the ST joint (Figure 14-8). The posterior tibiofibular ligament will be the superior landmark separating the ankle and ST joints and, for an isolated ST, arthroscopy can typically be left alone. Once the debridement is performed, distraction can be applied to aid in the diagnostic ST scope. The sheath of the FHL can be released and, using a probe with the ankle and big toe maximally flexed, much of the FHL can be inspected (Figure 14-9). In addition, the scope can be gently inserted into the sheath for further tendoscopy inspection.

Occasionally, a third accessory portal can be made: the posterolateral ventral portal.[10] This is typically used for ST fusions to aid in distraction of the joint by placing a blunt trocar through this portal and into the joint. Create this portal under direct visualization to ensure the trocar will line up perfectly with the ST joint and perform its desired distraction function. The landmarks are typically 1 cm proximal and 1 cm posterior to the tip of the lateral malleolus. It will lie directly posterior to the peroneal tendons and anterior to the sural nerve. Due to the proximity of these structures, careful blunt technique is mandatory to establish this portal. With the use of this portal, sufficient distraction is usually achieved to accomplish joint preparation for ST fusion (Figure 14-10). Closure of the portals is with 3-0 nylon if desired, although the authors prefer to leave them open for routine procedures, and the patient is placed in a soft dressing.

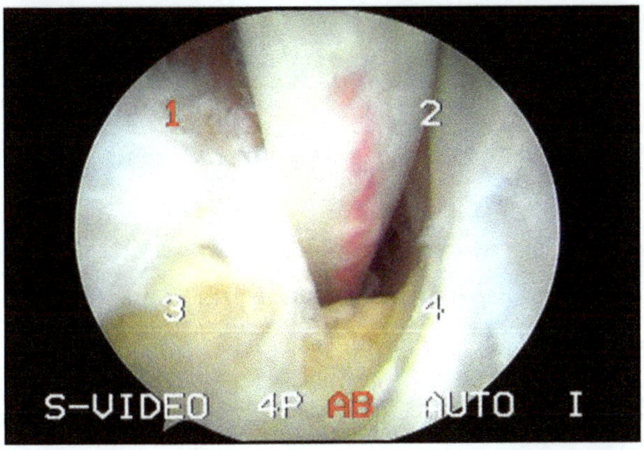

Figure 14-9. FHL and sheathe inspected.

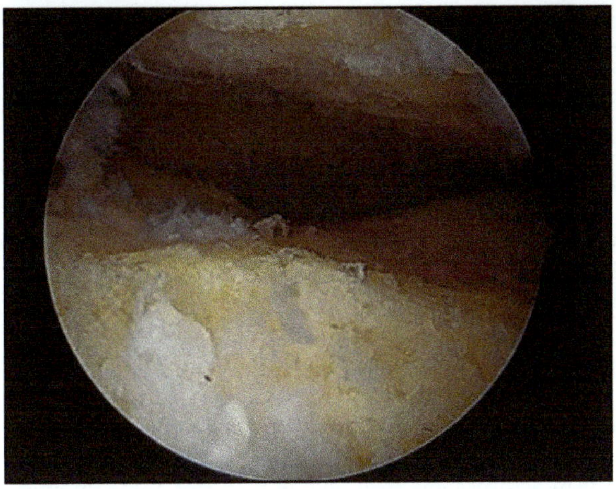

Figure 14-10. ST joint preparation for anticipated fusion.

Postoperative Protocol

Typically, for an isolated diagnostic hindfoot arthroscopy, the patient is placed in a boot and allowed to bear weight as tolerated. The patient can come out of the boot for range of motion exercises. Sutures are removed in 10 to 14 days and the patient can wean out of the boot at that time. Any variations to this protocol will depend on other procedures that were performed at the time of surgery.

Potential Complications

The most common reported complication from the posterior ankle/ST arthroscopy is injury to a nerve, usually the sural nerve.[18-20] The anatomy and safe zones have been studied and show that the sural nerve and small saphenous vein are closest to the portal sites.[21-23] The FHL tendon is also a risk if careful identification and resection is not performed. Medial to the FHL lays the tibial nerve and posterior tibial artery. If dissection strays too far laterally, the peroneal tendons and lateral ligaments can be injured. Other complications related to posterior scope include Achilles tightness, complex regional pain syndrome, infection, and cyst formation.[24] Although not specific to posterior ST arthroscopy, complications associated with tourniquet and traction can also occur, and the surgeon should be aware of these.[25,26]

Top Technical Pearls for the Procedure

1. Preoperative planning is essential with appropriate imaging and portal placement.
2. Prone patient positioning is required, as well as set-up with traction if needed.
3. Use blunt dissection and careful tissue spreading when creating portals; stay central.
4. Identify the FHL tendon early to protect it and use it as medial landmark.
5. Use accessory posterolateral ventral portal as an adjunct for distraction.

References

1. van Dijk CN, Scholten PE, Krips R. A 2-portal endoscopic approach for diagnosis and treatment of posterior ankle pathology. *Arthroscopy*. 2000;16(8):871-876.
2. Scholten PE, Sierevelt IN, van Dijk CN. Hindfoot endoscopy for posterior ankle impingement. *J Bone Joint Surg Am*. 2008;90(12):2665-2672.
3. Amendola A, Lee KB, Saltzman CL, et al. Technique and early experience with posterior arthroscopic subtalar arthrodesis. *Foot Ankle Int*. 2007;28(3):298-302.
4. Smyth N, Zwiers R, Wiegerinck J, et al. Posterior hindfoot arthroscopy: a review. *Am J Sports Med*. 2014;42(1):225-234.
5. Ogut T, Ayhan E, Irgit K, Sarikaya A. Endoscopic treatment of posterior ankle pain. *Knee Surg Sports Traumatol Arthrosc*. 2011;19:1355-1361.
6. Smyth N, Murawski C, Levine D, Kennedy J. Hindfoot arthroscopic surgery for posterior ankle impingement. *Am J Sports Med*. 2013;41(8):1869-1876.
7. Galla M, Lobenhoffer P. Technique and results of arthroscopic treatment of posterior ankle impingement. *Foot Ankle Surg*. 2011;(17):79-84.
8. Hsu A, Gross C, Lee S, Carreira D. Extended indications for foot and ankle arthroscopy. *J Am Acad Orthop Surg*. 2014;22:10-19.
9. De Leeuw P, van Sterkenburg M, van Dijk N. Arthroscopy and endoscopy of the ankle and hindfoot. *Sports Med Arthrosc Rev*. 2009;17:175-184.
10. Phisitkul P, Tochigi Y, Saltzman CL, et al. Arthroscopic visualization of the posterior subtalar joint in the prone position: a cadaver study. *Arthroscopy*. 2006;22(5):511-515.
11. Willits K, Sonneveld H, Amendola A, Giffin JR, Griffin S, Fowler PJ. Outcome of posterior ankle arthroscopy for hindfoot im-pingement. *Arthroscopy*. 2008;24(2):196-202. Epub 2007 Nov 8.
12. Guo Q, Hu Y, Jiao C, et al. Open versus endoscopic excision of a symptomatic os trigonum: a comparative study of 41 cases. *Arthroscopy*. 2010;26(3):384-390.
13. Beals TC, Junko JT, Amendola A, Nickisch F, Saltzman CL. Minimally invasive distraction technique for prone posterior ankle and subtalar arthroscopy. *Foot Ankle Int*. 2010;31(4):316-319.
14. van Dijk CN, Verhagen RA, Tol HJ. Technical note: resterilizable noninvasive ankle distraction device. *Arthroscopy*. 2001;17(3):E12.
15. Yoshimura I, Naito M, Kanazawa K, et al. Assessing the safe direction of instruments during posterior ankle arthroscopy using an MRI model. *Foot Ankle Int*. 2013;34:434-438.
16. Carro LP, Golanó P, Vega J. Arthroscopic subtalar arthrodesis: the posterior approach in the prone position. *Arthroscopy*. 2007;23(4):445.e1-e4. Epub 2007 Feb 20.
17. Phisitkul P, Amendola A. False FHL: a normal variant posing risks in posterior hindfoot endoscopy. *Arthroscopy*. 2010;26(5):714-718. Epub 2010 Jan 25.
18. Ferkel RD, Small HN, Gittins JE. Complications in foot and ankle arthroscopy. *Clin Orthop Relat Res*. 2001;391:89-104.
19. Abramowitz Y, Wollstein R, Barzilav Y, et al. Outcome of resection of a symptomatic os trigonum. *J Bone Joint Surg Am*. 2003;85-A(6):1051-1057.

20. Donnenwerth M, Roukis T. The incidence of complications after posterior hindfoot endoscopy. *Arthroscopy.* 2013;29(12):2049-2054.
21. Sitler DF, Amendola A, Bailey CS, Thain LMF, Spouge A. Posterior ankle arthroscopy: an anatomic study. *J Bone Joint Surg Am.* 2002;84:763-769.
22. Heck J, Mendicino RW, Stasko P, Shadrick D, Catanzariti AR. An anatomic safe zone for posterior ankle arthroscopy: a cadaver study. *J Foot Ankle Surg.* 2012;51(6):753-756. Epub 2012 Sep 21.
23. Mouilhade F, Oger P, Roussignol X, Boisrenoult P, Sfez J, Duparc F. Risks relating to posterior 2-portal arthroscopic arthrodesis and articular surfaces abrasion quality achievable with these approaches: a cadaver study. *Orthop Traumatol Surg Res.* 2011;97(4):396-400. Epub 2011 May 13.
24. Nickisch F, Barg A, Saltzman C, et al. Postoperative complications of posterior ankle and hindfoot arthroscopy. *J Bone Joint Surg Am.* 2012;94(5):439-446.
25. Carlson M, Ferkel R. Complications in ankle and foot arthroscopy. *Sports Med Arthrosc Rev.* 2013;21:135-139.
26. Ferkel R, Small H, Gittins J. Complications in foot and ankle arthroscopy. *Clin Orthop Relat Res.* 2001;(391):89-104.

Please visit www.routledge.com/9781617119989 to access additional material.

SECTION IV

Arthrodesis

15

Anatomic Arthroscopic Ankle Arthrodesis

Mark Glazebrook, MD

Introduction

End-stage ankle arthritis (ESAA) has a severe effect on patients' health-related quality of life.[1] When nonoperative treatments fail, ankle arthrodesis surgery or total ankle arthroplasty can improve pain, function, and health-related quality of life.[2,3] Arthrodesis remains the mainstay of operative treatment for patients with isolated ESAA and no ipsilateral periarticular arthritis (Canadian Orthopaedic Foot and Ankle Score [COFAS] type 1), intra-articular deformity, and isolated (COFAS type 2) and extra-articular deformity (COFAS type 3).[4]

The goal of an ankle arthrodesis is to fuse the talus and tibia to remove the majority of pain while sacrificing motion at the ankle joint. Current surgical treatment for ankle arthrodesis includes an open or arthroscopic technique fixed with rigid internal fixation. Arthroscopic ankle arthrodesis allows the surgical goals of ankle fusion to be achieved without extensive dissection that often results in excessive pain, swelling, and discomfort.[5,6]

The evidence-based indications for ankle arthroscopy demonstrate consistent level II and III studies, allowing a grade B recommendation supporting the surgical procedure of arthroscopic ankle arthrodesis for the treatment of end-stage ankle arthritis.[7] Recently, a prospective level III study[8] that compared outcomes for open and arthroscopic ankle arthrodesis demonstrated that both techniques were associated with significant improvement in patients' pain and function, while arthroscopic arthrodesis resulted in shorter hospital stays and better outcomes. Furthermore, arthroscopic arthrodesis may be performed as an outpatient procedure and thus be less costly to patients and third-party providers. Finally, arthroscopic arthrodesis is an anatomic sparing procedure with minimal bone resection, preserving anatomy for future options.

The purpose of this chapter is to describe an anatomic arthroscopic ankle arthrodesis that is safe and less technically demanding for surgeons with experience in ankle arthroscopy.

Indications

- Treatment of end-stage ankle arthritis (especially COFAS types 1 and 3) in those patients who have failed nonoperative treatments

Stone JW, Kennedy JG, Glazebrook M, eds. *The Foot and Ankle: AANA Advanced Arthroscopic Surgical Techniques* (pp 143-148).

Table 15-1. Indications and Contraindications for Anatomic Arthroscopic Ankle Arthrodesis

Indications	Absolute Contraindications	Relative Contraindications
Patients with ESAA (COFAS type 1 or 2) who failed nonoperative treatments and have minimal intra-articular deformity	Active untreated infection	Smokers not willing to quit smoking
	Charcot arthropathy	
	Severe bone loss	Diabetics with elevated hemoglobin A1C (HbA1C)
	Severe intra-articular deformity (COFAS type 2)	
	Severe extra-articular deformity requiring osteotomy (COFAS type 4)	

- Patients who have significant intra-articular ankle deformity associated with their ankle arthritis (COFAS type 2) may not be appropriate for the arthroscopic technique and may best be treated with an open technique.
- Patients with increased risks of healing complications may be most appropriate for arthroscopic ankle arthrodesis. (Table 15-1 lists indications and absolute and relative contraindications.)

Pertinent Physical Findings

Key findings that are common on the clinical history of patients with ESAA include the following:

- Severe pain at the ankle joint that is worse with weightbearing activity and relieved with nonweightbearing
- Patients may complain of start-up pain.
- Pain may be improved with analgesics, anti-inflammatory agents, weight reduction, activity modification, bracing, physical therapy, and other nonoperative treatments.

Key findings that are commonly elicited upon physical examination include the following:

- Pain to palpation directly over the anterior portion of the ankle joint. It is important to palpate and move the subtalar and other joints around the ankle to rule out ipsilateral periarticular arthritis.
- Pain with ankle range of motion
- Deformity in the coronal, sagittal, and axial planes. This should be noted to assist in deciding whether the deformity is correctable with an arthroscopic vs open arthrodesis.

Pertinent Imaging

- The diagnostic imaging of the patients should begin with standing anteroposterior and lateral views of the ankle.
- Computed tomography scans are helpful in detailing the bone structure and extent of arthritis.

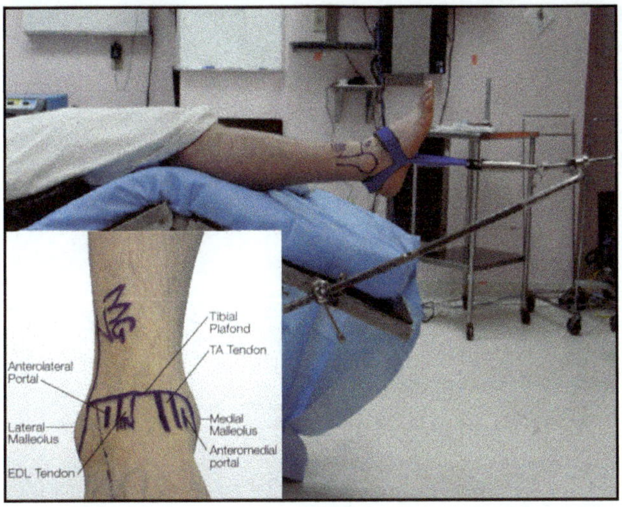

Figure 15-1. Patient positioning and anatomic landmarks for portal placement.

- The best test would be a computed tomography spec scan, where bone activity and detailed bone structure is revealed, to assist with diagnosing the severity of any arthritis in the hind- and midfoot.

Equipment

Suggested instrumentation for arthroscopic ankle arthrodesis are as follows:

- Standard arthroscopic equipment
- Noninvasive arthroscopic ankle distractor system
- 4.0-mm, 30-degree, high-definition arthroscope and sheath set or similar
- Motorized arthroscopic full radius shavers 4.5 mm or similar
- Motorized arthroscopic bony burr tips
- Arthroscopic hand instruments including probe, curettes, osteotomes grasper, and chondral picks
- Power driver to insert guide wires and overdrill for cannulated large fragment screws
- Arthroscopic drill guide system to allow rapid and precise arthroscopic placement of guide wires
- Large fragment (7 mm or similar) cannulated drill set and screws appropriate for percutaneous fixation
- Fluoroscopy (mini C-arm sufficient)

Positioning and Portals

After administration of anesthesia and application of the tourniquet, the lower leg is prepped and draped, leaving the calf, ankle, and foot exposed (Figure 15-1). The patient is then placed in the semi-beach chair position (see Figure 15-1) with the bed flexed at the hips and knees to allow a working space for posterolateral and posteromedial portals if necessary. A sandbag positioned under the ipsilateral hip assists with positioning the foot and ankle, with toes straight up. The procedure is best described as a 5-step process.

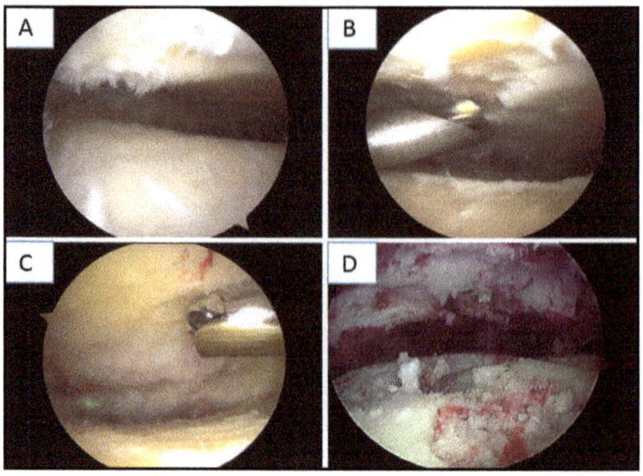

Figure 15-2. Ankle arthroscopic intra-articular views of (A) arthritic talar and tibial joints surface confirming diagnosis of ESAA; (B) motorized shaver removing remaining arthritic cartilage; (C) ball-tipped burr removing subchondral bone; and (D) foraged cancellous bone with guide wires in position.

Step-by-Step Description of the Procedure

The surgical technique of anatomic ankle arthroscopic arthrodesis begins with the patient awake and able to voluntarily contract muscular landmarks. This assists the surgeon in drawing all required anatomic landmarks on the patient's skin prior to anesthesia (see Figure 15-1). The bony landmarks are drawn first, including the distal edge of the tibial plafond and the medial and lateral malleolus. Next, the extensor digitorum longus tendon and the tibialis posterior tendon with the medial portal site just medial to the tibialis posterior tendon and the lateral portal site just lateral to the extensor digitorum longus tendon are each marked. Then, the margins of the Achilles tendon to the calcaneal insertion to define the posterior landmarks are marked. Lastly, the medial and lateral posterior portals are marked directly adjacent to the Achilles, at a level approximately 1 cm above the tip of the fibula.

Step 1: Diagnostic Ankle Arthroscopy to Confirm Diagnosis

Sterile saline (approximately 15 cc) is injected into the ankle joint through the marked medial portal site. The tip of a #10 scalpel blade is used to create an incision, taking care to protect neural structures, using a hemostat spreading technique for dissection. A cannula is inserted through the medial portal site and directed at the anterior border of the distal fibula, followed by an arthroscope, to establish the medial portal. The lateral portal (and posterior portals if necessary) is established using the same neurovascular protection technique. An initial systematic inspection is conducted to grade the arthritis and confirm the diagnosis (Figure 15-2A). The accessibility of all areas of the talar and tibial surfaces is determined to assure suitability for an arthroscopic approach. It is important that both the patient and surgeon understand that, at any point during the procedure, an arthroscopic arthrodesis can be converted to an open arthrodesis and may be required if technical difficulties are encountered.

Step 2: Debridement of Remaining Articular Cartilage to Expose Subchondral Bone

After confirmation of ESAA diagnosis, the remaining cartilage is removed using a combination of hand instruments and mechanical shavers, removing all cartilage on the talar dome and tibial plafond (Figure 15-2B). The cartilage should be removed in a systematic fashion starting with the talus, working from the anterolateral to posteromedial side and alternating to the tibial surface, as exposure allows. Rarely, there may be difficulty encountered in accessing the posterior portions of the joint that will be opposed when the ankle is placed in its final fusion position. If this occurs, a posterior portal may be established to gain better exposure to this area.

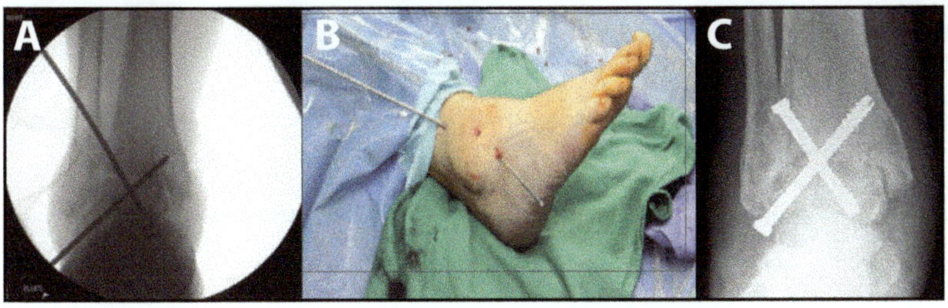

Figure 15-3. Diagnostic imaging and clinical photo showing guide wire and hardware positioning.

Step 3: Removal of Subchondral Bone

Once all cartilage has been removed and the subchondral bone has been exposed on both talar and tibial articular surfaces, a mechanical burr is used to remove the subchondral bone (Figure 15-2C) to expose underlying cancellous bone (Figure 15-2D). This is best done in a systematic fashion as well from anterolateral to posteromedial using posterior portals if necessary.

Step 4: Forage of Bone

Once all subchondral bone has been removed and the underlying cancellous bone has been exposed on both talar and tibial articular surfaces, a chondral pick is used to forage these surfaces (see Figure 15-2D), especially in areas where sclerotic bone remains.

Step 5: Percutaneous Rigid Internal Fixation

An arthroscopic drill guide system is used to allow rapid and precise arthroscopic placement of guide wires. The targeting arm of the arthroscopic drill guide is passed through the lateral portal and positioned on the posterior central portion of talar dome to allow passage of the guide wire into the sinus tarsi and penetration of the anterolateral surface of the talus (Figure 15-3). The second guide wire is inserted (see Figure 15-3) in a similar fashion through the tibia just anterior to the fibula, approximately 2 cm proximal to the tibial joint surface, and directed as such that it exits the tibial articular surface in the anterior central surface (see Figure 15-2D).

After removing all of the intra-articular arthroscopic instruments from the joint, the ankle is reduced to the anatomically neutral position (5-degree hindfoot valgus, slight external rotation, and neutral dorsiflexion) and guide wires are passed across the joint. Intraoperative fluoroscopy is then used to confirm adequate bone-to-bone reduction of the tibia and talus and guide wire positioning (see Figure 15-3).

The guide wires can be withdrawn enough to allow ankle joint motion and insertion of a bone graft or bone graft substitute, if the surgeon chooses to augment the procedure. The guide wires may then be reinserted across the joint to allow for internal fixation with large fragment cannulated screws. Wounds are closed after final fluoroscopic images are captured to confirm screw placement and anatomic reduction and dressed with sterile compression dressing and a U-slab plaster of Paris cast.

Postoperative Protocol

Patients are instructed to remain nonweightbearing on the operative limb for 6 weeks. Cast change and stitch removal is performed at 10 to 14 days postoperatively with cast removal at 6 weeks. Progressive weightbearing in a removable walker boot is commenced after 6 weeks of nonweightbearing at a rate of 25% body weight per week. Full weightbearing activities are allowed at 10 weeks postoperatively and should be adjusted according to pain and swelling experienced.

Potential Complications

Possible complications from this procedure include infection, neurovascular injury, healing problems, malunion, and nonunion.

Top Technical Pearls for the Procedure

1. Care and time must be taken to ensure appropriate portal positioning.
2. Patients should be consented for a possible open ankle arthrodesis in case technical difficulties are encountered with accessing the joint surfaces to allow for conversion to an open procedure.
3. When removing subchondral bone, extra effort should be dedicated to the removal of the medial and lateral shoulders of the talus to allow anatomic and congruent apposition of talar and tibial surfaces.
4. If anatomic and congruent apposition of talar and tibial surfaces is not possible, the lateral and medial walls of the talus may be debrided to provide room for reduction into the tibial ankle mortise.
5. If added stability is required for fixation, a percutaneous screw may be inserted into the posterior malleolus and directed toward the talar neck.

References

1. Glazebrook M, Daniels T, Younger A, et al. Comparison of health-related quality of life between patients with end-stage ankle and hip arthrosis. *J Bone Joint Surg Am.* 2008;90(3):499-505.
2. Haddad SL, Coetzee JC, Estok R, Fahrbach K, Banel D, Nalysnyk L. Intermediate and long-term outcomes of total ankle arthroplasty and ankle arthrodesis. A systematic review of the literature. *J Bone Joint Surg Am.* 2007;89(9):1899-1905.
3. Slobogean GP, Younger A, Apostle KL, et al. Preference-based quality of life of end-stage ankle arthritis treated with arthroplasty or arthrodesis. *Foot Ankle Int.* 2010;31(7):563-566.
4. Krause FG, Di Silvestro M, Penner MJ, et al. Inter- and intraobserver reliability of the COFAS end-stage ankle arthritis classification system. *Foot Ankle Int.* 2010;31(2):103-108.
5. Gougoulias NE, Agathangelidis FG, Parsons SW. Arthroscopic ankle arthrodesis. *Foot Ankle Int.* 2007;28(6):695-706.
6. Stone JW. Arthroscopic ankle arthrodesis. *Foot Ankle Clin.* 2006;11(2):361-368, vi-vii.
7. Glazebrook MA, Ganapathy V, Bridge MA, Stone JW, Allard JP. Evidence-based indications for ankle arthroscopy. *Arthroscopy.* 2009;25(12):1478-1490.
8. Townshend D, Di Silvestro M, Krause F, et al. Arthroscopic versus open ankle arthrodesis: a multicenter comparative case series. *J Bone Joint Surg Am.* 2013;95(2):98-102.

Please visit www.routledge.com/9781617119989 to access additional material.

VIDEO

16

Subtalar Arthrodesis by Arthroscopy Technique

Xavier Martin Oliva, PhD

Introduction

Isolated subtalar joint fusion is usually preferred rather than triple arthrodesis to preserve transverse tarsal joint motion and decrease the potential for degenerative joint disease in the ipsilateral periarticular joints. The main indications are calcaneal fracture nonunions, malunions, subtalar joint arthrosis, varus or valgus malalignment of the hindfoot, talocalcaneal coalitions, and neuromuscular/tendon disorders that lead to subtalar joint instability.

For many years, ankle arthroscopy has played a role in foot and ankle surgery. However, since 2000, when Van Dijk et al introduced the 2-portal posterior approach for hindfoot arthroscopy with the patient in the prone position,[1] an important change has taken place in the surgical treatment of ankle and subtalar pathology.

Until 2000, posterior soft tissue and bone impingements and tendinitis of the flexor hallucis longus (FHL) were only treated by open surgery. Further, subtalar arthrodesis was performed using an open lateral approach, mini-open treatments, or lateral arthroscopic procedures. The arthroscopic posterior approaches allow the treatment of posterior hindfoot pathologies[2] reducing morbidity, such as fewer soft tissue complications. This is optimal for patients who are smokers and those with diabetes or vascular diseases.

Indications

- The main indication for posterior arthroscopic arthrodesis of the subtalar joint is in patients with posttraumatic osteoarthritis. Sixty-eight percent of these cases are sequels of calcaneal fractures, and less represent talus fractures.[3,4]
- Painful talocalcaneal coalition
- Inflammatory and primary osteoarthritis of the subtalar joint

Stone JW, Kennedy JG, Glazebrook M, eds. *The Foot and Ankle: AANA Advanced Arthroscopic Surgical Techniques* (pp 149-156).

Contraindications

- Severe deformities in varus/valgus of the hindfoot such as some sequels of calcaneal fractures[5,6]
- Single- or multi-plane deformities are problematic for arthroscopic procedures.[7]
- Failed arthrodesis that requires an open approach and extended debridement[8]
- Valgus deformity secondary to coalition presents special difficulties when being corrected.[9]

Pertinent Physical Findings

The patient's clinical history is important, as is his or her height, weight, smoking status, occupation, and history of systemic illness at the time of subtalar arthrodesis. All of these factors must be taken into consideration.

Pertinent physical findings include the following:

- Determine the location of the pain by palpation of the subtalar joint at the sinus tarsi.
- Anesthetic diagnostic infiltration is also useful.
- Assess hindfoot alignment.

Pertinent Imaging

- Radiographic assessment includes the following:
  - Lateral and anteroposterior radiographs of the foot
  - Broden views
  - Anteroposterior radiograph of the ankle
  - Salzmann and Meary projections to evaluate the hindfoot axis
- Computed tomography scans
  - Magnetic resonance imaging scan
  - Positron emission tomography–computed tomography has become useful in the diagnosis of arthritis.

Equipment

- 4-mm arthroscope
- 2.7-mm arthroscope for tight joints
- Curettes, chisels, drill, and shaver

Positioning and Portals

The patient is placed in the prone position with the foot hanging off the operating table and a support under the tibia to allow plantarflexion, dorsiflexion, and eversion inversion of the ankle joint. This position is preferred to the lateral position. Skin traction is avoided.

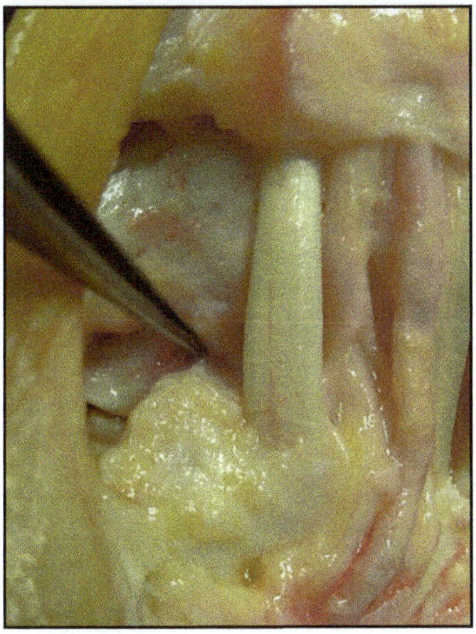

Figure 16-1. The distance between the FHL and posterior tibial nerve. (Reprinted with permission of X. Martin and A. Bravo.)

Step-by-Step Description of the Procedure

This procedure includes an isolated arthrodesis of the posterior facet since most publications report it is sufficient to limit subtalar movement.[7] Two posterior arthroscopic portals are recommended, while other authors recommend 3 portals.[10]

Precise placement of portals is important in order to avoid neurovascular bundle injury and to allow proper articular access during the arthrodesis procedure. The tibial nerve and vascular structures are an average distance of 6.8-mm from the FHL (Figure 16-1).

The posterolateral portal is first made 1 cm proximal to the distal point of the lateral malleolus and adjacent to the lateral edge of the Achilles tendon. The posteromedial portal is made at the same level on the medial edge of the Achilles tendon. The scope is introduced through the posterolateral portal directed toward the second metatarsal until the posterior part of the talus bone can be felt.

If the instruments are introduced through the posteromedial portal in the same direction, damage to the posterior tibial nerve is possible (Figure 16-2). To avoid this, the blunt trocar is introduced through the posteromedial incision and, after reaching the Achilles tendon, the instrumentation is turned 90 degrees (Figure 16-3) until the sheath of the optical device can be felt. Keeping this metallic contact, the author slides the instrumentation along the sheath until arriving to the posterior part of the tibiotalar articulation or talus bone (Figure 16-4).

This posterior part of the ankle joint is often obscured with fatty tissue, and it is important to spend time clearing away this fat with a shaver and blunt trocar using gentle movements. The main objective is to visualize the FHL tendon, posterior intermalleolar ligament, posterior tibioperoneal ligament, and tibiotalar and subtalar articular surfaces. It is important to stay lateral to the FHL tendon because it protects the posterior tibial vascular and nerve bundle.

The resection of the talocalcaneal ligament allows optical visualization of the subtalar articular surfaces (Figure 16-5). In patients presenting with traumatic sequels, identification of the subtalar articulation may be difficult. To make this easier, the blunt trocar can be used to open the joint. In case of doubt, use scan control.

After making sure the position is correct, the author starts with the resection of the joint surfaces using a shaver, burr, chisel (Figure 16-6), or curette, according to the characteristics or

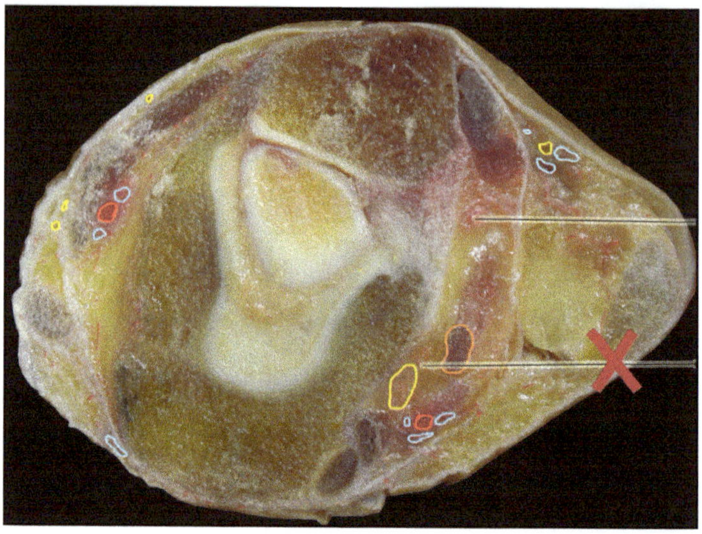

Figure 16-2. Introducing the instruments through the posteromedial portal in the same direction as the posterolateral approach may damage the posterior tibial nerve. (Reprinted with permission of X. Martin and A. Bravo.)

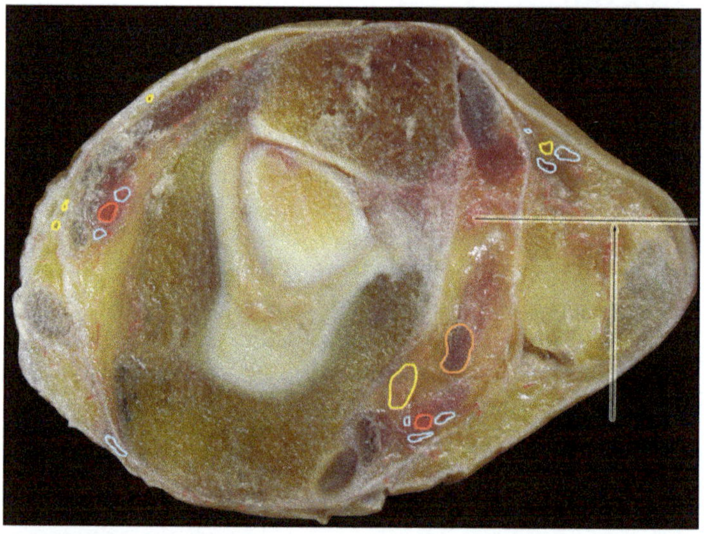

Figure 16-3. To avoid damage of the nerve, introduce the trocar blunt through the posteromedial incision and, after reaching the Achilles tendon, turn the instrumentation 90 degrees until the sheath of the optical device can be felt. (Reprinted with permission of X. Martin and A. Bravo.)

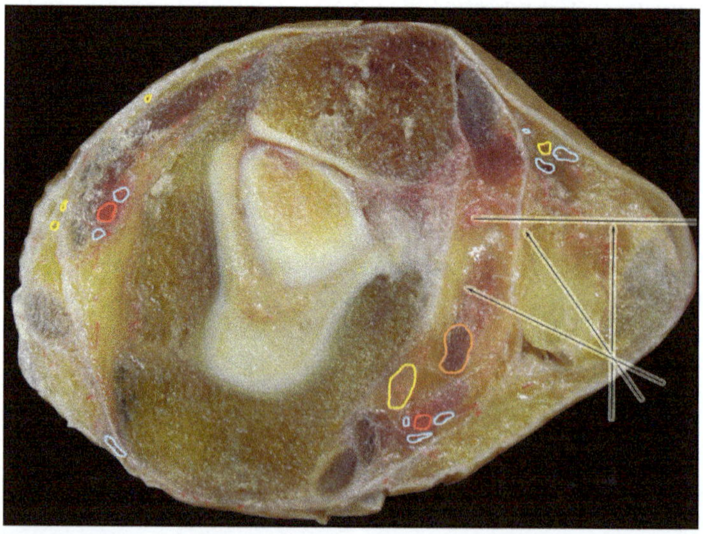

Figure 16-4. Slide the instrumentation along the sheath until arriving to the posterior part of the tibiotalar articulation or talus bone. (Reprinted with permission of X. Martin and A. Bravo.)

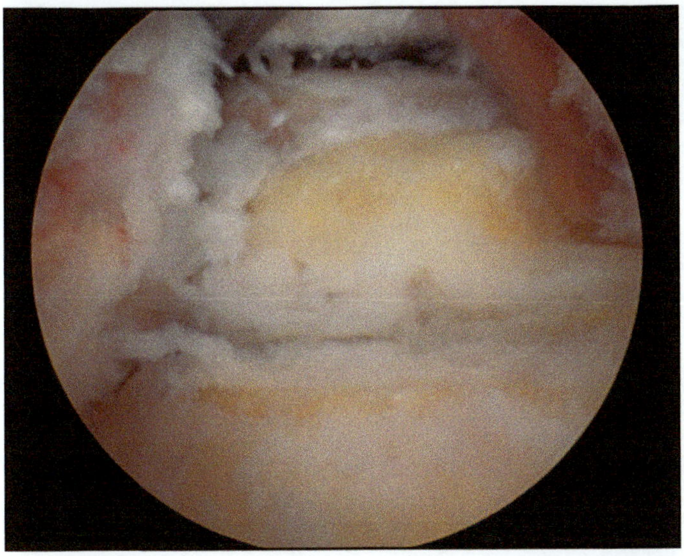

Figure 16-5. After resecting the posterior fat tissue, one can observe the tibiotalar articulation and the subtalar articulation.

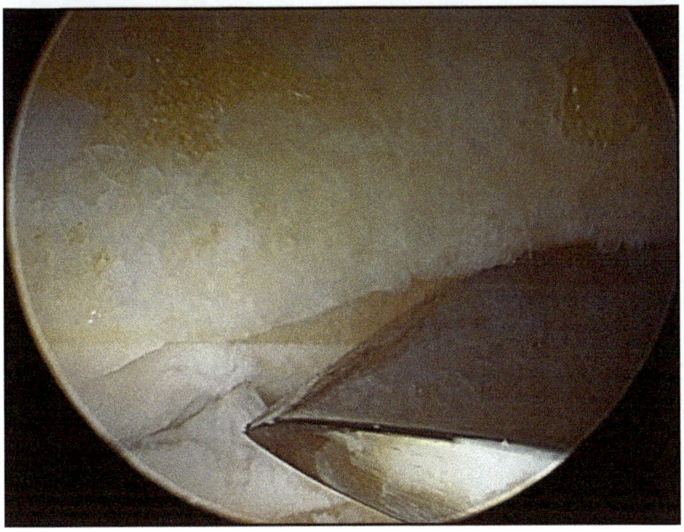

Figure 16-6. Start the cartilage resection using a chisel.

difficulties of the procedure. The author starts the resection of the articular surfaces with the shaver and also with the chisel, and when there is enough space, the author uses a burr or curette (Figure 16-7) and progresses until the anterior edge of the posterior subtalar facet is reached.

A complete cartilage resection of the articular surfaces must be carried out (Figure 16-8). The most critical part is in the medial and lateral edge of the posterior subtalar joint in order to achieve optimum surface contact for the correct consolidation of the fusion. Finally, the author places 2 cannulated screws in the posterior facet of the subtalar joint (Figure 16-9). Bone graft is not routinely used as studies available on arthroscopic subtalar arthrodesis using bone graft have not shown better results for the rate of fusion compared to studies not using bone grafting.[11]

Some authors recommend a lateral accessory portal in order to introduce instrumentation with the aim of mobilizing the articulation and to facilitate the arthrodesis technique.[1] The author of this chapter never uses this third approach because it is not necessary and also avoids the possible risk of vascular damage, which can occur because of manipulation in the sinus tarsi space.

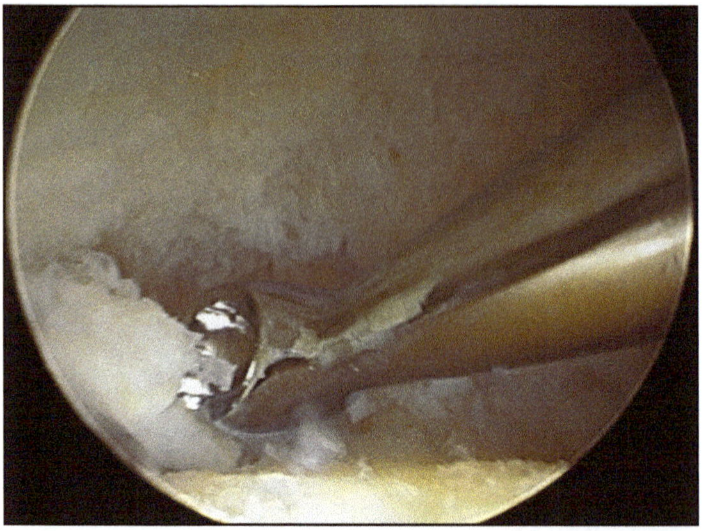

Figure 16-7. Once enough space is achieved, a burr or curette is used to remove cartilage.

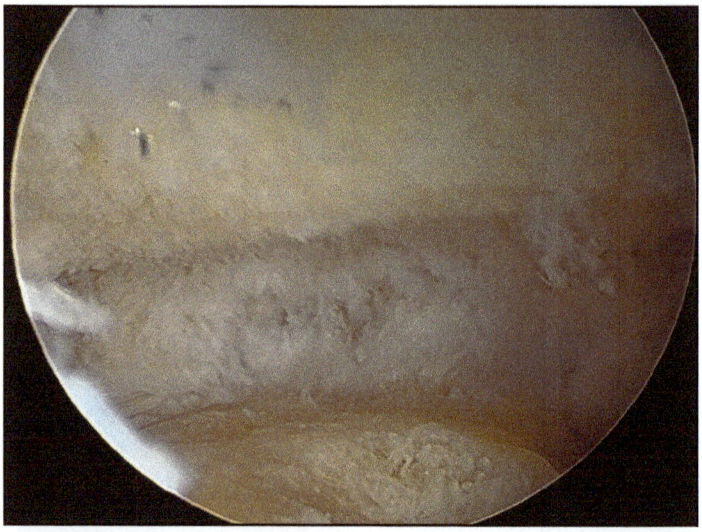

Figure 16-8. A complete cartilage resection of the articular surfaces prior to osteosynthesis.

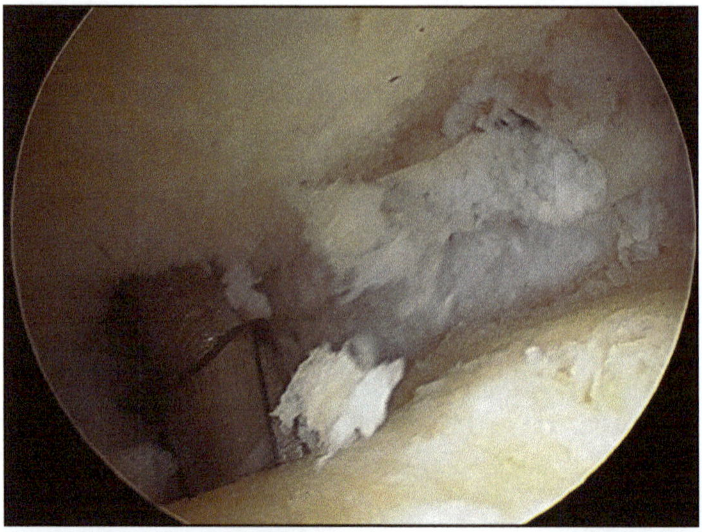

Figure 16-9. Two cannulated screws are placed in the posterior facet of the subtalar joint.

Postoperative Protocol

The ankle joint is immobilized for 4 weeks and the total time for nonweightbearing should be approximately 6 weeks. After this period, the patient can start with partial and progressive weightbearing. In the author's series, the average time until complete fusion was 8 to 9 weeks (range of 7 to 15 weeks), similar to the publications of Tasto[12] and Perez Carro et al.[13]

Potential Complications

In the author's patients, there is an incidence of 4% nonunion and 8% superficial infections. Other possible complications may be malalignment, deep infection, or long-term secondary inflammation.[14]

Top Technical Pearls for the Procedure

1. It must be emphasized that the main limitation to the use of arthroscopic techniques is that the patient must not present with severe varus/valgus deformity.
2. Normally, 2 posterior approaches are used to perform subtalar arthrodesis.
3. It is important to identify the FHL with the aim of protecting the posterior tibial nerve.
4. The complete resection of the cartilage of the subtalar articulation is important, especially taking into consideration the lateral and medial part of the joint.
5. For the correct stabilization of the arthrodesis, 2 cannulated screws are always used.

References

1. Van Dijk CN, Scholten PE, Krips R. A 2-portal endoscopic approach for diagnosis and treatment of posterior ankle pathology. *Arthroscopy.* 2000;16:871-876.
2. Frey C. Surgical advancements: arthroscopic alternatives to open procedures: great toe, subtalar joint, Haglund's deformity, and tendoscopy. *Foot Ankle Clin N Am.* 2009;14:313-339.
3. Lee K, Park CH, Seon JK, et al. Arthroscopic subtalar arthrodesis using a posterior 2-portal approach in the prone position. *Arthroscopy.* 2010;26(2):230-238.
4. Beimers L, De Leeuw P, Van Dijk N. A 3-portal approach for arthroscopic subtalar arthrodesis. *Knee Surg Sports Traumatol Arthrosc.* 2009;17:830-834.
5. Tasto JP, Mcginty JB, Burkhart SS, et al, eds. *Subtalar Arthroscopy: Operative Arthroscopy.* 3rd ed. New York, NY: Lippincott, Williams & Wilkins; 2003:944-952.
6. Ferkel RD. Subtalar arthroscopy. In: Ferkle RD, Whipple TL, eds. *Arthroscopic Surgery: The Foot and Ankle.* Philadelphia, PA: Lippincott-Raven; 1996:231-254.
7. Radnay C, Clare M, Sanders R. Subtalar fusion after displaced intra-articular calcaneal fractures: does initial operative treatment matter? *J Bone Joint Surg Am.* 2010;92(Suppl 1, Pt 1):32-43.
8. Beimers L, de Leeuw PA, van Dijk CN. A 3-portal approach for arthroscopic subtalar arthrodesis. *Knee Surg Sports Traumatol Arthrosc.* 2009;17:830-834.
9. Glanzmann MC, Sanhueza-Hernandez R. Arthroscopic subtalar arthrodesis for symptomatic osteoarthritis of the hindfoot: a prospective study of 41 cases. *Foot Ankle Int.* 2007;28:2-7.

10. Lee KB, Saltzman CL, Suh JS, Wasserman L, Amendola A. A posterior 3 portal arthroscopic approach for isolated subtalar arthrodesis. *Arthroscopy.* 2008;24:1306-1310.
11. Amendola A, Lee KB, Saltzman CL, Suh JS. Technique and early experience with posterior arthroscopic subtalar arthrodesis. *Foot Ankle Int.* 2007;28:298-302.
12. Tasto JP. Arthroscopic subtalar arthrodesis. *Tech Foot Ankle Surg.* 2003;2:122-128.
13. Perez Carro L, Golano P, Vega J. Arthroscopic subtalar arthrodesis: the posterior approach in the prone position. *Arthroscopy.* 2007;23:445.e1-4.
14. Cobb TK, Gabrielsen TA, Campbell DC II, Wallrichs SL. Cigarette smoking and nonunion after ankle arthrodesis. *Foot and Ankle Int.* 1994;15:64-67.

Please visit www.routledge.com/9781617119989 to access additional material.

Section V

Tendinopathy

17

Tendoscopy

Ruben Zwiers, MSc, PhD-candidate and C. Niek van Dijk, MD, PhD

Introduction

In the absence of intra-articular pathology, ankle complaints are often caused by disorders of the surrounding tendons. Degeneration of the Achilles tendon is being found in a considerable part of the asymptomatic tendons. Therefore, it is questionable whether degeneration of the tendon itself is the main cause of the pain. It is suggested that neovascularization, enhanced neurovascular growth in the peritendineum, and scarring and shrinkage of peritendinous tissue are the main causes of pain. Denervation of the Achilles tendon by releasing the peritendineum from the Achilles tendon may therefore be sufficient to resolve the complaints.

Pathology of the peroneal tendons consists of tenosynovitis, tendon dislocation or subluxation, and (partial) tears. Peroneal tendon pathology is not always recognized as a cause of lateral ankle pain. As the lateral ankle stabilizes, more strain is placed on these muscles in chronic ankle instability, possibly resulting in hypertrophic tendinopathy, tenosynovitis, and tears.

In posterior tibial tendon pathology, 2 main groups can be distinguished. The first group consists of younger patients who present with a form of systematic inflammation. The other group consists of older patients with a dysfunction of the tendon as a result of chronic overuse.

In this chapter, the indications and surgical techniques of tendoscopy of the Achilles, peroneal, and posterior tibial tendons will be addressed.

Indications

Tendoscopy (literally, endoscopy of the tendon sheath) can be performed for the diagnosis and treatment of various pathologic conditions of tendons around the ankle.[1-6] If nonoperative treatment fails, surgical treatment is indicated.[7-9]

- Achilles tendoscopy is indicated when combined tendinopathy and paratendinopathy exists.[10]
- Peroneal tendoscopy is indicated for the treatment of synovitis; adhesions and suspected longitudinal rupture of the peroneal tendons play a role.[11]

Stone JW, Kennedy JG, Glazebrook M, eds. *The Foot and Ankle: AANA Advanced Arthroscopic Surgical Techniques* (pp 159-166).

- Posterior tibial tendoscopy is indicated for tenosynovitis, tendon sheath release, adhesions, and debridement in partial rupture.[12]

Contraindications

- An absolute contraindication for endoscopic ankle surgery is a localized soft tissue infection.
- Relative contraindications are severe edema or vascular diseases.

Pertinent Physical Findings

- Achilles tendon
  - Stiffness after a period of rest
  - Painful swelling
  - When paratendinopathy is present, there is local thickening or inflammation of the paratenon at the level of the nodular thickening in the tendon. The tendon swelling will move along during ankle plantar-dorsiflexion movement in tendinopathy but not in Achilles paratendinopathy.[2,13,14]
  - Patients with chronic tendinopathy experience the pain, especially on the medial side.[15]
- Posterior tibial tendon
  - In the early phase of dysfunction, the main complaint of the patient is persisting ankle pain medially along the course of the tendon.
  - Patients may complain of fatigue and aching on the plantar medial aspect of the ankle.
  - When a tenosynovitis is present, swelling is common.[3,16]
  - Observation of the shoes may show typical excessive wear on the medial side.
  - Valgus angulation of the hindfoot is frequently seen with accompanying abduction of the forefoot (ie, "too many toes" sign).[16]
- Peroneal tendons
  - Crepitus and recognizable tenderness over the tendons are present in tendinopathy.
  - Peroneal tendon tendinopathy frequently coexists with a lateral ankle sprain. The diagnosis in a patient with a recent painful lateral ankle trauma can therefore be difficult.[17] Careful history taking must focus on the trauma mechanism. Other conditions associated with (peroneal) tendon problems must be taken into account. These include rheumatoid arthritis, psoriasis, hyperparathyroidism, diabetic neuropathy, calcaneal fractures, fluoroquinolone use, and local steroid injections.[18]

Pertinent Imaging

- Achilles tendon
  - Magnetic resonance imaging (MRI) and ultrasonography (US) can provide useful information to differentiate between the various forms of Achilles tendinopathy.[19]
- Posterior tibial tendon
  - Conventional radiography may show abnormal alignment, plantar arch flattening, or bony changes. US is known as a cost-effective and accurate method to evaluate posterior tibial tendon disorders. MRI, however, is considered the gold standard for assessing posterior

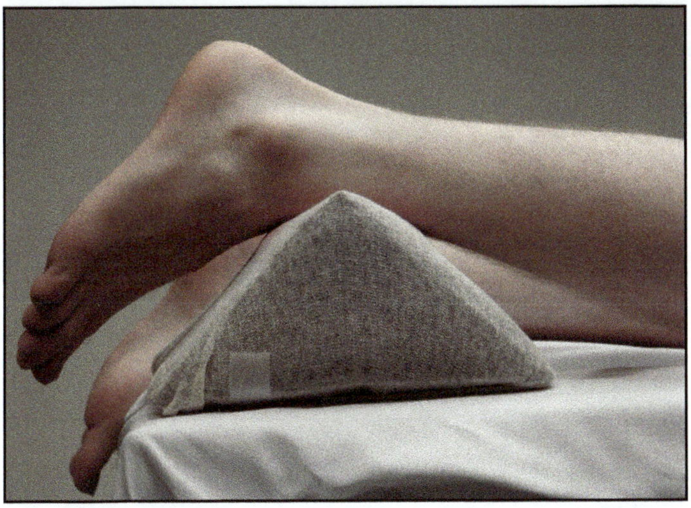

Figure 17-1. Patient is placed in the prone position with a support placed under the ankle. The foot is positioned just over the end of the table.

tibial tendon dysfunction. A major advantage over US is the ability to detect bony edema. Other findings can be fluid or synovitis around the tendon, hypertrophy of tendon, intrasubstance tears showing increased signal, longitudinal tears, and complete tendon tears.[20,21]

- Peroneal tendons
  - As multiple pathological conditions can coexist, routine weightbearing radiographs in the anteroposterior and lateral direction are made if posterolateral ankle pain persists after a trauma.
  - Additional radiographic imaging, such as MRI and US, may be helpful in diagnosing (partial) tears of the peroneal tendons. Both are considerably accurate and precise.[22,23]

Equipment

- Standard endoscopic equipment with a 2.7-mm arthroscope
- A pressurized bag or pump device is sometimes used for inflow with the 2.7-mm arthroscope. When a 4-mm arthroscope is used, gravity inflow is usually sufficient.
- Additional instruments include blunt probes, a retrograde knife, a spinal needle, scissors, and an endoscopic shaver system.[10-12,24]

Positioning and Portals

Tendoscopy procedures can be performed in an ambulatory setting under local regional or general anesthesia.

- Achilles tendoscopy: The patient is in the prone position with a support placed under the ankle. The foot is positioned just over the end of the table so the surgeon is able to obtain full plantar- and dorsiflexion (Figure 17-1).[10]
- Posterior tibial tendoscopy: The patient is placed in the supine position. To better be able to palpate the posterior tibial tendon, the patient is asked to actively invert the foot so the portals can be marked on the skin.[12]

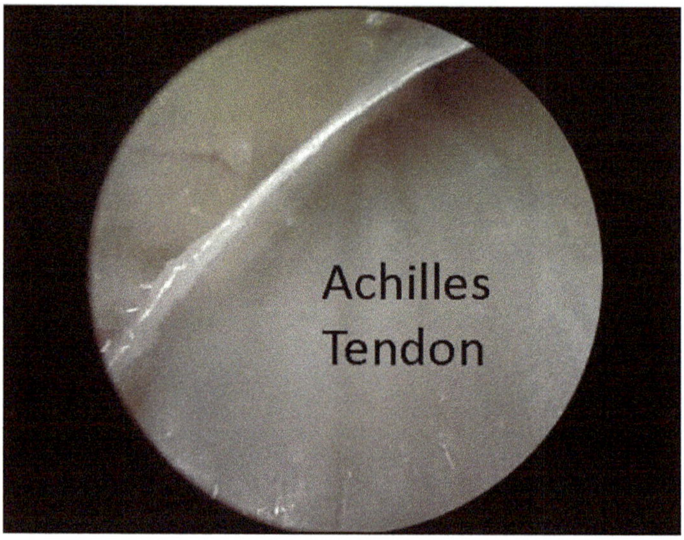

Figure 17-2. Endoscopic view of the Achilles tendon.

- Peroneal tendoscopy: The patient is placed in the lateral decubitus position. Alternatively, the patient can also be placed in the supine position with the foot in internal rotation. The patient is asked to actively evert the affected foot, enabling a better view and palpation of the peroneal tendon. A support is placed under the affected leg, making it possible to move the ankle freely.[11]

Step-by-Step Description of the Procedure

Achilles Tendon

To visualize the complete surface of the tendon, the distal portal is located on the lateral border of the Achilles tendon 2 to 3 cm distal to the pathologic nodule, and the proximal portal is located medial to the border of the Achilles tendon 2 to 4 cm proximal to the nodule. The procedure starts with the distal portal. After making the skin incision, the mosquito clamp is introduced, followed by the blunt trocar in a craniomedial direction. With this blunt trocar, the paratenon is approached and is blindly released from the tendon by moving around it. The 2.7-mm, 30-degree arthroscope is then introduced. To minimize the risk of iatrogenic damage, the arthroscope should be kept on the tendon. At this time, the correct position of the scope between the deepest layer of the paratenon and Achilles tendon should be confirmed. If the correct position cannot be confirmed, a further release may be performed (Figure 17-2).

The proximal portal is made by introducing a spinal needle, followed by a mosquito clamp and probe. The plantaris tendon can be identified at the anteromedial border of the Achilles tendon.

In a typical case of local paratendinopathy, the plantaris tendon, Achilles tendon, and paratenon may be tight together due to the inflamed process. Removal of local thickened paratenon on the posterior and posteromedial side of the Achilles tendon at the level of the nodule and release of the plantaris tendon can be performed. Fibrotic adhesions and neovessels accompanied by small nerve fibers can be found in this area and are removed with a 2.7-mm, full radius resector (Figure 17-3).

Changing portals can be helpful. At the end of the procedure, it must be possible to move the arthroscope over the complete symptomatic area of the Achilles tendon.[2]

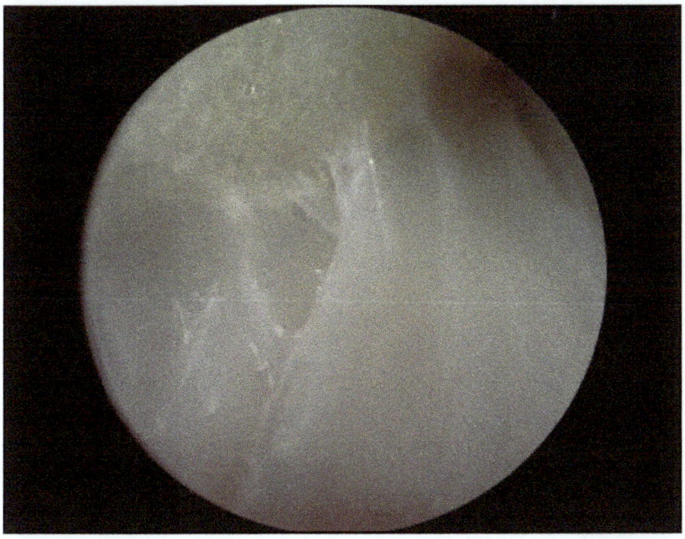

Figure 17-3. Endoscopic view of the Achilles tendon showing adhesions.

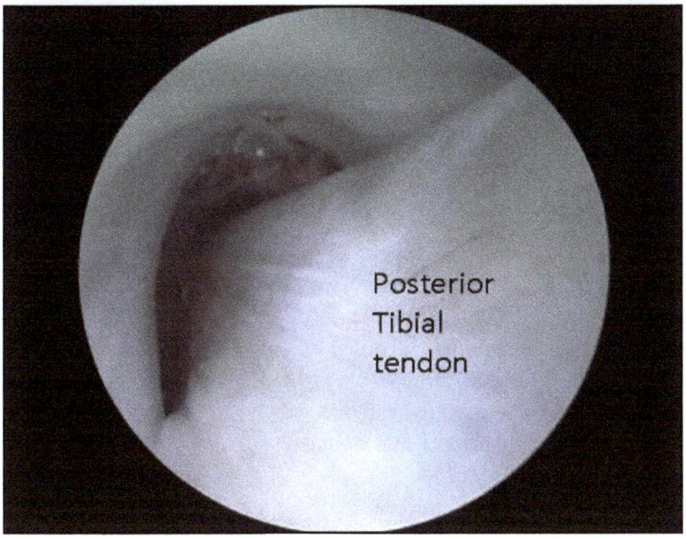

Figure 17-4. Endoscopic view of the posterior tibial tendon.

Posterior Tibial Tendon

Tendoscopy of the posterior tibial tendon is performed using 2 portals directly over the tendon 2 to 3 cm distal and 2 to 3 cm proximal to the posterior edge of the medial malleolus. First, the distal portal is created. A skin incision is made, after which blunt dissection of the peritenon is performed using a mosquito clamp. The tendon sheath is opened using the arthroscopic shaft and blunt trocar. A 2.7-mm, 30-degree arthroscope is introduced and the tendon sheath is filled with saline. The proximal portal is made under direct vision by introducing a spinal needle; subsequently, an incision is made into the tendon sheath. By creating the portal under direct vision, iatrogenic damage is prevented. The complete sheath can be inspected by rotating the arthroscope around the tendon.

From the distal portal, a synovectomy can be performed from the insertion of the navicular bone to approximately 6 cm above the tip of the medial malleolus (Figure 17-4). Special attention

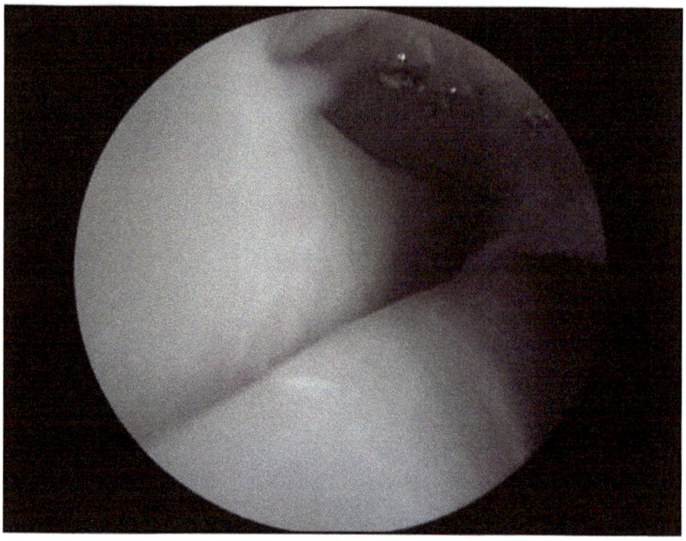

Figure 17-5. Endoscopic view of the peroneal tendons.

must be given to the posterior ankle joint capsule, the posterior aspect of the medial malleolar surface, and the tendon sheath. Because the tendon sheath between the posterior tibial tendon and the flexor digitorum longus is relatively thin, one should always check if the correct tendon is inspected. This can be done by passively flexing and extending the toes. A tendon length rupture can be repaired through a mini-open approach.[25]

Peroneal Tendons

The distal portal is made first, 2 to 2.5 cm distal to the posterior edge of the lateral malleolus. An incision is made through the skin and the tendon sheath is opened with a blunt trocar. Subsequently, the 2.7-mm, 30-degree arthroscope is introduced. The inspection starts approximately 6 cm proximal to the posterior tip of the fibula. Here, a thin membrane splits the tendon compartment into 2 separate tendon chambers. More distally, the tendons lie in one compartment. The peroneus brevis tendon is situated closest to the lateral malleolus.

Under direct vision, a second portal is made. A spinal needle is introduced approximately 2 to 2.5 cm proximal to the posterior edge of the lateral malleolus.

Through the distal portal, a complete overview of both tendons can be obtained. By rotating the arthroscope over and in between both tendons, the whole compartment can be inspected (Figure 17-5).

For a total synovectomy of the tenon sheath, a third portal can be created more proximal or distal. In case a rupture of one of the peroneal tendons is seen, endoscopic synovectomy is performed and the rupture is repaired through a mini-open approach.[1]

Postoperative Protocol

Postoperative management consists of a compressive dressing and partial weightbearing for 2 to 3 days. Full weightbearing is allowed as tolerated, and the patient is instructed to elevate the foot when not walking. Active range of motion exercises are advised to start directly after surgery, at least 3 times per day for 10 minutes each time.

Potential Complications

The complication rates after tendoscopy are low. In several studies reporting on tendoscopy, no single complication was reported.[2,3,26-28] Zengerink and van Dijk reported damage to the saphenous nerve after release of the posterior tibial tendon.[29] Potential complications are similar to standard ankle arthroscopy, which includes neurological injury and superficial wound infections.

Top Technical Pearls for the Procedure

1. It is important to identify the location of the peroneal tendons before creating the portals. Ask the patient to actively evert the foot, identify the tendon, and mark the location of the portals on the skin.
2. Place a support under the affected ankle prior to surgery so the ankle can be moved freely.
3. It is important to identify the location of the posterior tibial tendon before creating the portals. Ask the patient to actively invert the foot, identify the tendon, and mark the location of the portals on the skin.
4. In cases where the tendon sheath of the flexor digitorum longus is entered, the tendons are easily seen moving up and down when the toes are passively flexed and extended.
5. To prevent iatrogenic damage, keep the trocar onto the tendon when blindly releasing the peritendineum from the Achilles tendon.

References

1. van Dijk CN, Kort N. Tendoscopy of the peroneal tendons. *Arthroscopy.* 1998;14(5):471-478.
2. Steenstra F, van Dijk CN. Achilles tendoscopy. *Foot Ankle Clin.* 2006;11(2):429-438, viii.
3. Bulstra GH, Olsthoorn PG, Niek van DC. Tendoscopy of the posterior tibial tendon. *Foot Ankle Clin.* 2006;11(2):421-427, viii.
4. Bigony L. Arthroscopic surgery: a historical perspective. *Orthop Nurs.* 2008;27(6):349-354.
5. Myerson MS, Quill G. Ankle arthrodesis. A comparison of an arthroscopic and an open method of treatment. *Clin Orthop Relat Res.* 1991;(268):84-95.
6. Guhl JF. Operative arthroscopy. *Am J Sports Med.* 1979;7(6):328-335.
7. Lui TH. Endoscopic assisted posterior tibial tendon reconstruction for stage 2 posterior tibial tendon insufficiency. *Knee Surg Sports Traumatol Arthrosc.* 2007;15(10):1228-1234.
8. Maffulli N, Ferran NA. Management of acute and chronic ankle instability. *J Am Acad Orthop Surg.* 2008;16(10):608-615.
9. Kvist M. Achilles tendon injuries in athletes. *Ann Chir Gynaecol.* 1991;80(2):188-201.
10. van Dijk CN. Achilles tendoscopy. In: *Ankle Arthroscopy.* New York, NY: Springer; 2014:335-355.
11. van Dijk CN. Peroneal tendoscopy. In: *Ankle Arthroscopy.* New York, NY: Springer; 2014:355-365.
12. van Dijk CN. Posterior tibial tendoscopy. In: *Ankle Arthroscopy.* New York, NY: Springer; 2014:375-387.
13. Maffulli N, Walley G, Sayana MK, Longo UG, Denaro V. Eccentric calf muscle training in athletic patients with Achilles tendinopathy. *Disabil Rehabil.* 2008;30(20-22):1677-1684.
14. Williams JG. Achilles tendon lesions in sport. *Sports Med.* 1993;16(3):216-220.
15. Segesser B, Goesele A, Renggli P. [The Achilles tendon in sports]. *Orthopade.* 1995;24(3):252-267.

16. Trnka HJ. Dysfunction of the tendon of tibialis posterior. *J Bone Joint Surg Br.* 2004;86(7):939-946.
17. Molloy R, Tisdel C. Failed treatment of peroneal tendon injuries. *Foot Ankle Clin.* 2003;8(1):115-129, ix.
18. Heckman DS, Reddy S, Pedowitz D, Wapner KL, Parekh SG. Operative treatment for peroneal tendon disorders. *J Bone Joint Surg Am.* 2008;90(2):404-418.
19. Aström M, Gentz CF, Nilsson P, Rausing A, Sjöberg S, Westlin N. Imaging in chronic achilles tendinopathy: a comparison of ultrasonography, magnetic resonance imaging and surgical findings in 27 histologically verified cases. *Skeletal Radiol.* 1996;25(7):615-620.
20. Kong A, Van der Vliet A. Imaging of tibialis posterior dysfunction. *Br J Radiol.* 2008;81(970):826-836.
21. Miller SD, Van HM, Boruta PM, Wu KK, Katcherian DA. Ultrasound in the diagnosis of posterior tibial tendon pathology. *Foot Ankle Int.* 1996;17(9):555-558.
22. Rosenberg ZS, Bencardino J, Astion D, Schweitzer ME, Rokito A, Sheskier S. MRI features of chronic injuries of the superior peroneal retinaculum. *AJR Am J Roentgenol.* 2003;181(6):1551-1557.
23. Rockett MS, Waitches G, Sudakoff G, Brage M. Use of ultrasonography versus magnetic resonance imaging for tendon abnormalities around the ankle. *Foot Ankle Int.* 1998;19(9):604-612.
24. van Dijk CN. Instrumentation. In: *Ankle Arthroscopy.* New York, NY: Springer; 2014:67-80.
25. van Dijk CN, Kort N, Scholten PE. Tendoscopy of the posterior tibial tendon. *Arthroscopy.* 1997;13(6):692-698.
26. Maquirriain J, Ayerza M, Costa-Paz M, Muscolo DL. Endoscopic surgery in chronic achilles tendinopathies: a preliminary report. *Arthroscopy.* 2002;18(3):298-303.
27. Vega J, Cabestany JM, Golano P, Perez-Carro L. Endoscopic treatment for chronic Achilles tendinopathy. *Foot Ankle Surg.* 2008;14(4):204-210.
28. Pearce CJ, Carmichael J, Calder JD. Achilles tendinoscopy and plantaris tendon release and division in the treatment of non-insertional Achilles tendinopathy. *Foot Ankle Surg.* 2012;18(2):124-127.
29. Zengerink M, van Dijk CN. Complications in ankle arthroscopy. *Knee Surg Sports Traumatol Arthrosc.* 2012;20(8):1420-1431.

Please visit www.routledge.com/9781617119989 to access additional material.

18

Achilles Tendon Repair and Gastrocnemius Recession

Phinit Phisitkul, MD and Chamnanni Rungprai, MD

Introduction: Endoscopic-Assisted Percutaneous Achilles Repair

Acute Achilles tendon rupture is a relatively common sports injury that can be treated with either nonoperative or operative treatments. However, the optimal treatment remains controversial.[1] The disadvantage of nonoperative treatment using cast immobilization or a brace is a higher re-rupture rate and elongation of the tendon. In contrast, wound complications and scar formation are the common complications following open surgical repair techniques.[2] Recently, percutaneous techniques have shown initial successful outcomes, but sural nerve entrapment is a risk due to the blind passing of sutures, as shown in previous studies.[3,4] Endoscopic-assisted surgery allows clear visualization of the tendon ends and suture passage at the tendinous part of the ruptured tendon, which may result in an improved quality of repair while minimizing complications.[3]

Indications

- An acute closed rupture of the Achilles tendon within 10 to 14 days from the onset of injury

Contraindications

- Duration of Achilles tendon rupture longer than 14 days
- Prior history of surgery at the Achilles tendon due to tendon retraction and scar adhesion, which limit endoscopic visualization and tendon mobilization

Stone JW, Kennedy JG, Glazebrook M, eds. *The Foot and Ankle: AANA Advanced Arthroscopic Surgical Techniques* (pp 167-176).

Pertinent Physical Findings

- Patients typically present with a history of sudden pain at the hindfoot accompanied by a snap and the inability to resume sporting activities.
- The clinical examination typically reveals a palpable gap at the site of the rupture, typically 2 to 6 cm proximal to the calcaneal tuberosity.
- The diagnosis is primarily clinical, including 2 or more of the following tests to establish the diagnosis:
  - Best test: clinical Thompson test (Simmonds squeeze test)
  - Decreased ankle plantarflexion strength
  - Presence of a palpable gap (defect, loss of contour)
  - Increased passive ankle dorsiflexion with gentle manipulation[5]

Pertinent Imaging

- Plain radiographs are usually normal in patients with an acute Achilles rupture but are important to rule out avulsion fracture of the calcaneus.
- Ultrasound and magnetic resonance imaging are adjunctive investigations that may be helpful when the diagnosis is uncertain or for the evaluation of the tendon approximation in conjunction with nonoperative treatment.[6]

Equipment

A 4.0-mm, 30-degree arthroscope with fluid irrigation system is used for endoscopic-assisted Achilles tendon repair. A penetrating-tip suture passer (BirdBeak, Arthrex) is a key instrument to puncture and introduce #2 nonabsorbable braided sutures through the tendon, and a blunt-tip suture grasper is helpful in passing the suture within the paratenon sheath.

Positioning and Portals

The operation is performed with the patient in the prone position under either general or spinal anesthesia. The bilateral lower extremities are prepped and draped (Figure 18-1A), and a thigh tourniquet is applied. Both feet slightly hang over the end of the operating table with adequate room for full dorsiflexion (see Figure 18-1A). The affected limb demonstrates less resting ankle plantarflexion in knee 90-degree flexion due to rupture of the Achilles tendon (Figure 18-1B), and this position will be useful for the confirmation of appropriate repair tension at the completion of the procedure.

Six portals are required for this procedure (Figure 18-1C). Distal medial (DM) and distal lateral (DL) portals are located just medial and lateral to the Achilles tendon border at the level of insertion to the posterior calcaneal tuberosity. Midmedial (MM) and midlateral (ML) portals are located medial and lateral to the rupture site level, and the distance between the 2 portals is approximately the width of the tendon at this level. The ML portal should not be placed too lateral or the sural nerve can be at risk. Proximal medial (PM) and proximal lateral (PL) portals are created 5 cm proximal to the palpable proximal tendon end. The PL portal is always created under arthroscopic guidance and clear tendon visualization. It is made as far away as possible from the palpable sural nerve.

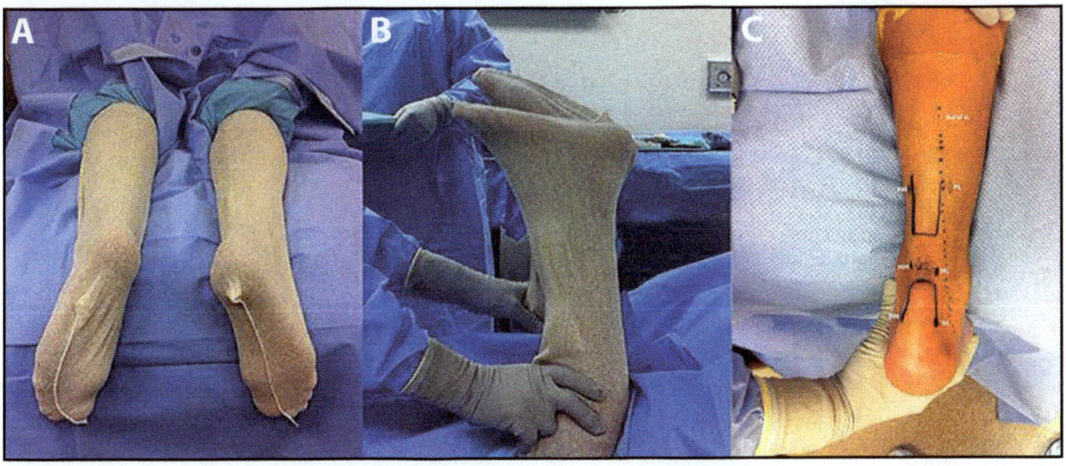

Figure 18-1. (A) Patient is placed into the prone position and both extremities are prepped and draped. (B) The right ankle demonstrates less ankle plantarflexion due to rupture of the Achilles tendon in knee 90-degree flexion. (C) Six endoscopic portals (5 black portals and 1 dashed portal [PL]) and sural nerve path. DL, distal lateral; DM, distal medial; ML, midlateral; MM, midmedial; PL, proximal lateral; PM, proximal medial portals.

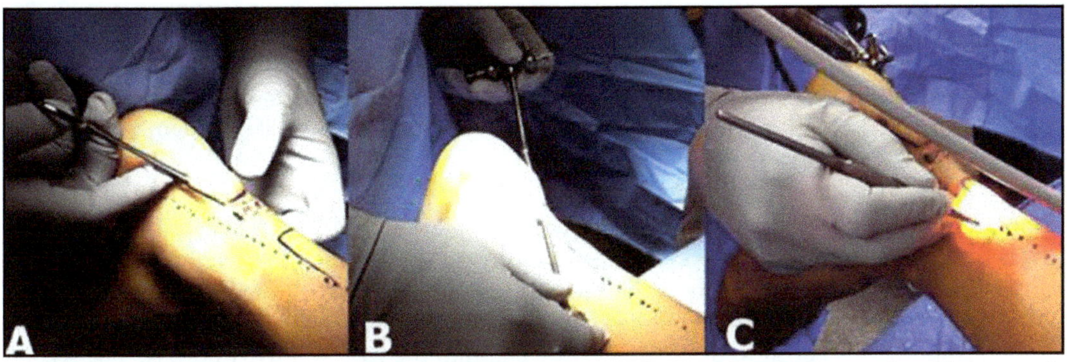

Figure 18-2. (A) A hemostat is utilized to create a space superficial to the Achilles tendon. (B) A cannula is introduced from the DM portal using a retrograde technique. (C) The PL portal is created under direct visualization using endoscopy to minimize the chance of injury to the sural nerve.

Step-by-Step Description of the Procedure

Five portals (all portals except the PL portal) and the location of the sural nerve are marked on the posterior aspect of the Achilles tendon (see Figure 18-1C). All 5 portals are made by using a #15 blade through the skin only and then bluntly dissecting down to the tendon with a hemostat, creating a working space in the paratenon plane (Figure 18-2A). A trocar for a 4.0-mm arthroscope or switching stick is subsequently introduced to create a plane through the paratenon from the rupture site (MM or ML portal) toward the DM portal. The endoscopic sheath is then introduced retrograde from the DM portal (Figure 18-2B). The rupture site is examined and organized hematoma is debrided if necessary using a shaver from the middle portals. The camera is advanced into the proximal aspect of the paratenon sheath along the dorsal aspect of the proximal Achilles tendon stump (Figure 18-2C). The sural nerve can be palpated by the surgeon's fingers against the cannula on the lateral aspect of the proximal Achilles tendon, which allows the PL portal to be made away from it. This portal is made by using a scalpel through the skin only and a curved

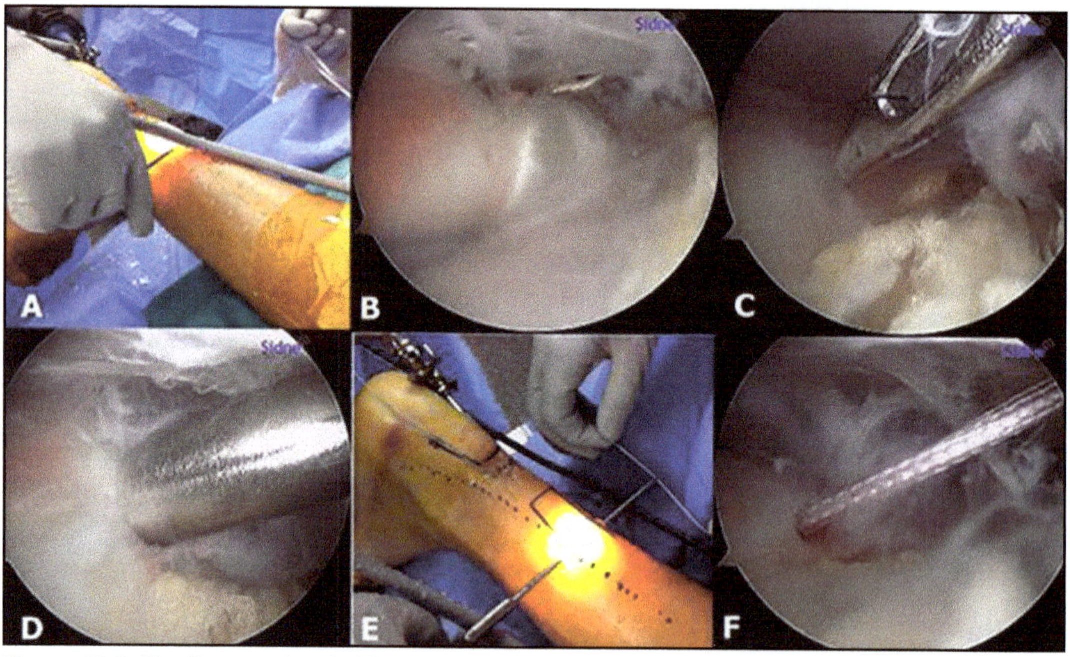

Figure 18-3. The first nonabsorbable suture is introduced using a suture passer. (A) The suture passer is initially inserted from the PL portal under endoscopic control and (B) the myotendinous part of the Achilles tendon is identified, ensuring that the sural nerve is not visible. (C, D) The suture passer is used to puncture through the myotendinous part and (E) exit at the PM portal and, thereafter, the suture is fed and pulled back to the PL portal. (F) The suture is securely passed through the Achilles tendon.

hemostat is used for the deep dissection under endoscopic visualization. A penetrating-tip suture passer is inserted from the PL portal under endoscopic control into the tendinous part of the proximal Achilles tendon and exits at the PM portal (Figures 18-3A through E). The #2 braided suture is fed into the passer tip and pulled back through the PL portal. A blunt suture grasper is inserted from the PL portal to place each suture end into the ML and MM portals. The second braided suture is placed through the proximal tendon in the same manner as the first one, while the first suture ends are held under some tension. Additionally, the suture end from the PL portal is passed through the tendon diagonally and exits at the MM portal (Figures 18-4A through D). The other end of the second suture from the PM portal is retrieved by a penetrating-tip suture passer inserted from the ML retrograde and diagonally through the proximal Achilles tendon (Figures 18-4E and F). At this stage, the proximal tendon has 2 sets of suture fixation: one in a box shape and the other in crisscross configuration (Figures 18-5A and B). For distal repair, the previously placed 2 suture sets are placed in the mirror-image fashion percutaneously and without endoscopic visualization (see Figures 18-5A and B). The sutures from the proximal box-shaped repair will make a crisscross repair distally and vice versa. The final suture ends are located in the DM and/or DL portals prior to the knot tying. The ankle is set in slightly greater plantarflexion than the normal side, and both sutures are tied after 10 to 15 rounds of ankle cycling into plantarflexion and dorsiflexion to remove the slack in the repair (Figure 18-5D). The continuity of the Achilles tendon without a gap should be appreciated by palpation (Figure 18-5C). All portals are closed using 3-0 nylon sutures and a postoperative anteroposterior splint is applied with the ankle in a position of 30 degrees equinus.

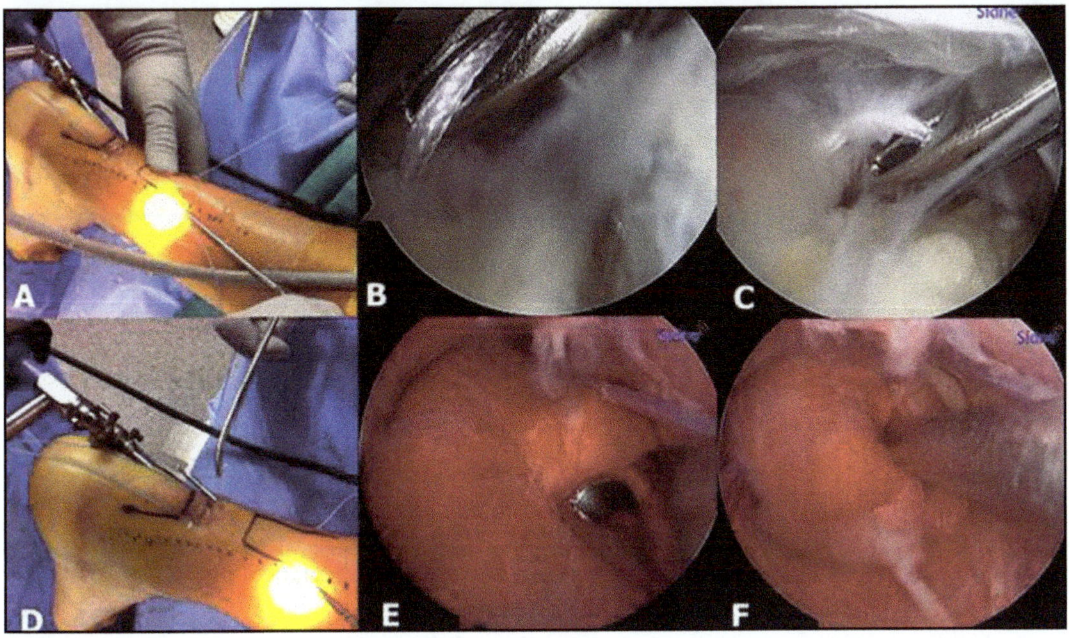

Figure 18-4. A second suture is introduced by the BirdBeak. (A, B) The suture is held by the BirdBeak from outside and introduced into the PL portal. (C) It is then used to puncture at the myotendinous portion of the Achilles tendon and (D) exit at the MM portal. (E, F) For the other end of suture, the BirdBeak is inserted from the ML portal, introduced into the proximal tendon end, and exited at the PM portal, after which the other end of suture is fed and pulled into the ML portal.

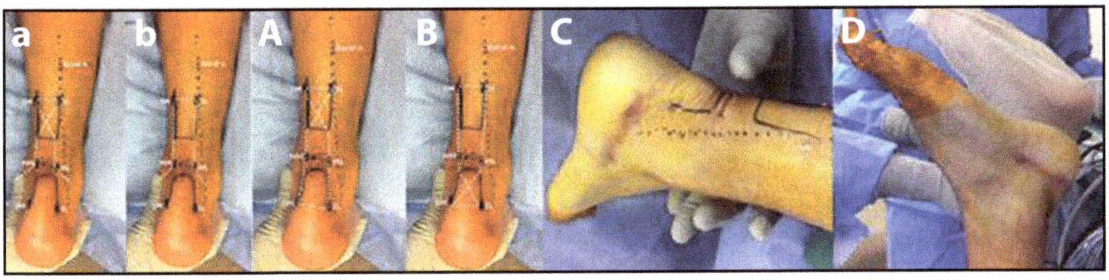

Figure 18-5. Demonstration of the suture configuration of the proximal part; (a) the first suture and (b) the second suture and distal portion of Achilles tendon; (A) the first suture and (B) second suture. (C) The continuity of Achilles tendon was stored and (D) the tension was set slightly greater plantarflexion compared to the normal side.

Postoperative Protocol

Patients are instructed to remain nonweightbearing for the first 4 weeks postoperatively. At the 2-week postoperative visit, the surgical wound is checked and the sutures are removed. The patient is placed into an immobilizing boot with a 1-inch heel wedge. From 2 to 4 weeks postoperatively, patients perform range of motion exercises in the sitting position, but dorsiflexion is limited to neutral. At 4 weeks postoperatively, the 1-inch heel wedge is exchanged for a 0.5-inch wedge, and progressive weightbearing is initiated while continuing to perform range of motion exercises. At the 6-week postoperative visit, patients are allowed to progress to full weightbearing as tolerated in the boot without a heel wedge and, subsequently, patients can wean themselves out of the boot when they can walk fully weightbearing without pain. Concentric strengthening with rubberbands is used during weeks 6 to 12 postoperatively.

Potential Complications

The complications of endoscopic-assisted percutaneous Achilles tendon repair have been reported, including wound complication (0% to 5.3%), re-rupture of Achilles tendon (0% to 1.8%), sural nerve entrapment (0% to 20%), and deep vein thrombosis (0% to 1.8%).[7-9]

Top Technical Pearls for the Procedure

1. All portals are made carefully with a sharp incision through the skin only, and portals are established by inserting a hemostat into the paratenon sheath.
2. The creation of the PL portal and all procedures through this portal need to be performed under arthroscopic control for the prevention of sural nerve injury.
3. Proximal repair must be performed through the tendinous part of the Achilles tendon and not the muscle belly to ensure maximal strength of the repair.
4. The distal part of the Achilles tendon can be repaired percutaneously without endoscopic control.
5. The immediate postoperative position of the Achilles tendon repair should be slightly more plantarflexed compared to the normal side.

Introduction: Endoscopic Gastrocnemius Recession

Isolated gastrocnemius contracture was reported to be present in 65% to 88% of patients presenting to a foot and ankle clinic for evaluation of non-neuropathic forefoot and midfoot symptoms. It is a common condition that is associated with several foot and ankle conditions including adult-acquired flatfoot deformities, hallux valgus, plantar fasciitis, metatarsalgia, and diabetic foot ulcer.[8,10,11] Open gastrocnemius and tendo-Achilles lengthening techniques have been used as the standard treatment for equinus contracture since the 19th century. However, potential wound complications and poor cosmesis can lead to patient dissatisfaction. Endoscopic gastrocnemius recession (EGR), first reported by Saxena in 2002,[12] has been demonstrated to be safe and efficacious as a treatment for patients with isolated gastrocnemius tightness.[8,10,13-16] In addition, it has led to improved functional outcomes, pain relief, and restoration of ankle dorsiflexion while minimizing wound complications.[8]

Indications

- Isolated gastrocnemius contracture, which is defined as limitation of ankle dorsiflexion with passive dorsiflexion greater than 10 degrees with the knee flexed, but less than or equal to 5 degrees of dorsiflexion with the knee extended[10]
- Failure to respond to nonoperative treatment including NSAIDs, orthotics, stretching, and physical therapy for at least 6 months[8]

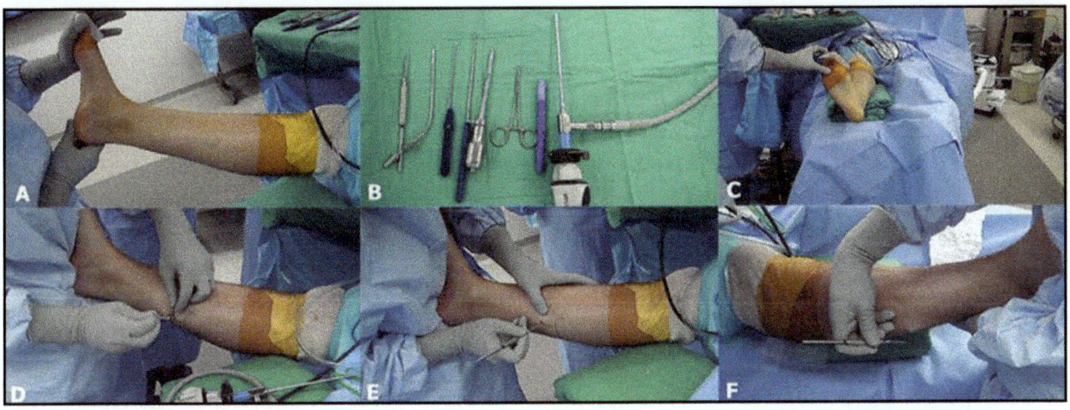

Figure 18-6. (A) Zero degrees of passive ankle dorsiflexion with the knee fully extended. (B) The instruments are used for the EGR procedure. (C) The heel should be at the distal edge of the operating table. (D) Sterile cotton swabs help clean the cannula and improve visualization. (E) The medial portal is created 2 cm distal to the palpable distal aspect of the gastrocnemius muscle and (F) the lateral portal is created at the same level of the medial portal but using an inside-out technique.

Contraindications

- Patients with a history of surgery in the musculotendinous area of the gastrocsoleus
- Patients with active infection overlying the soft tissue in the calf

Pertinent Physical Findings

- Patients with isolated gastrocnemius contracture may present with chronic midfoot and forefoot problems such as diabetic foot ulcers, hallux valgus,[11] metatarsalgia,[10] adult acquired flatfoot deformity,[10] and plantar fasciitis.[11]
- The diagnosis is based on the clinical examination, and radiographs are helpful for the evaluation of associated conditions.
- The Silfverskiöld test is commonly used to differentiate gastrocnemius equinus from a triceps surae contracture. A positive result is indicated when passive ankle dorsiflexion is less than 10 degrees with the knee extended and ankle dorsiflexion improves with the knee flexed (Figure 18-6A).[17]

Pertinent Imaging

- The diagnosis of isolated gastrocnemius or combined gastrocsoleus contracture without associated pathology is based on history and physical examination, and the imaging is not routinely required. However, imaging can be performed if there is associated pathology accompanied with gastrocnemius or gastrocsoleus contracture such as flatfoot deformity, cavovarus foot deformity, hallux valgus, or ankle arthritis.

Equipment

The 4.0-mm, 30-degree arthroscope is used for EGR performed without fluid irrigation throughout the procedure. A hemostat and a blunt trocar with slotted cannula (ECTRA II, Smith & Nephew) are used to create the correct plane for the procedure. Sterile cotton swabs (Figure 18-6D) help clean the cannula and improve visualization, while the retrograde knife is used to release the aponeurotic part of the gastrocnemius and soleus muscle (Figure 18-6B).

Positioning and Portals

The operation is performed with the patient in the supine position under either general or spinal anesthesia. The procedure can also be performed in the prone position. The lower extremity is prepped and draped with a thigh tourniquet. The heel should be at the distal edge of the operating table (Figure 18-6C).

Five-millimeter medial and lateral portals are necessary for the procedure. The medial portal (Figure 18-6E) is created 2 cm distal to the palpable distal aspect of the gastrocnemius muscle, and the lateral portal is created at the same level as the medial portal but using an inside-out technique (Figure 18-6F).

Step-by-Step Description of the Procedure

The medial portal is created and a curved hemostat is then used to puncture and dilate through the crural fascia overlying the superficial posterior compartment (Figure 18-7A). A blunt trocar with slotted cannula is then inserted superficial to the gastrocnemius aponeurosis but deep to the crural fascia. At this level, the sural nerve is typically located superficial to the fascia, and all attempts are made to keep the trocar in the correct plane to prevent injury to the sural nerve. In addition, the sural nerve and the lesser saphenous vein can almost always be palpated posterior to the trocar. Once the correct plane has been established, the trocar should be able to advance laterally and swivel from side to side with minimal force. A small counterincision is made laterally in an inside-out fashion to create the lateral portal (see Figure 18-6F). The trocar is thereafter removed, leaving the slotted cannula in place, and a 4.0-mm, 30-degree arthroscope is inserted for endoscopic examination from the medial portal (Figure 18-7B). Sterile cotton swabs are used as necessary to clear blood or fatty tissue from the cannula to enhance visualization (see Figure 18-6D). If the cannula is found to be just superficial to the crural fascia, a 3-mm suction tube or a switching stick can be introduced into the correct plane using a retrograde technique from the lateral portal under endoscopic guidance (Figure 18-7C). The gastrocnemius aponeurosis is thoroughly inspected and palpated with a probe to ensure the correct surgical plane and the absence of sural nerve trapped in this plane (Figure 18-7D). The camera and cannula are then rotated 180 degrees to evaluate the posterior compartment fascia and identification of the sural nerve along with the lesser saphenous veins (Figure 18-7E). The ankle is held in dorsiflexion by the body of the surgeon and an endoscopic retrograde knife is introduced from the lateral portal. As the gastrocnemius aponeurosis and the underlying soleal fascia are released from medial to lateral, separation of the transected tissue and the exposure of underlying soleus muscle is observed (Figure 18-7F). The medial part of the gastrocnemius aponeurosis and the plantaris tendon can be released from lateral to medial from the medial portal while observing from the lateral portal. The medial aspect of the release usually contributes to most of the range of motion gained. Adequacy of the tendon released is confirmed by having at least 10 to 15 degrees of ankle dorsiflexion when the knee is in extension.

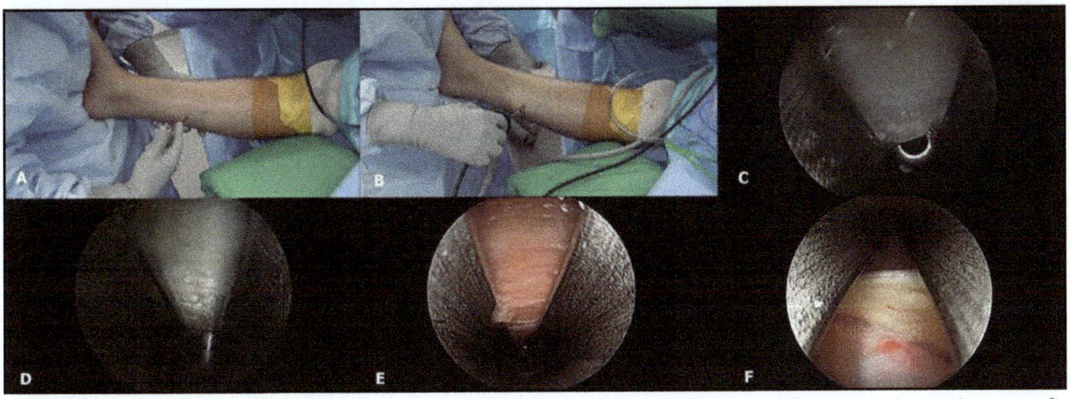

Figure 18-7. (A) A hemostat is used to puncture and dilate through the crural fascia overlying the superficial posterior compartment. (B) A 4.0-mm, 30-degree arthroscope is inserted for endoscopic examination from the medial portal. (C) A 3-mm suction tube or a switching stick can be introduced into the correct plane using a retrograde technique from the lateral portal. (D) A probe is used to ensure the correct surgical plane and the absence of sural nerve trapped in this plane. (E) The underlying soleus muscle is observed after complete release gastrocnemius aponeurosis and the underlying soleal fascia. (F) The cannula is rotated 180 degrees to evaluate the posterior compartment fascia and identify the sural nerve along with the lesser saphenous veins.

Postoperative Protocol

For an isolated procedure, immediate weightbearing in a boot is allowed. However, if concurrent reconstructive procedures were performed, the limb should be splinted at neutral dorsiflexion. A night splint is recommended to keep the ankle at neutral dorsiflexion during sleep for the first 6 weeks. The walking boot can be weaned off at 4 to 6 weeks postoperatively. Range of motion exercise of the ankle is encouraged starting on postoperative day 1. Rehabilitation regimes are tailored according to associated procedures.

Potential Complications

From the literature review, complications of EGR include sural nerve dysesthesia (0% to 11.1%),[8,14,16] weakness on plantarflexion (0% to 9.7%),[8,18] and wound complication (0% to 13%).[8,16] Sural nerve dysesthesia and plantarflexion weakness usually resolves within 1 year. A small percentage of patients had persistent mild weakness that did not substantially affect activities of daily living and sport activities.[8]

Top Technical Pearls for the Procedure

1. A tourniquet and sterile cotton swabs are utilized as an initial step in the EGR procedure to achieve a bloodless and clean operative field.
2. The sural nerve can be identified in most patients by palpation of the nerve posterior to the slotted cannula, or in some by turning the camera 180 degrees toward the crural fascia.
3. Clear visualization of the gastrocnemius aponeurosis without neurovascular structures is required prior to the release with a retrograde knife to minimize sural nerve injury.

(continued)

4. The complete release of the medial part of the gastrocnemius aponeurosis is important in order to achieve adequate ankle dorsiflexion. It can be released from lateral to medial from the medial portal while observing from the lateral portal.
5. The optimal ankle dorsiflexion should be 10 to 15 degrees intraoperatively for normal gait and prevention of overlengthening of the gastrocnemius muscle.

References

1. Lim J, Dalal R, Waseem M. Percutaneous vs. open repair of the ruptured Achilles tendon—a prospective randomized controlled study. *Foot Ankle Int.* 2001;22(7):559-568.
2. Nistor L. Surgical and non-surgical treatment of Achilles tendon ruptures. *J Bone Joint Surg Am.* 1981;63:394-399.
3. Lui TH. Endoscopic-assisted Achilles tendon repair with plantaris tendon augmentation. *Arthroscopy.* 2007;23:556.e1-e5.
4. Ma GW, Griffith TG. Percutaneous repair of acute closed ruptured Achilles tendon: a new technique. *Clin Orthop Relat Res.* 1977;(128):247-255.
5. Chiodo CP1, Glazebrook M, Bluman EM, et al; American Academy of Orthopaedic Surgeons. Diagnosis and treatment of acute Achilles tendon rupture. *J Am Acad Orthop Surg.* 2010;18(8):503-510.
6. Calleja M, Connell DA. The Achilles tendon. *Semin Musculoskelet Radiol.* 2010;14(3):307-322.
7. Halasi T, Tallay A, Berkes I. Percutaneous Achilles tendon repair. *Am J Sports Med.* 1993;21:724-727.
8. Phisitkul P, Rungprai C, Femino JE, Arunakul M, Amendola A. Endoscopic gastrocnemius recession for the treatment of isolated gastrocnemius contracture: a prospective study on 320 consecutive patients. *Foot Ankle Int.* 2014;35(8):747-756.
9. Thermann H, Tibesku CO, Mastrokalos DS, Pässler HH. Endoscopically assisted percutaneous Achilles tendon suture. *Foot Ankle Int.* 2001;22(2):158-160.
10. DiGiovanni CW, Kuo R, Tejwani N, et al. Isolated gastrocnemius tightness. *J Bone Joint Surg Am.* 2002;84-A:962-970.
11. Downey MS, Banks AS. Gastrocnemius recession in the treatment of nonspastic ankle equinus: a retrospective study. *J Am Podiatr Med Assoc.* 1989;79(4):159-174.
12. Saxena A. Endoscopic gastrocnemius tenotomy. *J Foot Ankle Surg.* 2002;41(1):57-58.
13. Grady JF, Kelly C. Endoscopic gastrocnemius recession for treating equinus in pediatric patients. *Clin Orthop Relat Res.* 2010;468(4):1033-1038.
14. Saxena A, Widtfeldt A. Endoscopic gastrocnemius recession: preliminary report on 18 cases. *J Foot Ankle Surg.* 2004;43(5):302-306.
15. Tashjian RZ, Appel AJ, Banerjee R, DiGiovanni CW. Endoscopic gastrocnemius recession: evaluation in a cadaver model. *Foot Ankle Int.* 2003;24:607-613.
16. Trevino S, Gibbs M, Panchbhavi V. Evaluation of results of endoscopic gastrocnemius recession. *Foot Ankle Int.* 2005;26(5):359-364.
17. Silfverskiöld N. Reduction of the uncrossed two-joint muscles in spastic conditions. *Acta Chiropractic Scandinavia.* 1924;56:315-330.
18. DiDomenico LA, Adams HB, Garchar D. Endoscopic gastrocnemius recession for the treatment of gastrocnemius equinus. *J Am Podiatr Med Assoc.* 2005;95(4):410-413.

Please visit www.routledge.com/9781617119989 to access additional material.

19

Noninsertional Achilles Tendinosis

Richard Freeman, MBBS, FRCS(Tr & Ortho) and
James D. F. Calder, MD, FRCS(Tr & Orth), FFSEM(UK)

Introduction

Noninsertional Achilles tendinopathy is a common complaint. In most cases, conservative treatment is successful, but when this fails, surgery can be highly effective.

A protracted period of conservative therapy is advised before considering surgery. The relative avascularity of the tendon, while allowing the tendon to perform incredible feats of tensile strength, does not allow for rapid healing.

Conservative treatments include the following:

- Rest with or without immobilization
- Shoe modifications: Heel raise, eversion control
- Eccentric strengthening exercises
- Extracorporeal shock wave therapy
- Injection therapy

Shoe modifications are safe and effective. Strategies include shock absorption, control of eversion, and heel raises to offload the tendon.[1] Eccentric (more so than concentric) strengthening and stretching have been shown to produce clinical and radiological improvements in a high percentage of patients, although in some series, almost one-third of patients failed to improve.[2-4] Extracorporeal shock wave therapy is gaining favor as a treatment for both insertional and noninsertional Achilles pathology, although studies often fail to isolate these groups.[5] Caution must be exercised when injecting corticosteroid into or around tendons[6,7] as it is possible that this may increase the risk of tendon rupture.

Other injected agents have been studied, including hyperosmolar dextrose and platelet-rich plasma.[8-11] Studies of platelet-rich plasma have thus far been mixed; one randomized, controlled trial[12] showed no difference compared to saline, and a recent meta-analysis[13] appears to show a beneficial effect following Achilles rupture but not in tendinopathy.

Stone JW, Kennedy JG, Glazebrook M, eds. *The Foot and Ankle: AANA Advanced Arthroscopic Surgical Techniques* (pp 177-183).

Indications

- Tender Achilles tendon 2 to 7 cm proximal to insertion
- Failed conservative treatment
- Significant symptoms

Controversial Indications

- Medial-sided tenderness

Recent evidence has pointed to the plantaris tendon as a source for some Achilles tendinopathy.[14] The plantaris has been shown to be stiffer and stronger than the Achilles and has a differential movement to it.[15] This may generate friction with subsequent inflammation and adhesion formation at the interface between the tendons as they lie in a shared paratenon. Small studies have shown good results with plantaris release and excision.[16-18]

Pertinent Physical Findings

- Noninsertional pathology is typically 2 to 7 cm proximal to the insertion.
- Tenderness and swelling are typical findings.
- Predominantly medial tenderness suggests a plantaris effect.

Pertinent Imaging

- Ultrasound is useful in detecting inflamed bursae and for assessing for tendon involvement.
- Magnetic resonance imaging can also be useful.[19]
- Ultrasonographic tissue characterization[20] is a promising new imaging modality.

Equipment

A basic orthopedic set including the following is required:

- A #15 and #10 blade
- Gillies and Adson forceps
- McIndoe or tenotomy scissors
- Cat's paw retractors
- Small hemostat clip
- Needle holders

Positioning and Portals

The ideal positioning for access to the Achilles is prone; however, this increases the demands on anesthetic colleagues and operating room staff. The "sloppy lateral" allows good exposure of the posterior aspect of the leg and is more convenient for the operating room team.[21]

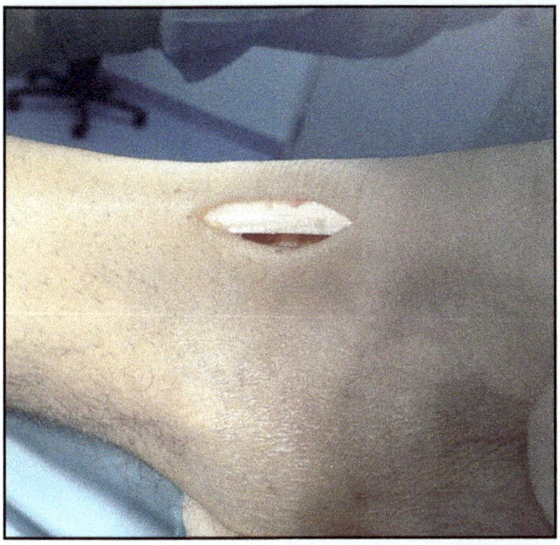

Figure 19-1. Medial paramedian incision.

Step-by-Step Description of Noninsertional Tendinopathy Resection Procedure

Tendonoscopic[22-24] and minimally invasive[25,26] procedures have been described; however, open procedures are still the gold standard.[27,28]

- A medial paramedian incision is centered over the diseased tendon (often a nodular swelling is palpable; Figure 19-1).
- The paratenon is incised in the line of the skin incision.
- The Achilles tendon is identified and carefully dissected from the paratenon.
- Adhesions, particularly ventral neovascularization, are released.
- The Achilles is incised and any degenerate tissue is removed.
- The Achilles is closed with buried sutures (3/0 polydioxanone) in a tubular fashion.
- The paratenon is closed as a distinct layer (3/0 Monocryl), then fat (2/0 Monocryl) and skin (3/0 Monocryl).

Postoperative Protocol

Elevation is strongly encouraged and the patient is allowed to fully bear weight in a prefabricated boot. The dressings are taken down and the wounds are inspected at 2 weeks. After this, eccentric exercises begin. Sports are prohibited for 6 weeks.

Step-by-Step Description of Plantaris Excision

- At the point of maximal tenderness/swelling, make a medial paramedian incision that is 2 to 3 cm long.
- Open the paratenon and identify the plantaris and Achilles tendons.
- Release any adhesions, particularly any ventral neovascularization.

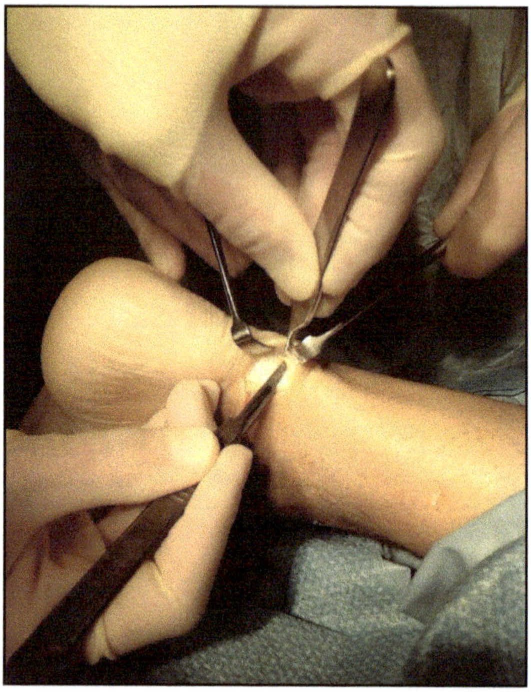

Figure 19-2. Release of the plantaris tendon at its distal attachment.

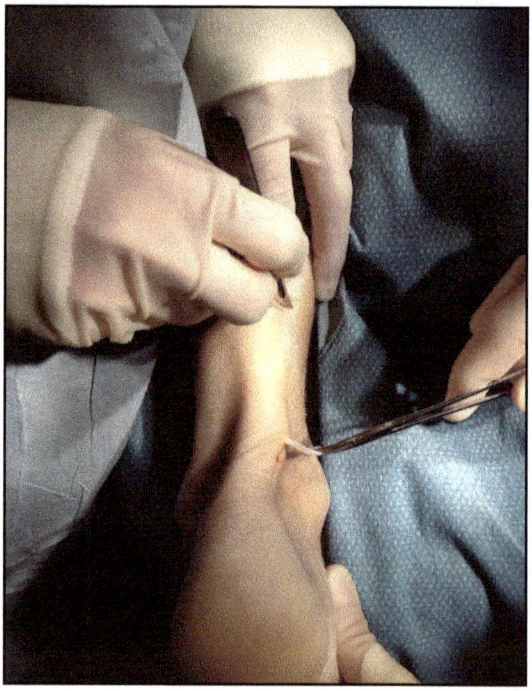

Figure 19-3. Passing of the plantaris stump subcutaneously.

- Release the plantaris distally (Figure 19-2).
- Using a hemostat, pass the stump within the paratenon 10 to 15 cm proximally (Figure 19-3).
- Retrieve and excise the tendon through a separate stab incision (Figures 19-4 and 19-5).
- The paratenon is closed as a distinct layer (3/0 Monocryl), then fat (2/0 Monocryl) and skin (3/0 Monocryl).

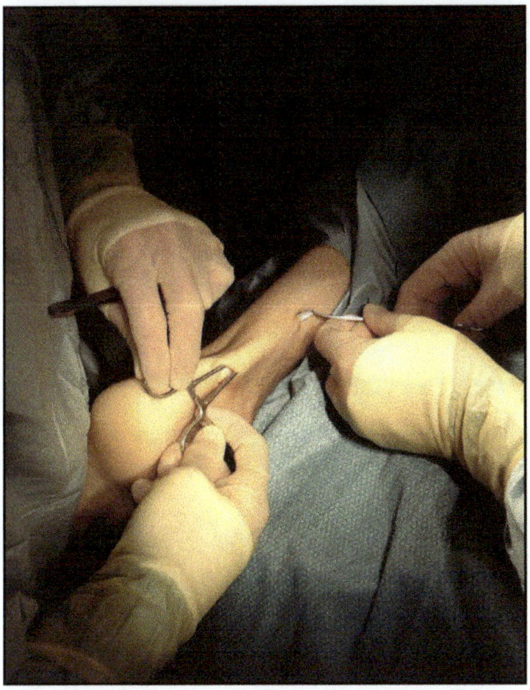

Figure 19-4. Retrieval of the plantaris stump proximally.

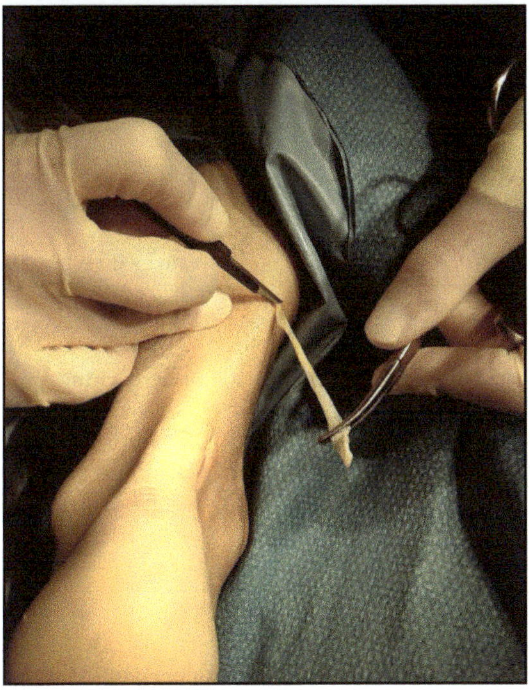

Figure 19-5. Excision of the plantaris.

Postoperative Protocol

A firm compressive bandage is applied to the operative site and elevation is encouraged for 10 days. Weightbearing with crutches is allowed and ankle range of motion exercises are commenced from 48 hours postoperatively after reducing the dressings to a double Tubigrip

(Mölnlycke Health Care). An Achilles strengthening program is introduced at 2 weeks once wound healing has been ensured.

Potential Complications

Overall, complications have been reported as 11%.[29] Wound breakdown is the greatest fear and can be expected in approximately 5% of open repairs.[25] Venous thromboembolism is comparatively high following Achilles surgery, with clinically apparent cases occurring in up to 7%.[30] Patients who are diabetic[31] or who smoke[32] are at particular risk.

Top Technical Pearls for the Procedure

1. Use the sloppy lateral position.
2. Take meticulous care of the soft tissue, especially during retraction.
3. Use sharp dissection to avoid traumatizing the soft tissues.
4. Bury knots to avoid adhesion formation.
5. Close the paratenon as a separate layer.

References

1. Gross ML, Davlin LB, Evanski PM. Effectiveness of orthotic shoe inserts in the long-distance runner. *Am J Sports Med.* 1991;19:409-412.
2. Fahlström M, Jonsson P, Lorentzon R, Alfredson H. Chronic Achilles tendon pain treated with eccentric calf-muscle training. *Knee Surg Sports Traumatol Arthrosc.* 2003;11:327-333.
3. Alfredson H, Pietilä T, Jonsson P, Lorentzon R. Heavy-load eccentric calf muscle training for the treatment of chronic Achilles tendinosis. *Am J Sports Med.* 1998;26:360-366.
4. Mafi N, Lorentzon R, Alfredson H. Superior short-term results with eccentric calf muscle training compared to concentric training in a randomized prospective multicentre study on patients with chronic Achilles tendinosis. *Knee Surg Sports Traumatol Arthrosc.* 2001;9(1):42-47.
5. Al-Abbad H, Simon JV. The effectiveness of extracorporeal shock wave therapy on chronic Achilles tendinopathy: a systematic review. *Foot Ankle Int.* 2013;34:33-41.
6. Mahler F, Fritschy D. Partial and complete ruptures of the Achilles tendon and local corticosteroid injections. *Br J Sports Med.* 1992;26:7-14.
7. Chechick A, Amit Y, Israeli A, Horoszowski H. Recurrent rupture of the Achilles tendon induced by corticosteroid injection. *Br J Sports Med.* 1982;16:89-90.
8. Monto RR. Platelet rich plasma treatment for chronic Achilles tendinosis. *Foot Ankle Int.* 2012;33:379-385.
9. Sofka CM, Adler RS, Positano R, Pavlov H, Luchs JS. Haglund's syndrome: diagnosis and treatment using sonography. *HSS J.* 2006;2:27-29.
10. Checa A, Chun W, Pappu R. Ultrasound-guided diagnostic and therapeutic approach to retrocalcaneal bursitis. *J Rheumatol.* 2011;38:391-392.
11. Ryan M, Wong A, Taunton J. Favorable outcomes after sonographically guided intratendinous injection of hyperosmolar dextrose for chronic insertional and midpor- tion achilles tendinosis. *Am J Roentgenol.* 2010;194:1047-1053.
12. de Vos RJ, Weir A, van Schie HT, et al. Platlet-rich plasma injection for chronic Achilles tendinopathy: a randomized controlled trial. *JAMA.* 2010;303(2)144-149.

13. Sadoghi P, Rosso C, Valderrabano V, Leithner A, Vavken P. The role of platelets in the treatment of Achilles tendon injuries. *J Orthop Res.* 2013;31(1):111-118.
14. Andersson G, Danielson P, Alfredson H, Forsgren S. Nerve-related characteristics of ventral paratendinous tissue in chronic Achilles tendinosis. *Knee Surg Sports Traumatol Arthrosc.* 2007;15:1272-1279.
15. Lintz F, Higgs A, Millett M, et al. The role of plantaris longus in Achilles tendinopathy: a biomechanical study. *Foot Ankle Surg.* 2011;17:252-255.
16. Pearce CJ, Carmichael J, Calder JD. Achilles tendinoscopy and plantaris tendon release and division in the treatment of non-insertional Achilles tendinopathy. *Foot Ankle Surg.* 2012;18:124-127.
17. van Sterkenburg MN, Kerkhoffs GM, van Dijk CN. Good outcome after stripping the plantaris tendon in patients with chronic mid-portion Achilles tendinopathy. *Knee Surg Sports Traumatol Arthrosc.* 2011;19:1362-1366.
18. Calder JD, Freeman R, Pollock N. Plantaris excision in the treatment of non-insertional Achilles tendinopathy in elite athletes. *Br J Sports Med.* do:10.1136/bjsports-2014-093827.
19. Wijesekera NT, Calder JD, Lee JC. Imaging in the assessment and management of Achilles tendinopathy and paratendinitis. *Semin Musculoskelet Radiol.* 2011;15(1):89-100.
20. van Schie HT, de Vos RJ, de Jonge S, et al. Ultrasonographic tissue characterisation of human Achilles tendons: quantification of tendon structure through a novel non-invasive approach. *Br J Sports Med.* 2010;44(16):1153-1159.
21. Gougoulias N, Dawe E, Sakellariou A. The recovery position for posterior surgery of the ankle and hindfoot. *Bone Joint J.* 2013;95-B:1317-1319.
22. Thermann H, Benetos IS, Panelli C, Gavrlilidis I, Feil S. Endoscopic treatment of chronic mid-portion Achilles tendinopathy: novel technique with short-term results. *Knee Surg Sports Traumatol Arthrosc.* 2009;17(10):1264-1269.
23. Vega J, Cabestany JM, Golanó P, Pérez-Carro L. Endoscopic treatment for chronic achilles tendinopathy. *Foot Ankle Surg.* 2008;14:204-210.
24. Steenstra F, van Dijk CN. Achilles tendoscopy. *Foot Ankle Clin.* 2006;11:429-438.
25. Maffulli N, Testa V, Capasso G, Bifulco G, Binfield PM. Results of percutaneous longitudinal tenotomy for Achilles tendinopathy in middle- and long-distance runners. *Am J Sports Med.* 1997;25:835-840.
26. Longo UG, Ramamurthy C, Denaro V, Maffulli N. Minimally invasive stripping for chronic Achilles tendinopathy. *Disabil Rehabil.* 2008;30:1709-1713.
27. Nelen G, Martens M, Burssens A. Surgical treatment of chronic Achilles tendinitis. *Am J Sports Med.* 1989;17:754-759.
28. Schepsis AA, Leach RE. Surgical management of Achilles tendinitis. *Am J Sports Med.* 1987;15:308-315.
29. Paavola M, Orava S, Leppilahti J, Kannus P, Järvinen M. Chronic Achilles tendon overuse injury: complications after surgical treatment: an analysis of 432 consecutive patients. *Am J Sports Med.* 2000;28:77-82.
30. Saragas NP, Ferrao PNF. The incidence of venous thromboembolism in patients undergoing surgery for acute Achilles tendon ruptures. *Foot Ank Surg.* 2011;17:263-265.
31. Wukich DK, McMillen RL, Lowery NJ, Frykberg RG. Surgical site infections after foot and ankle surgery: a comparison of patients with and without diabetes. *Diabetes Care.* 2011;34(10):2211-2213.
32. Lee JJ, Patel R, Biermann JS, Dougherty PJ. The musculoskeletal effects of cigarette smoking. *J Bone Joint Surg Am.* 2013;95(9):850-859.

Please visit www.routledge.com/9781617119989 to access additional material.

20

Haglund's Deformity
Endoscopic Calcaneoplasty

Youichi Yasui, MD; Ethan J. Fraser, MD, MBBS;
and John G. Kennedy, MD, MCh, FRCS

Introduction

Haglund's deformity is characterized as an enlarged prominence of the superior aspect of the posterior calcaneus. Alone, this bony prominence may be asymptomatic. However, the described Haglund's syndrome involves a painful osseous prominence with the addition of retrocalcaneal bursitis and Achilles tendinosis.[1] This is a mechanically induced pathology caused by the repetitive stress both between the Achilles tendon and the calcaneal prominence, and also from direct pressure from footwear with the formation of a callus, a common finding. This mechanical stimulus leads to a biological deterioration initially at the calcaneal insertion of the Achilles tendon. Conservative treatments are useful in the early stages of this pathology and are aimed at reducing the mechanical strain on the tendon. These include limited immobilization, modification of shoe wear, orthotics, heel lifts, and eccentric stretching. More controversial modalities can also be used to improve the biological environment. These include the judicious use of corticosteroid injection into the inflamed retrocalcaneal bursa alone, shock wave therapy, and platelet-rich plasma (PRP) injection.[2-4] While good basic science evidence exists for both PRP and shock wave therapies, these modalities will require more level I evidence before they are universally adopted. Corticosteroids are controversial and, in the senior author's practice, are only used infrequently and then in selected cases of an inflamed bursa. Small amounts can be delivered under ultrasound guidance, but great care should be taken to avoid injecting into the tendon itself. Despite many patients responding to conservative therapies, over 20% of patients ultimately require surgical treatment due to persistent hindfoot pain and decreased function.[3,4]

In a subset of these surgical candidates, endoscopic calcaneoplasty represents an attractive option. This procedure is usually performed via a 2-portal approach, utilizing posteromedial and posterolateral portals.[5-9] Recently, a systematic review by Wiegerinck and colleagues showed that this procedure had more than 90% good to excellent clinical outcomes and lower complication rates than traditional open procedures.[10] Despite excellent outcomes, endoscopic calcaneoplasty should be used judiciously in patients with advanced disease or with signs of Achilles calcifications or extensive tendinopathy as these pathologies are more difficult to address using a minimally invasive approach.[11,12] In this text, the authors review the use of endoscopic calcaneoplasty for Haglund's syndrome with a step-by-step operative technique outlined.

Stone JW, Kennedy JG, Glazebrook M, eds. *The Foot and Ankle: AANA Advanced Arthroscopic Surgical Techniques* (pp 185-195).

Indications

- Patients with Haglund's deformity who have failed 6 months of conservative treatment[9,11]
- High-demand athletes with Haglund's deformity who have persistent pain following failed conservative treatment for 3 months
- Patients with moderate to severe tendon degeneration
  - Less than 20% of total cross-sectional tendon area involved
    - Comparative studies performed by Kondreddi and colleagues suggest that patients with degenerative change in the Achilles tendon show inferior clinical outcomes following endoscopic calcaneoplasty.[12]

Controversial Indications

- Massive Haglund's bony prominence with overgrowth over the tendon
- Low-demand patients with Haglund's deformity who have persistent pain following failed conservative treatment for 6 months
- Patients at higher risk of wound complications (eg, smokers, diabetics)
- Patients with mild degenerative change (more than 20% per tendon area) of insertion of the Achilles tendon can be treated with endoscopic calcaneoplasty.
  - However, if degenerative change is located deep in the tendon, open surgery should be considered.

Pertinent Physical Findings

- Best test: Palpation typically reveals tenderness and swelling over the insertion of the Achilles as well as proximal to its insertion.[3] This is not usually accompanied by rubor or erythema unless tight-fitting footwear is worn.
- Enlarged prominence can be found over the heel.
- Deep palpation of the anterolateral or anteromedial Achilles may produce pain from an inflamed retrocalcaneal bursa.[6]
- Pain may be reproduced with passive and active ankle dorsiflexion and plantarflexion.[6]
- Positive Silfverskiöld test indicates tightness of gastrocnemius, with the possibility of causing increased stress at the insertion of the Achilles tendon.
- Posterior ankle impingement test: Pain on excessive passive plantarflexion typically indicates posterior ankle impingement syndrome. It is important to distinguish it from a Haglund's deformity.[13]
- Restriction of range of motion and neurological deficit are rare.

Pertinent Imaging

Radiography

- Lateral ankle view (weightbearing)
  - Kager's fat pad: Inflammation of the retrocalcaneal bursa may result in lack of definition of Kager's fat pad[10]

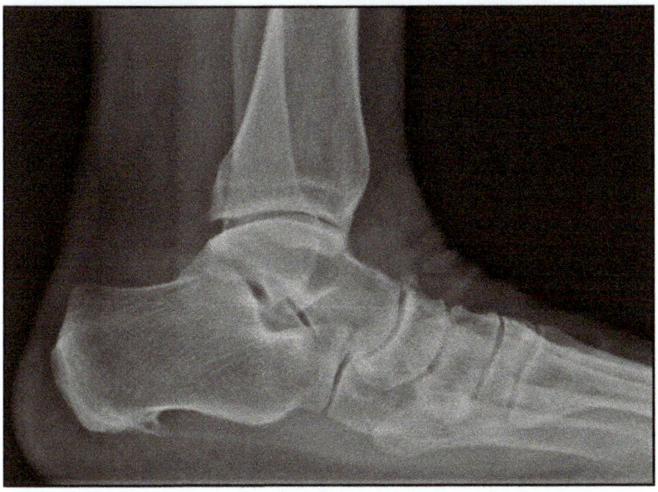

Figure 20-1. Lateral radiograph showing abnormalities of the insertion of the Achilles tendon, including spurs and calcification of tendon.

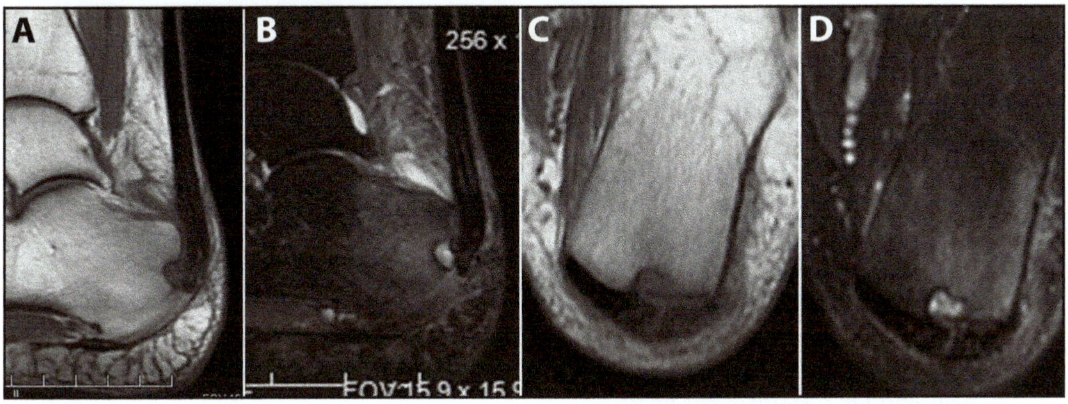

Figure 20-2. Preoperative magnetic resonance images of a Haglund's deformity. (A) T1-weighted sagittal image with Haglund's and pathological change in Achilles tendon and insertion site. (B) T2-weighted image with bony edema in the calcaneus, retrocalcaneal bursitis, and heterogeneous signal in the Achilles representing degenerative change. (C, D) Axial T1 and T2-weighted images with similar pathologic change appreciated.

  - Effective for evaluation of the posterior calcaneal exostosis
  - Abnormalities of the insertion of Achilles tendon, including spurs and calcification of the Achilles tendon (Figure 20-1)
    - The size of bony prominence is evaluated using the Fowler and Philips angle (normal values 45 to 70 degrees) and calcaneal pitch angle (normal values 17 to 32 degrees)[14]
- Standard anteroposterior, lateral, and mortise weightbearing radiographs
  - Classically obtained for all ankle and hindfoot pathologies

Magnetic Resonance Imaging

- Sagittal view
  - Showing soft and bony pathological lesion: enlarged exostosis, bone marrow edema, cyst in calcaneal bone, the extent of retrocalcaneal bursa, and partial tear of Achilles tendon itself. Excessive signal change around the tendon and in adjacent bone would be a typical finding (Figure 20-2).

- Axial view
  - Useful to evaluate abnormalities of the Achilles tendon and cross-sectional tendon area with degenerative change. As aforementioned, moderate to severe tendinosis should be treated with open procedure.
  - Potential concomitant osteochondral lesions, posterior ankle impingement syndrome, and involvement of other tendons can be investigated.

Ultrasound

- Local anesthetic injection using guided ultrasound imaging is utilized as a confirmatory test.
- Corticosteroid injection for retrocalcaneal bursitis may be useful as conservative treatment. However, steroids increase the risk of Achilles tendon rupture and are rarely used in the senior author's practice.

Equipment

- Thigh tourniquet
- General arthroscopy equipment required for endoscopic calcaneoplasty mirrors that which is used in anterior ankle arthroscopy, with some exceptions.
- A monitor, light source, and control unit for both the camera and motorized shaver and other instruments are required in all cases. The monitor should be at the surgeon's eye line.
- A distractor is not necessary.
- Irrigation system (pressure: 50 to 60 mm Hg; fluid flow: 0.5 to l/min)
- A 2.7- or 4.0-mm arthroscope with 30- or 70-degree viewing angle; 70-degree arthroscopy can be useful but usually is not necessary.
- A 3.5- and 4.5-mm shaver for soft tissue debridement
- A 4.0-mm aggressive shaver or burr for bony resection
- A 1.8-mm Kirschner wire (K-wire)
- Fluoroscopy
- Elastic bandage

Positioning and Portals

The patient is placed in the prone or sloppy lateral position and prepped and draped in the normal fashion. The foot should be either overhanging the end of the table or supported with an angular cushion placed underneath the distal tibia so that the leg is raised approximately 15 cm above the contralateral leg to facilitate the movement of arthroscopic instruments (Figure 20-3). Ensure that there are no focal pressure points and that all neurovascular structures are protected with well-padded supports.

Supine positioning has also been reported. However, it is less commonly utilized.[15]

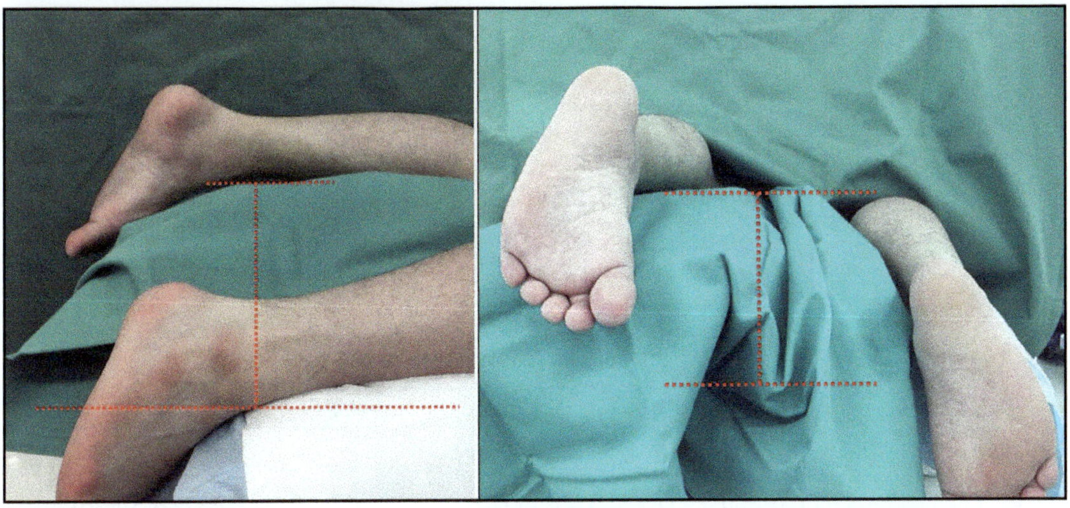

Figure 20-3. Patient positioning for endoscopic calcaneoplasty. With the patient supine, the foot should be overhanging the end of the table or supported with an angular cushion placed underneath the distal tibia. Red broken line showing the height difference between operative limb and contralateral limb (operative limb approximately 15 cm higher than other side).

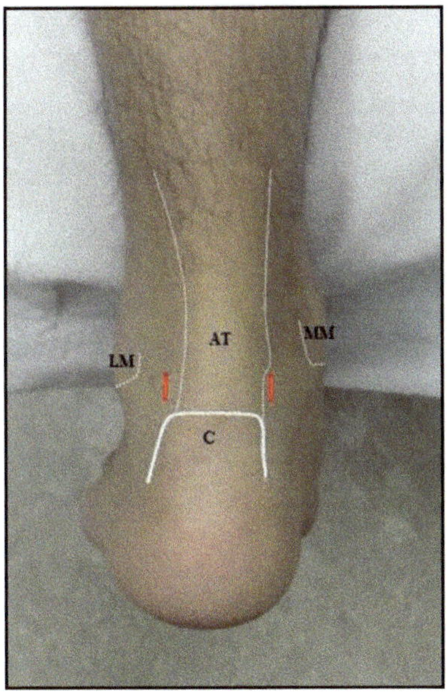

Figure 20-4. Anatomic landmarks and location for portals. Red lines represent location of portals. AT, Achilles tendon; C, calcaneus shown; LM, lateral malleolus; MM, medial malleolus.

Step-by-Step Description of the Procedure

- Step 1: Marking anatomic landmarks and portal sites (Figure 20-4)
  - The anteromedial and anterolateral edges of the Achilles tendon and superoposterior edges of the calcaneal tuberosity should be marked on the skin using a sterile surgical marker.
  - The tip of the fibula and tibia should also be marked.
  - The posteromedial portal site is next identified and should be located 5.0 mm medial to the anteromedial edge of the Achilles tendon and 7.0 mm proximal to the superoposterior edge of the calcaneal tuberosity.

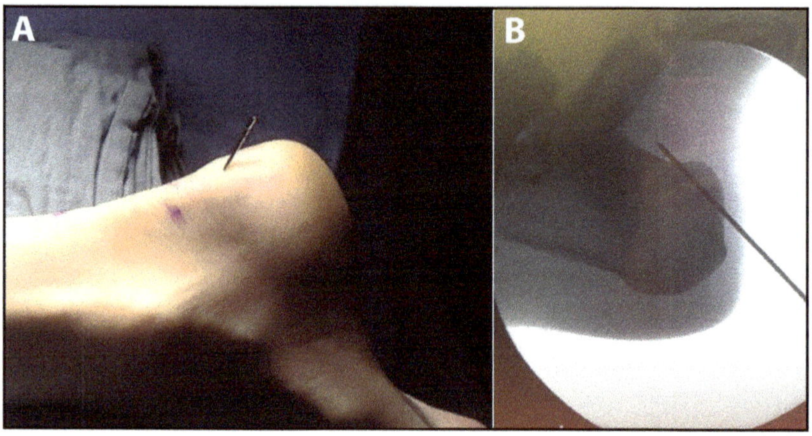

Figure 20-5. Insertion of K-wire. (A) Percutaneous placement of K-wire to guide resection. (B) Insertion starting from an inferior, posterior position and advanced superiorly and anteriorly under fluoroscopic guidance.

- ▹ The posterolateral portal is marked 5.0 mm lateral to the anterolateral edge of the Achilles tendon and 7.0 mm proximal to the superoposterior edge of the calcaneal tuberosity.
- ▹ Portals are more distal than those used in a standard posterior hindfoot arthroscopy.
- ▹ Ensure that portal sites are created above the level of the superior tip of the calcaneal prominence as this will allow the surgeon to achieve a better view of the Haglund's prominence and ensures that complete debridement is possible.[16]
- ▹ The sural nerve should be palpated and its course marked to avoid iatrogenic nerve injury.
  - ◆ The sural nerve can be found 7.0 mm lateral and 4 cm proximal to the posterior calcaneal tuberosity, coursing laterally and distally to be found 17.5 mm laterally at the level of the posterior calcaneal tuberosity.[17,18]

- ▸ Step 2: Inserting K-wire (Figure 20-5)
  - ▹ A K-wire (1.8 mm) is inserted from the posterior aspect of calcaneal tuberosity to the anterior edge of the Haglund's deformity prominence under fluoroscopy.
  - ▹ After confirming the proper position of the K-wire, the end of the K-wire is cut.
- ▸ Step 3: Making portals
  - ▹ Vertical skin incisions 7.0 mm in length are made over the posteromedial and posterolateral portals marked previously. Care should be taken to avoid damage to the sural nerve by only incising the superficial tissues.
  - ▹ Subcutaneous blunt dissection using a mosquito clamp is performed via both portals. Of note, the soft tissue around the superior edge of calcaneal bone and the anterior surface of the Achilles tendon should be dissected as well, which will facilitate the next steps.
- ▸ Step 4: Creating working space
  - ▹ The arthroscope sleeve with trocar is introduced via a posterolateral portal and carefully advanced into the space anterior to the Achilles tendon and superior to Haglund's prominence.
  - ▹ Once calcaneal bone can be palpated with the trocar, it is switched for the arthroscope.
  - ▹ Initial visualization may be poor as a result of soft tissue cicatrization and the presence of a fat pad in this area (Figure 20-6). Debridement of soft tissue with the shaver positioned in the posteromedial portal is performed to create a working space and expose the K-wire.
  - ▹ The shaver blade must always be visible to avoid iatrogenic injury to healthy tissue.
  - ▹ We prefer to use a 2.7-mm arthroscope as the working space is limited.

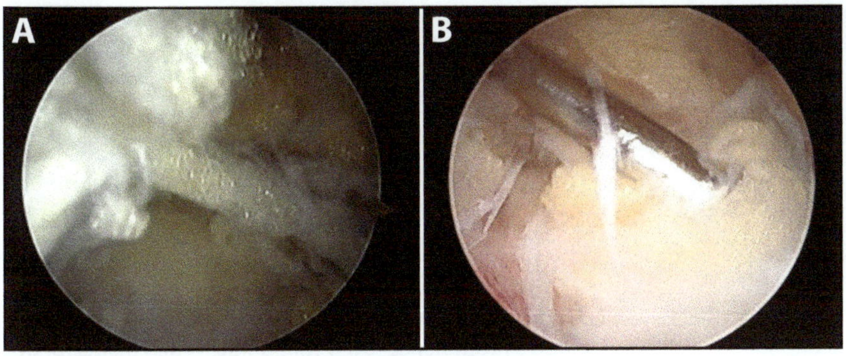

Figure 20-6. Endoscopic images showing poor visualization due to the presence of (A) a fat pad in this area and (B) soft tissue cicatrization, which is often present.

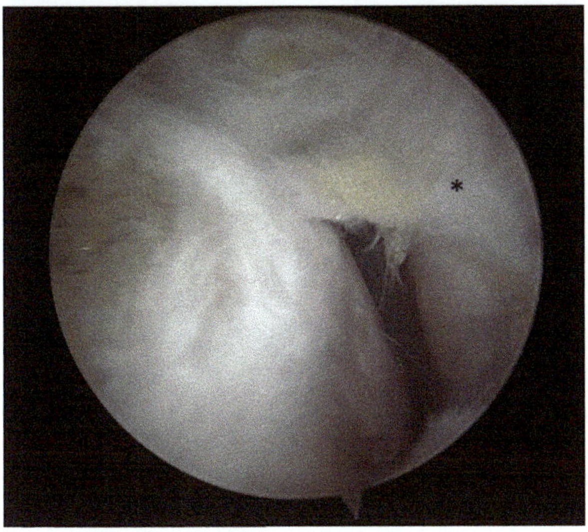

Figure 20-7. Endoscopic image showing post-debridement state with Achilles tendon insertion being visible. *, Achilles tendon.

- Step 5: Debridement of soft tissue
  - Soft tissue, including inflamed retrocalcaneal bursa and inflamed and cicatrized soft tissue, are debrided using a 3.5- or 4.5-mm shaver via the posteromedial portal.
  - Portals for the arthroscope and shaver may be switched in order to gain optimal access to all pathology and achieve adequate debridement.
  - Once appropriate debridement for soft tissue is achieved, the Achilles tendon insertion can be exposed (Figure 20-7).
- Step 6: Debridement for Haglund's deformity
  - The Haglund's prominence is debrided using a 3.5- or 4.0-mm aggressive shaver or bone cutter via the posterolateral portal using the previously inserted K-wire as a guide for the resection (Figure 20-8).
  - Once appropriate debridement of the bony prominence is achieved under arthroscopic and fluoroscopic views, the K-wire can be removed.
  - The authors prefer to debride calcaneal bone from the anterior calcaneus toward the Achilles tendon. In this way, the working space is larger, which facilitates improved debridement (see Figure 20-8).
- Step 7: Debridement of paratenon and Achilles tendon
  - Paratenon surrounding the Achilles tendon as well as the tendon itself are debrided according to preoperative radiological evaluation and intraoperative findings.

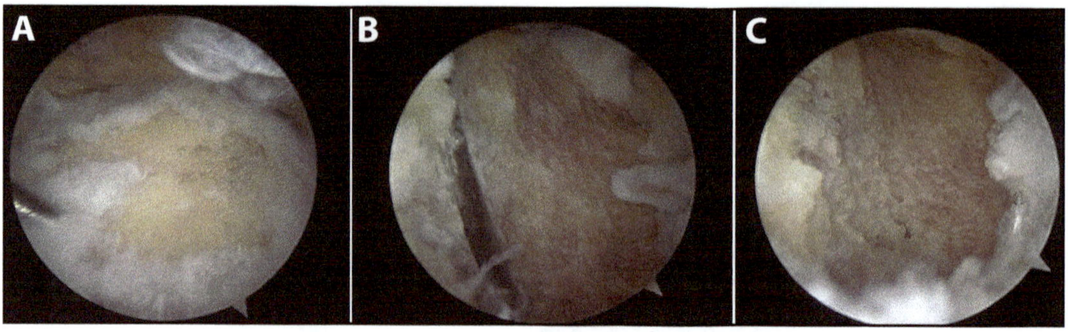

Figure 20-8. Sequential debridement of the Haglund's prominence. (A) K-wire guide, which marks (B) the point where debridement should be ceased, following which (C) the K-wire can be removed.

Figure 20-9. Postoperative image confirming adequate resection of the calcaneus.

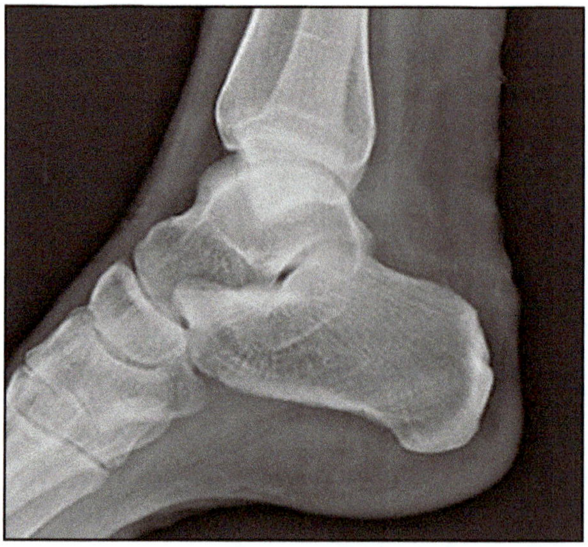

  - The location and size of degenerative tissue must be measured preoperatively in order to avoid iatrogenic Achilles tendon rupture postoperatively.
- Step 8: Evaluation following debridement
  - Fluoroscopy is used to evaluate the adequacy of the resection (Figure 20-9).
- Step 9: Skin closure
  - A 4-0 nylon is used to suture skin incision.
- Step 10 (optional): Biologic enhancement with PRP or bone marrow concentrate
  - PRP or bone marrow concentrate can be injected into the degenerative Achilles tendon.
  - PRP can be used on superficial wounds after skin closure and may enhance wound healing and decrease wound complications.
- Step 11: Immobilization immediately postoperatively
  - Compressive bandage immobilization alone is utilized after Haglund's resection without Achilles debridement, while a posterior splint is applied in cases where debridement of the Achilles tendon has been performed.

Postoperative Protocol

Endoscopic calcaneoplasty is typically performed as an outpatient procedure, with most patients returning home the day of surgery. Wound healing must be carefully monitored and steps taken to prevent early wound complications as the skin around the hindfoot has poor healing potential. Patients are instructed to keep the operative limb elevated with regular application of ice to reduce pain and swelling. Nonsteroidal anti-inflammatory medications may be useful in the acute phase. Suture removal can be done 10 to 14 days postoperatively. Physiotherapy can be commenced at 2 to 3 weeks after surgery.

Specific postoperative care includes the following:

- Minimal debridement of the Achilles tendon
    - Early range of motion and full weightbearing as tolerated can be advised soon after surgery, typically 10 to 14 days.
    - Returning to sports activity can be permitted once the wound has healed, strength is restored, and balance and proprioceptive goals are attained. Typically, this is 4 to 6 weeks postoperatively.
- Moderate or extensive Achilles debridement
    - A postoperative splint is maintained until 2 weeks after surgery.
    - A controlled ankle movement (CAM) boot is then applied and utilized until 4 to 6 weeks postoperatively.
    - Range of motion exercises are permitted from 2 weeks after surgery.
    - Patients should be kept nonweightbearing for the first 2 weeks. Weightbearing should be progressed from 2 to 4 weeks at 10% of body weight each day. Full weightbearing is allowed at 4 weeks postsurgery.
    - Return-to-sports activity can be advised when patients have no further hindfoot symptoms.
    - The CAM boot occasionally causes skin irritation even after complete wound healing. Caution must be paid to skin irritation, and a well-padded CAM boot heel is useful in this regard.

Potential Complications

The potential complications are wound complications, nerve injury, scar formation, Achilles tendon rupture, deep venous thrombosis (DVT), and pulmonary embolism.

Leitze and colleagues performed a prospective cohort study comparing 31 patients who underwent endoscopic decompression with 14 patients treated with open techniques.[11] The authors found that the endoscopic procedure resulted in fewer complications (infection: 3% vs 12%; altered sensation: 10% vs 18%; scar tenderness: 7% vs 18%).[11]

Wiegerinck and colleagues found a 2.0% complication rate in patients undergoing the endoscopic procedure.[10] In another study by Ortmann and McBryde, 1 patient out of 30 suffered an Achilles tendon rupture within 3 weeks of endoscopic surgery.[6]

Regarding DVT and pulmonary embolism, there is a dearth of information regarding arthroscopic debridement of Haglund's, but as with any surgery around the Achilles tendon, DVT prophylaxis may be used at least in the initial postoperative period. Each institution will have its own clinical practice guidelines regarding DVT prophylaxis. Early mobilization following this procedure may reduce the risk of DVT.

Top Technical Pearls for the Procedure

1. The primary indication for endoscopic calcaneoplasty is the presence of a Haglund's deformity without significant Achilles tendinosis in a patient who has failed nonoperative treatment.
2. K-wire insertion before making portals facilitates endoscopic calcaneoplasty.
3. The portals are marked 5.0 mm anterior to the anterior edge of the Achilles tendon and 7.0 mm proximal to superior edge of calcaneal tuberosity.
4. The shaver blade must always be under endoscopic view.
5. Biologic adjuncts may improve the quality of the Achilles tendon repair tissue following debridement and may reduce scar tissue and inflammation.

References

1. Haglund P. Beitrag zur Klinik der Achillessehne [Article on clinical pathology of the Achilles tendon]. *Zeitschr Orthop Chir.* 1928;49:49-58. [in German].
2. Lohrer H, Nauck T. Retrocalcaneal bursitis but not Achilles tendinopathy is characterized by increased pressure in the retrocalcaneal bursa. *Clin Biomech (Bristol, Avon).* 2014;29(3):283-238.
3. Irwin TA. Current concepts review: insertional Achilles tendinopathy. *Foot Ankle Int.* 2010;31(10):933-939.
4. Roche AJ, Calder JD. Achilles tendinopathy: a review of the current concepts of treatment. *Bone Joint J.* 2013;95-B(10):1299-1307.
5. Scholten PE, van Dijk CN. Endoscopic calcaneoplasty. *Foot Ankle Clin.* 2006;11(2):439-446, viii.
6. Ortmann FW, McBryde AM. Endoscopic bony and soft-tissue decompression of the retrocalcaneal space for the treatment of Haglund deformity and retrocalcaneal bursitis. *Foot Ankle Int.* 2007;28(2):149-153.
7. Jerosch J, Schunck J, Sokkar SH. Endoscopic calcaneoplasty (ECP) as a surgical treatment of Haglund's syndrome. *Knee Surg Sports Traumatol Arthrosc.* 2007;15(7):927-934.
8. Kaynak G, Öğüt T, Yontar NS, Botanlıoğlu H, Can A, Ünlü MC. Endoscopic calcaneoplasty: 5-year results. *Acta Orthop Traumatol Turc.* 2013;47(4):261-265.
9. Jerosch J. Endoscopic calcaneoplasty. *Foot Ankle Clin.* 2015;20(1):149-165.
10. Wiegerinck JI, Kok AC, van Dijk CN. Surgical treatment of chronic retrocalcaneal bursitis. *Arthroscopy.* 2012;28(2):283-293.
11. Leitze Z, Sella EJ, Aversa JM. Endoscopic decompression of the retrocalcaneal space. *J Bone Joint Surg Am.* 2003;85-A(8):1488-1496.
12. Kondreddi V, Gopal RK, Yalamanchili RK. Outcome of endoscopic decompression of retrocalcaneal bursitis. *Indian J Orthop.* 2012;46(6):659-663.
13. Smyth NA, Zwiers R, Wiegerinck JI, et al. Posterior hindfoot arthroscopy: a review. *Am J Sports Med.* 2014;42(1):225-234.
14. Bulstra GH, van Rheenen TA, Scholtes VA. Can we measure the heel bump? Radiographic evaluation of Haglund's deformity. *J Foot Ankle Surg.* 2015;54(3):338-340.
15. van Dijk CN, van Dyk GE, Scholten PE, Kort NP. Endoscopic calcaneoplasty. *Am J Sports Med.* 2001;29(2):185-189.
16. Carmont MR, Fawdington RA, Mei-Dan O. Endoscopic debridement of the Achilles insertion, bursa, and the calcaneal tubercle with an accessory postero-lateral portal: technique tip. *Foot Ankle Int.* 2011;32(6):648-650.

17. Webb J, Moorjani N, Radford M. Anatomy of the sural nerve and its relation to the Achilles tendon. *Foot Ankle Int*. 2000;21(6):475-477.
18. Lohrer H, Nauck T, Dorn NV, Konerding MA. Comparison of endoscopic and open resection for Haglund tuberosity in a cadaver study. *Foot Ankle Int*. 2006;27(6):445-450.

21

Posterior Ankle Impingement
Os Trigonum, Posterior Talar Process, Flexor Hallucis Longus

Andrew W. Ross, BA; Ethan J. Fraser, MD, MBBS; and John G. Kennedy, MD, MCh, FRCS

Introduction

Posterior ankle impingement (PAI) comprises a spectrum of anatomic and pathologic conditions that results in posterior ankle pain during plantarflexion.[1,2] The origin of PAI can be multifactorial and include both osseous structures and soft tissues. Typical anatomic osseous causes of PAI are compression of an os trigonum or posterior talar process (Stieda process).[1,2] Compression of either bony feature between the calcaneus and talus can lead to osseous damage, surrounding inflammation, and irritation of the synchondrosis.[3] Hypertrophy of the flexor hallucis longus (FHL) tendon, the presence of a tendon nodule, and inferior extension of the FHL muscle belly have been shown to be associated with PAI and are considered soft tissue causes of PAI.[4] Not surprisingly, PAI often occurs in athletic populations competing in sports that demand repeated forceful hyperplantarflexion as observed in ballet dancers, soccer players, and runners.[5-8] Often, a concomitant anatomic abnormality in conjunction with microtrauma can exacerbate the condition.[4,6] Conservative treatments including rest, bracing, and anti-inflammatories are often helpful in alleviating symptoms and can be successful in some patients, particularly in early stages of posterior impingement.[9,10] However, a symptomatic os trigonum or posterior talar process indicates surgical removal of the bony abnormality, as symptoms are unlikely to resolve from conservative treatments alone. For FHL etiologies, conservative measures do not always completely reduce pain and require extended treatment. Thus, for athletes with osseous or FHL involvement aiming to make a rapid return to competition, surgical intervention is typically indicated.[4]

Indications

- Compression of os trigonum or posterior talar process
- FHL tenosynovitis
- Inferior extension of FHL muscle belly
- Failure of conservative therapies

Stone JW, Kennedy JG, Glazebrook M, eds. *The Foot and Ankle: AANA Advanced Arthroscopic Surgical Techniques* (pp 197-206).

Pertinent Physical Findings

- Pain on passive plantarflexion is considered a positive test for PAI; however, it is important to ascertain the precise source of the pain.
- Palpation reproduces pain at the posterior ankle and along the subtalar joint margin both medial and lateral to the Achilles tendon.
- Ultrasound-guided local anesthetic injection (1% lidocaine) into the posterior hindfoot adjacent to the FHL tendon or pathologic osseous structure provides symptomatic relief upon passive plantarflexion.[11,12]
- FHL tenosynovitis pain typically occurs posterior to the medial malleolus and can be induced by hallux dorsiflexion or isometric plantarflexion of the hallux against resistance.[13]
- An FHL tendon nodule may be identified by palpation or seen on ultrasound.
- Imaging is essential to confirming a pathologic os trigonum or posterior talar process diagnosis.

Pertinent Imaging

- Radiography: Imaging techniques are employed prior to surgery to confirm or reject the diagnosis made during the physical exam. Standard anteroposterior, lateral, and oblique (mortise) weightbearing radiographs are classically obtained for ankle pathologies. For osseous causes of PAI, lateral radiographs are most effective.[14] Additionally, placing the patient in 25 degrees of external rotation can aid in differentiating between a posterior talar process and an os trigonum. Differentiation between an osseous fragment and an os trigonum can be made by observing a smooth, oval structure for an os trigonum vs an irregular fragment seen in bone fractures.[3]
- Magnetic resonance imaging (MRI): Soft tissue injuries are best observed using MRI.[4] This can be especially helpful in detecting surrounding edema and fluid within the tendon sheath of the FHL. MRI allows for an investigation of potential concomitant osteochondral lesions (OCLs); this is crucial considering that up to 50% of ankle inversion injuries result in chondral lesions.[15] Soft tissue PAI is often characterized by intermalleolar, posterior inferior tibiofibular, or posterior talofibular ligament impingement. Inflammation, surrounding edema, and potential impingement of these structures can be observed. Furthermore, peroneal tendinopathy can be ruled out using MRI. For examination of OCL and FHL pathologies, T2-weighted images are recommended.[16]
- Ultrasound: Ultrasound imaging for PAI is primarily utilized to guide local anesthetic injections as a confirmatory test during the physical exam. In conjunction with MRI, ultrasound can be used to examine the FHL tendon undergoing plantarflexion and dorsiflexion movements.
- Computed tomography (CT): For suspected symptomatic osseous structures, spiral CT is often utilized. Helical CT is a commonly employed diagnostic method for ascertaining the extent of OCLs and has been shown to be superior to radiographs and equivalent to MRI for OCL diagnosis.[17]

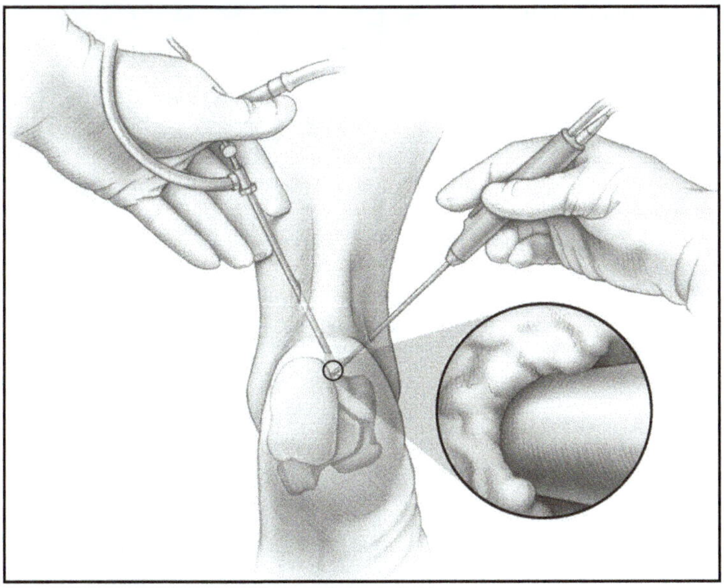

Figure 21-1. Short-barreled arthroscope used for greater control. Picture and intraoperative view.

Equipment

- The general arthroscopy equipment required for posterior ankle arthroscopy mirrors that which is used in anterior ankle arthroscopy with some exceptions.
- A monitor, light source, and control unit for both the camera and motorized shaver and other instruments are required in all cases. The monitor should be at the surgeon's eye line and will vary depending on whether he or she is sitting or standing for the case.
- In contrast to the anterior ankle scope, a short-barreled scope should be used as it allows the operator's hands to be closer to the joint, allowing for more controlled movement (Figure 21-1).
- A distractor is generally not required as the majority of the procedure is extra-articular.
- A short probing hook is required for accurate palpation of soft tissue structures as well as cartilage surfaces.
- An inflow and outflow fluid pump is attached to the arthroscopic port with a pressure of 30 to 40 mm Hg adequate for most cases.
- 3.5- and 4.5-mm shavers are used sequentially to debride any cicatrized tissue, inflamed soft tissue, and posterior fat pad to allow adequate visualization.
- A 0.25-inch straight and curved osteotome may be required to remove a Stieda process.
- A Freer elevator is useful in determining a fibrous union of an os process.
- A curette is used to remove pathological or unstable areas of cartilage at the rim if an osteochondral defect is found on the posterior joint surface.
- A microfracture awl of a smaller diameter than that used in the knee is required. A large awl will compress the subchondral bone, closing trabecular channels and not allowing for mesenchymal stem cell migration to the area of the lesion.
- A simple mosquito clamp or arthroscopic loose body forceps are often used to grasp the arthroscopic graspers to remove the os once liberated from the talus.

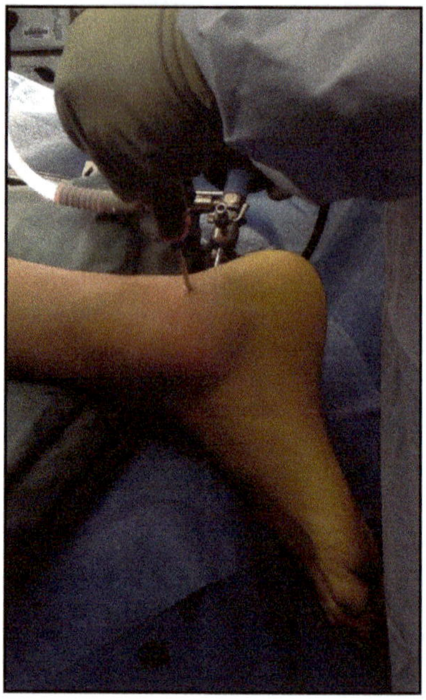

Figure 21-2. Patient position with foot overhanging the end of the operating table.

Positioning and Portals

The patient is placed in the prone position with the foot either overhanging the end of the table or supported with an angular cushion placed underneath the distal tibia (Figure 21-2).[18] A proximal leg tourniquet is applied while ensuring that the ankle joint is free for manipulation during the procedure. Frequently, dorsiflexion is adequate for allowing access to the posterior talus, but distraction can be utilized to allow further visualization if necessary.[19] Arthroscopic PAI surgery can be offered on an outpatient basis and is performed with the patient under general or spinal anesthesia, often with an additional regional block.[4]

Step-by-Step Description of the Procedure

After proper patient positioning is achieved, careful attention must be directed toward correct arthroscopic portal placement. A horizontal line from the tip of the medial malleolus is made using a marking pen. The lateral and medial borders of the Achilles tendon should also be palpated and marked. The posterolateral portal can be marked 5 mm lateral to the Achilles at the level of the horizontal line (Figure 21-3). A small 10-mm skin incision should be made initially, followed by subcutaneous blunt dissection using a mosquito clamp. A 2.7-mm arthroscope sleeve with trocar is then introduced and judiciously advanced to touch the posterior aspect of the talus by directing it toward the first interdigital web space. Care should be taken to avoid damage to the sural nerve while advancing the trocar. Once bone can be palpated with the trocar, it is switched out for a 2.7-mm arthroscope. Poor visualization of the posterior facet is a common finding as a result of the soft tissue cicatrization and the presence of a fat pad in this area; this requires careful debridement with the shaver once the medial portal has been established.

After placement of the lateral portal, attention should be turned to the medial portal. The medial portal should be created under direct visualization to avoid the neurovascular structures. The skin incision can be made at the level of the horizontal line 5 mm medial to the Achilles tendon, and blunt dissection is once again carried out using a mosquito clamp. Under direct

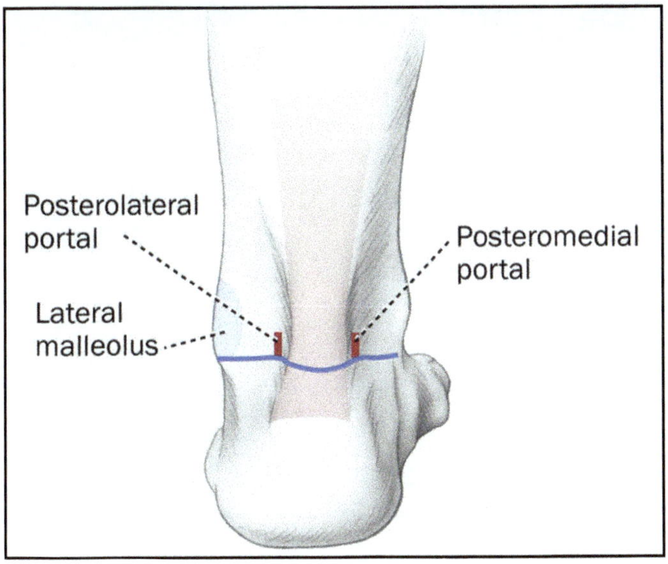

Figure 21-3. Portal sites.

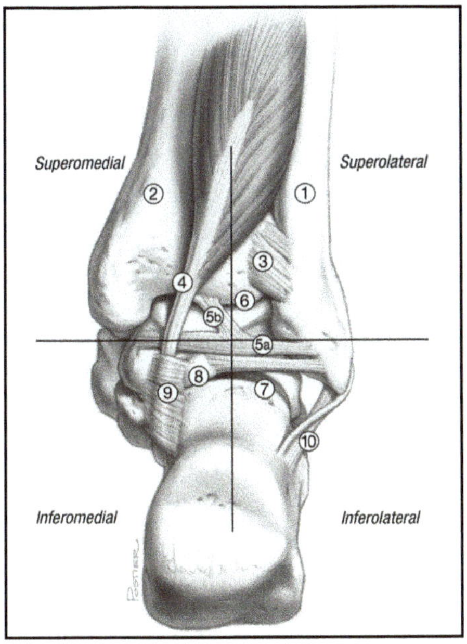

Figure 21-4. 4-quadrant approach to posterior arthroscopy. Hindfoot extra-articular structures divided into quadrants as defined by the intermalleolar ligament. (1) Fibula. (2) Tibia. (3) Posterior inferior tibiofibular ligament. (4) FHL tendon. (5a) Intermalleolar ligament. (5b) Superior tibial insertion of the intermalleolar ligament. (6) Tibiotalar joint. (7) Subtalar joint. (8) Posterolateral talar process. (9) FHL retinaculum. (10) Calcaneofibular ligament. (Illustration copyright of and reproduced with permission from J. G. Kennedy, MD. Reproduction without express written consent is prohibited. From Smyth NA, Murawski CD, Levine DS, Kennedy JG. Hindfoot arthroscopic surgery for posterior ankle impingement: a systematic surgical approach and case series. *Am J Sports Med.* 2013;41(8):1869-1876.)

visualization, a 2.7-mm arthroscope sleeve and trocar can be advanced to touch the posterior aspect of the talus. Once confident that correct portal placement has been achieved, a 3.5-mm followed by a 4.5-mm resector can be introduced via the medial portal, and cautious debridement of soft tissue will allow for adequate visualization prior to proceeding with the indicated surgical procedure.

Posterior ankle arthroscopy is best approached in a systematic way. A suggested 4-quadrant approach (superolateral, superomedial, inferomedial, and inferolateral) allows full assessment of all structures at the posterior ankle and subtalar joints (Figure 21-4).[20]

The anatomic landmark for defining the quadrants is the intermalleolar ligament along with its superior tibial insertion. The main portion of the intermalleolar ligament is a horizontal structure that delineates the superior quadrants from the inferior quadrants. The tibial attachment of the ligament lies obliquely and further divides the quadrants into the medial and lateral orientation.

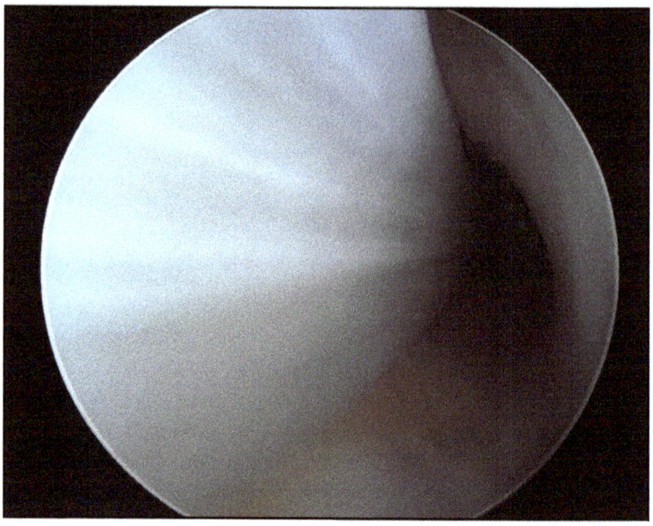

Figure 21-5. Arthroscopic view of the FHL in tunnel.

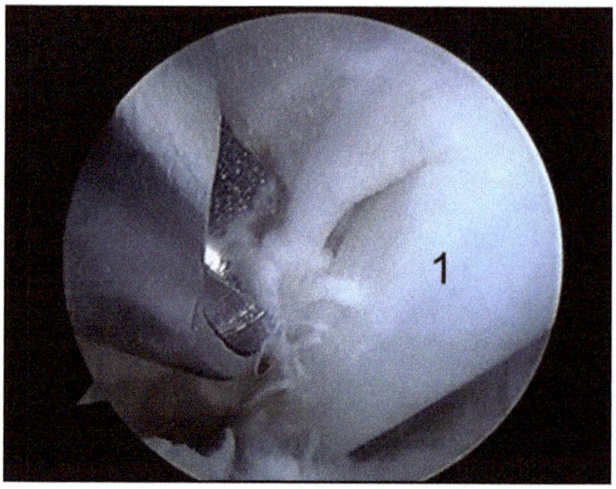

Figure 21-6. Debridement of the FHL tendon. (1) FHL. (Illustration copyright of and reproduced with permission from J. G. Kennedy, MD. Reproduction without express written consent is prohibited. From Smyth NA, Murawski CD, Levine DS, Kennedy JG. Hindfoot arthroscopic surgery for posterior ankle impingement: a systematic surgical approach and case series. *Am J Sports Med.* 2013;41(8):1869-1876.)

Inspection starts in the superolateral quadrant, which contains the posterior tibiofibular ligament. This area must be carefully inspected in cases of suspected high ankle sprains. Visualization of the intermalleolar ligament is then required, looking for any thickening or impingement, and confirmed by plantarflexing the ankle under direct visualization to assess for impingement of the ligament with the osseous structures.

The impinging areas can be resected, but otherwise the intermalleolar ligament is left intact. The landmark for the superomedial quadrant is the FHL tendon and its associated fibro-osseous tunnel (Figure 21-5). Tenosynovitis is a common finding in patients with ankle pain. By flexing the great toe, impingement of the tendon in its sheath can be identified and resected using a 4.5-mm resector if required (Figure 21-6). The inferomedial quadrant can then be inspected for a prominent Stieda process or separate os trigonum (Figure 21-7) and, if present, these can be removed using a 0.25-inch osteotome with care taken to avoid the subtalar joint. The FHL sheath is then able to be accessed with an arthroscope to allow full visualization of the tendon along its length with debridement as needed for vincula and cicatrization.

The final extra-articular quadrant to be inspected is the inferolateral region, which contains the posterior talofibular ligament and which may be thickened in the presence of posterior impingement requiring debridement. The calcaneofibular ligament is also able to be visualized at this time, and its integrity should be assessed.

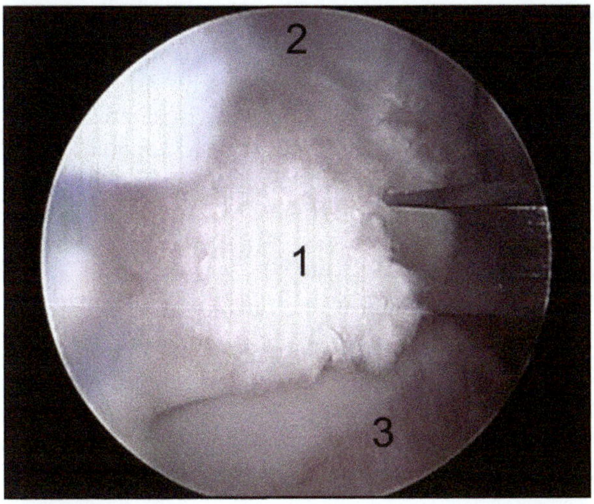

Figure 21-7. Stieda process being removed with an osteotome. (1) Stieda process. (2) Talus. (3) Calcaneus. (Illustration copyright of and reproduced with permission from J. G. Kennedy, MD. Reproduction without express written consent is prohibited. From Smyth NA, Murawski CD, Levine DS, Kennedy JG. Hindfoot arthroscopic surgery for posterior ankle impingement: a systematic surgical approach and case series. *Am J Sports Med.* 2013;41(8):1869-1876.)

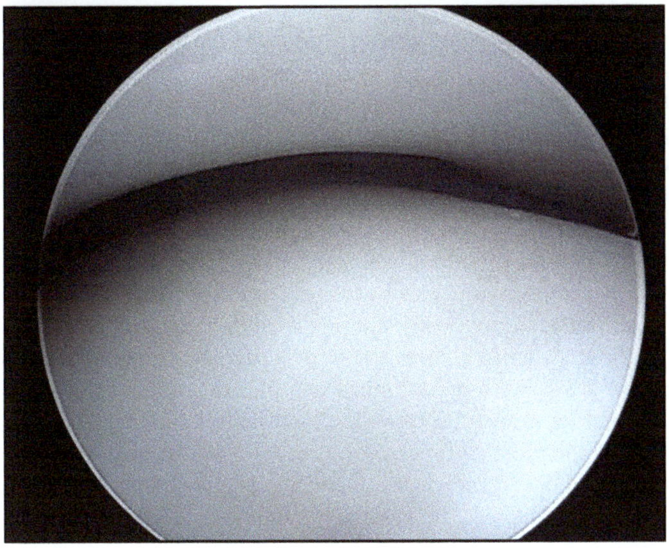

Figure 21-8. Subtalar joint.

Once the extra-articular structures have been systematically assessed and any pathology addressed, the articular surfaces of the ankle and subtalar joints must be examined. The tibial plafond and talar dome are able to be visualized by manually dorsiflexing the ankle joint. Any chondral lesions should be debrided and bone marrow stimulation techniques employed to encourage mesenchymal stem cell migration and chondral healing. Subtalar articular surfaces are assessed and treated in the same manner, and both can be visualized using the same standard portals as described (Figure 21-8).

Postoperative Protocol

PAI arthroscopic surgeries are typically outpatient procedures with patients returning home the same day without ankle immobilization. For the following 7 to 10 days, patients are instructed to keep the lower limb elevated and are put on a 10-day course of nonsteroidal anti-inflammatory drugs to reduce pain and swelling. Icing the ankle allows for additional pain relief and aids in reducing inflammation as well. Many surgeons suggest patients begin weightbearing with assistance from crutches as tolerated from day 1 of the operation with progressive increases in weightbearing by the end of week 1.[21,22] Early mobilization and range of motion exercises including ankle pumps, up to 10 minutes repeated multiple times per day, aids in preventing cicatrization.[4] From the second day postoperatively, weightbearing is allowed as tolerated by the patient. It is expected that the patient should be fully weightbearing by 1 week postoperatively. It is recommended that patients begin a physical therapy regimen with emphasis on restoring full ankle range of motion and FHL flexion if tendon pathology was addressed during the procedure. Early weightbearing is not always advised to patients who underwent significant removal of bony structures. Standard suture removal can be done at week 2 and previous activity level can be resumed once pain subsides.[23,24] In addition, if the patient underwent concomitant procedures at the time of surgery, such as lateral ligament reconstruction, then the postoperative course must be modified accordingly. This includes the use of a postoperative splint, nonweightbearing for 2 weeks, followed by a 2-week period of protected weightbearing at 10% of weight body. Over the following 2 weeks, weightbearing is increased so that the patient is full weightbearing by 6 weeks postoperatively, at which time he or she can transition into a functional physical therapy program.

Potential Complications

Complication rates for posterior ankle arthroscopies for PAI have been shown to be between 2.3% and 8.5%, which compares favorably to an open approach complication rate of 15.9%.[9,13,25,26] The 2 primary sites of potential complications during the 2-portal technique are damage to the sural nerve on the lateral side and neurovascular bundle (tibial nerve, posterior tibial artery, and vein) on the medial side. In a cadaveric MRI study, the sural nerve was found to be located 3.2 mm from the posterolateral portal and the neurovascular bundle was located 6.4 mm medial to the posteromedial portal.[27] Thus, the proximity of both structures to the surgical sites demands an intimate knowledge of hindfoot anatomy and experience performing arthroscopic procedures.[18] Despite the proximity of these structures, a review of 311 posterior ankle arthroscopies revealed a total complication rate of 2.3%, with neurological complications being the most common.[25] Another study including 189 ankles found the complication rate to be higher at 8.5%, with neurological complications again being the most common.[26] In the same study, postoperative Achilles tendon tightness was reported in 2.1% of procedures. Smyth and colleagues examined 7 case series totaling 385 posterior ankle arthroscopies and found a complication rate of 6.2%.[4] Not surprising given the close proximity of the sural nerve to the posterolateral portal, it has been shown that neurological complications are most common.[25] In the Nickisch and colleagues study of 189 ankles noted previously,[26] sural nerve dysesthesia and plantar numbness accounted for 19% and 25% of postoperative complications, respectively. For this reason, it is recommended that the initial incision should be made no deeper than the skin and blunt dissection through the subcutaneous tissue and should proceed using a hemostat. Care should be taken when exchanging instruments through portals and during surgical manipulation.[26]

Infection rates during arthroscopic surgery in general are relatively low, ranging from 0.01% to 0.48%, and have been reported to be as low as 0.6% for posterior ankle arthroscopies. However, reports have been as high as 1.1%.[25,28]

A relatively uncommon and poorly understood process is the development of complex regional pain syndrome (CRSP), also known as *reflex sympathetic dystrophy*, following arthroscopic surgery. Nickisch and colleagues, in the same study noted previously, reported the development of CRSP in 1.1% of PAI procedures.[26,29] A study analyzing CRSP at 4 European hospitals found that, of all CRSP diagnoses, surgery accounted for 24.8% of the cases.[29] It has been reported that physiotherapy, local anesthetics, corticosteroids, and gamma-Aminobutyric acid analogs can offer treatment with resolution of symptoms.[26,29,30] CRSP is a complicated pathology with unknown etiology and no definitive treatment course, warranting further investigation.[31]

Conclusion

A posterior ankle arthroscopic approach is a safe procedure once the anatomy is known and approached in a systematic fashion. The open approach by comparison can have a complication rate of up to 24%; therefore, open surgery is rarely indicated for these procedures.[32]

Top Technical Pearls for the Procedure

1. The patient is placed in the prone position with the foot either overhanging the end of the table or supported with an angular cushion placed underneath the distal tibia.
2. Correct portal placement is key to visualization.
3. A 4-quadrant approach (superolateral, superomedial, inferomedial, and inferolateral) allows full assessment of all structures at the posterior ankle and subtalar joints.
4. The shaver blade must always be under endoscopic view.
5. Keep lateral to the FHL tendon to avoid damaging neurovascular structures.

References

1. Van Dijk CN. Anterior and posterior ankle impingement. *Foot Ankle Clin.* 2006;11(3):663-683.
2. Brodsky AE, Khalil MA. Talar compression syndrome. *Foot Ankle.* 1987;7(6):338-344.
3. Rogers J, Dijkstra P, Mccourt P, et al. Posterior ankle impingement syndrome: a clinical review with reference to horizontal jump athletes. *Acta Orthop Belg.* 2010;76(5):572-579.
4. Smyth NA, Zwiers R, Wiegerinck JI, et al. Posterior hindfoot arthroscopy: a review. *Am J Sports Med.* 2014;42(1): 225-234.
5. Hamilton WG, Geppert MJ, Thompson FM. Pain in the posterior aspect of the ankle in dancers. Differential diagnosis and operative treatment. *J Bone Joint Surg Am.* 1996;78(10):1491-1500.
6. Sammarco GJ, Cooper PS. Flexor hallucis longus tendon injury in dancers and nondancers. *Foot Ankle Int.* 1998;19:356-362.
7. Hedrick MR, McBryde AM. Posterior ankle impingement. *Foot Ankle Int.* 1994;15:2-8.
8. Roche AJ, Calder JD, Lloyd Williams R. Posterior ankle impingement in dancers and athletes. *Foot Ankle Clin.* 2013;18(2):301-318.
9. Zwiers R, Wiegerinck JI, Murawski CD, Smyth NA, Kennedy JG, van Dijk CN. Surgical treatment for posterior ankle impingement. *Arthroscopy.* 2013;29(7):1263-1270.
10. Pearce CJ, Calder JDF. Posterior ankle arthroscopy in sports: Posterior impingement/os trigonum. *Oper Tech Orthop.* 2008;18:271-276.
11. Rockett MS, Waitches G, Sudakoff G, Brage M. Use of ultrasonography versus magnetic resonance imaging for tendon abnormalities around the ankle. *Foot Ankle Int.* 1998;19:604-612.
12. Waitches GM, Rockett M, Brage M, Sudakoff G. Ultrasonographic surgical correlation of ankle tendon tears. *J Ultrasound Med.* 1998;17:249-256.
13. Van Dijk CN. Hindfoot endoscopy. *Foot Ankle Clin.* 2006;11(2):391-414.
14. Theobald P, Bydder G, Dent C, Nokes L, Pugh N, Benjamin M. The functional anatomy of Kager's fat pad in relation to retrocalcaneal problems and other hindfoot disorders. *J Anat.* 2006;208(1):91-97.
15. Loomer R, Fisher C, Lloyd-Smith R, Sisler J, Cooney T. Osteochondral lesions of the talus. *Am J Sports Med.* 1993;21(1):13-19.
16. Lüsse S, Claassen H, Gehrke T, et al. Evaluation of water content by spatially resolved transverse relaxation times of human articular cartilage. *Magn Reson Imaging.* 2000;18(4):423-430.

17. Verhagen RA, Maas M, Dijkgraaf MG, Tol JL, Krips R, van Dijk CN. Prospective study on diagnostic strategies in osteochondral lesions of the talus: is MRI superior to helical CT? *J Bone Joint Surg Br.* 2005;87:41-46.
18. Van Dijk CN, Scholten PE, Krips R. A 2-portal endoscopic approach for diagnosis and treatment of posterior ankle pathology. *Arthroscopy.* 2000;16(8):871-876.
19. Beals TC, Junko JT, Amendola A, Nickisch F, Saltzman CL. Minimally invasive distraction technique for prone posterior ankle and subtalar arthroscopy. *Foot Ankle Int.* 2010;31:316-319.
20. Smyth NA, Murawski CD, Levine DS, Kennedy JG. Hindfoot arthroscopic surgery for posterior ankle impingement: a systematic surgical approach and case series. *Am J Sports Med.* 2013;41(8):1869-1876.
21. Willits K, Sonneveld H, Amendola A, Giffin JR, Griffin S, Fowler PJ. Outcome of posterior ankle arthroscopy for hindfoot impingement. *Arthroscopy.* 2008;24(2):196-202.
22. Yilmaz Cl, Eskandari MM. Arthroscopic excision of the talar Stieda's process. *Arthroscopy.* 2006;22(2):225.
23. Calder JD, Sexton SA, Pearce CJ. Return to training and playing after posterior ankle arthroscopy for posterior impingement in elite professional soccer. *Am J Sports Med.* 2010;38:120-124.
24. Scholten PE, Sierevelt IN, van Dijk CN. Hindfoot endoscopy for posterior ankle impingement. *J Bone Joint Surg Am.* 2008;90:2665-2672.
25. Zengerink M, van Dijk CN. Complications in ankle arthroscopy. *Knee Surg Sports Traumatol Arthrosc.* 2012;20:1420-1431.
26. Nickisch F, Barg A, Saltzman CL, et al. Postoperative complications of posterior ankle and hindfoot arthroscopy. *J Bone Joint Surg Am.* 2012;94(5):439-446.
27. Sitler DF, Amendola A, Bailey CS, Thain LM, Spouge A. Posterior ankle arthroscopy: an anatomic study. *J Bone Joint Surg Am.* 2002;84:763-769.
28. Babcock HM, Matava MJ, Fraser V. Postarthroscopy surgical site infections: review of the literature. *Clin Infect Dis.* 2002;34(1):65-71.
29. Freedman M, Greis AC, Marino L, Sinha AN, Henstenburg. Complex regional pain syndrome: diagnosis and treatment. *J Phys Med Rehabil Clin N Am.* 2014;25(2):291-303.
30. De Boer RD, Marinus J, van Hilten JJ, et al. Distribution of signs and symptoms of complex regional pain syndrome type I in patients meeting the diagnostic criteria of the International Association for the Study of Pain. *Eur J Pain.* 2011;15(8):830.
31. Borchers AT, Gershwin ME. Complex regional pain syndrome: a comprehensive and critical review. *Autoimmun Rev.* 2014;13(3):242-265.
32. Abramowitz Y, Wollstein R, Barzilay Y, et al. Outcome of resection of a symptomatic os trigonum. *J Bone Joint Surg Am.* 2003;85:1051-1057.

Please visit www.routledge.com/9781617119989 to access additional material.

22

First Metatarsophalangeal Joint Arthroscopy

Youichi Yasui, MD; Ethan J. Fraser, MD, MBBS;
Alberto Marangon, MD; and John G. Kennedy, MD, MCh, FRCS

Introduction

Hallux metatarsophalangeal (MTP) joint pain is caused by various pathological conditions, including hallux valgus, hallux rigidus, osteochondral lesions, soft tissue impingement, loose bodies, gout, and osteoarthritis.[1] Although these represent separate, distinct pathological conditions, all may be caused by a combination of mechanical stress and/or biological deterioration and can coexist as concomitant pathology in many cases. Conservative treatments are therefore aimed to improve mechanical and/or biologic components and relieve symptoms. Included in the conservative management of first MTP joint pathologies are footwear modifications, orthotics, physiotherapy, steroid injection, shock wave therapy, and the use of biological adjuncts including platelet-rich plasma (PRP) injection and hyaluronic acid. However, if patients fail a 3- to 6-month trial of conservative therapy, then operative treatment is often indicated, particularly in the setting of worsening pain or function.[2,3]

First MTP joint arthroscopic procedures are being increasingly utilized as a means to treat a variety of pathologies. Typically, MTP joint arthroscopy is performed using a 2-portal approach with dorsomedial and dorsolateral portals. These are positioned on either side of the extensor hallux longus (EHL) tendon over the MTP joint.[2-5] Although still a relatively new technique, an increasing number of clinical studies suggest a favorable outcome and low complication rates when using first MTP joint arthroscopy to treat soft tissue, osseous, and cartilage pathology.[2,6,7] To optimize outcomes using this procedure, careful clinical assessment and patient selection are required to identify those patients who are suitable candidates for an arthroscopic approach, as some patients may be more appropriately treated using a traditional open approach. In addition, surgeon skill and experience are likely to play a role in outcomes, particularly given the relatively high technical difficulty associated with this procedure.

In this text, the authors review the hallux MTP joint arthroscopic procedure and describe the step-by-step operative technique.

Stone JW, Kennedy JG, Glazebrook M, eds. *The Foot and Ankle: AANA Advanced Arthroscopic Surgical Techniques* (pp 207-219).

Indications

Patient selection for first MTP joint arthroscopy is important. Although the general indications for an arthroscopic technique are the same as for an open technique, advanced disease, concomitant pathology, and certain patient factors may direct the surgeon to perform an open procedure in favor of an arthroscopic approach. Additionally, caution needs to be exercised when applying first MTP joint arthroscopy as most evidence for its use is based solely on level IV studies.

- General indications
  - Patients with first MTP joint pain who have failed 3 to 6 months of conservative therapy
  - High-demand athletes with persistent MTP joint pain or decreased function failing 6 weeks to 3 months of conservative treatment
  - Patients at risk of wound complications with open procedure
- Indicated pathology
  - Hallux rigidus (Coughlin and Shurnas grade I or II)[8]
  - Chondral or osteochondral lesion (lesion size < 50 mm^2)
    - Osteochondral lesion can be treated with bone marrow stimulation (BMS) under arthroscopy if the lesion size is less than 50 mm^2. Kim and colleagues found the 50 mm^2 area to be a critical size, beyond which clinical scores following BMS in osteochondral lesion of first MTP joint dropped significantly.[9]
  - Synovitis and soft tissue impingement
  - Loose bodies

Controversial Indications

- Hallux valgus under certain conditions
  - An arthroscopic approach may be indicated when the hallux valgus angle is less than 40 degrees and the first intermetatarsal angle is less than 25 degrees.[3,10-12]
- Gout and gouty tophi[13]
- Osteoarthritis with diminishing joint space[14]

Contraindications

- Cosmesis with no associated symptoms of pain or decreased function
- Severe osteoarthritis
- Poor vascular status
- Unacceptable surgical/anesthetic risk

Pertinent Physical Findings

- Inspection
  - Gait
  - Footwear (modifications etc)
  - Skin (intact, erythema, gouty tophi, callous formation [dorsal-hallux rigidus; medial MTP joint-hallux valgus; plantar aspect of lesser metatarsal heads suggesting overloading of lateral forefoot])

  - Calor with rubor may be found in gout or joint infection.
  - Swelling
  - Heel alignment
  - Forefoot pronation or supination
  - Hallux valgus
  - Associated clawing or hammertoe deformity may be present.
  - Dorsal MTP joint protuberance (hallux rigidus)
- Palpation
  - Joint line tenderness (first MTP joint)
  - Pain over lesser MTP joint
  - Crepitus with movement
  - Planovalgus alignment-associated Achilles or plantar fascia pain may be present.
  - Effusion
  - Positive Tinel's test may accompany most first MTP joint pathology from capsular swelling and dorsal osteophytes. This is critical to map out and record before any surgical intervention.
- Range of motion
  - Hallux rigidus/osteoarthritis
    - Pain and limitation of motion with MTP joint dorsiflexion
    - Limitation of movement may be a mechanical block and/or soft tissue impingement.
    - Crepitus
    - Pain during push phase of gait noted
    - Pain with "grind test" (passive movement with axial load)
  - Hallux valgus
    - Hypermobility of first ray often present
    - Pain with passive and active motion
    - Pain with movement of the lateral MTP joint may be present.
    - Important to examine for pes planus and hindfoot, midfoot, and forefoot range of motion

Pertinent Imaging

Radiography

- Recommended views include standard anteroposterior, oblique, and lateral foot views with weightbearing and medial oblique (sesamoid view).
  - First-line imaging in suspected first MTP joint pathology
  - Joint incongruity
  - Narrowing of joint space
  - Sclerotic change of joint surface
  - Osteophyte formation
  - Bipartite sesamoid, sesamoid retraction (turf toe), or fracture
    - Comparison to contralateral anatomy is helpful.

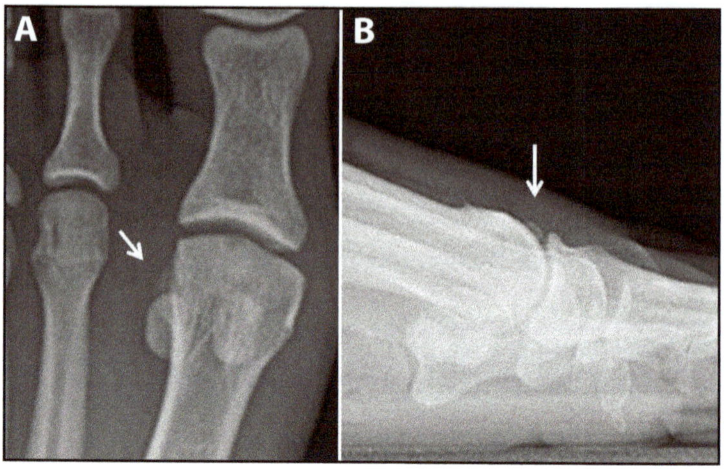

Figure 22-1. (A) Anteroposterior and (B) lateral radiographs showing loose bodies in the first MTP joint space.

- ▹ Loose bodies in the joint space (Figure 22-1)
- ▹ May show osteochondral lesion, although not a sensitive diagnostic modality for this purpose
- ▹ Calcification and fractures
- ▹ Hallux valgus angle, intermetatarsal angle, and talonavicular angle in standard anteroposterior view must be evaluated for a diagnosis of hallux valgus deformity.
- ▹ Talar-first metatarsal and calcaneal inclination angles in lateral view must be evaluated. These angles show whether abnormal foot morphology exists.
- ▹ Grading in hallux rigidus is dependent on radiograph findings as well as physical examination findings.[15]

Magnetic Resonance Imaging

- Useful in assessing soft tissue involvement osseous abnormalities and cartilage lesions
- "Gold standard" for most first MTP joint pathology
- Useful in the detection of the following:
  - ▹ First MTP joint effusion
  - ▹ Osteophyte formation and associated soft tissue impingement
  - ▹ Osteochondral lesion
- Location and size of osteochondral lesion must be evaluated (Figure 22-2A)
  - ▹ Bursitis
  - ▹ Bone marrow edema
  - ▹ Isolated soft tissue impingement
  - ▹ Degenerative joint changes (cartilage loss, bone cyst, subchondral sclerosis)
  - ▹ Plantar plate tear (helpful in grading turf toe I through III, and also grading reliant on physical examination findings)
  - ▹ Loose body (Figure 22-2B)
  - ▹ Surrounding ligament injury, tendon injury, neuritis, neuroma, or fracture

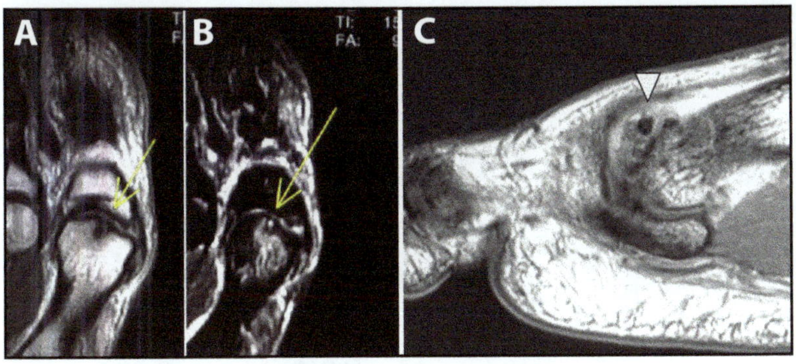

Figure 22-2. MRI of the first MTP joint. On the axial view, (A) the T1 image shows an osteochondral defect, while (B) the T2 image demonstrates significant bony edema. (C) The sagittal image shows a loose osteochondral fragment associated with lesion.

Computed Tomography

- Less useful modality than magnetic resonance imaging for most first MTP joint pathologies
- Effective to evaluate whether osseous loose body exists
- May be used to assess osteochondral lesions with extensive osseous involvement (uncommon)

Equipment

- Thigh tourniquet
- General arthroscopy equipment
- A monitor, light source, and control unit for both the camera and motorized shaver and other instruments are required in all cases. The monitor should be at the surgeon's eye line.
- Finger trap with holder apparatus and 3 to 5 kg of weight (optional) is useful to distract the first MTP joint
- Irrigation system (pressure: 30 to 60 mm Hg; fluid flow: 0.5 to l/min)
- A 1.9-, 2.5-, or 2.7-mm arthroscope with a 30- or 70-degree viewing angle. A 70-degree arthroscope can be useful but is usually not necessary.
- 2.5-mm shaver for soft tissue debridement
- 2.0-mm curette
- Small, curved, and straight hemostats
- A 2.5-mm bone resector for debridement of osseous structures/osteophytes
- Small microfracture awl or Kirschner wire (1.0 mm)
- 22-gauge needle
- Fluoroscopy
- Elastic bandage

Positioning and Portals

The patient is placed into the supine position. A finger trap is applied to the great toe and secured with sterile elastic wrap. Gravity distraction allows access to the joint. Careful positioning of the hanging distractor will prevent issues with portal access once the surgery is underway (Figure 22-3).

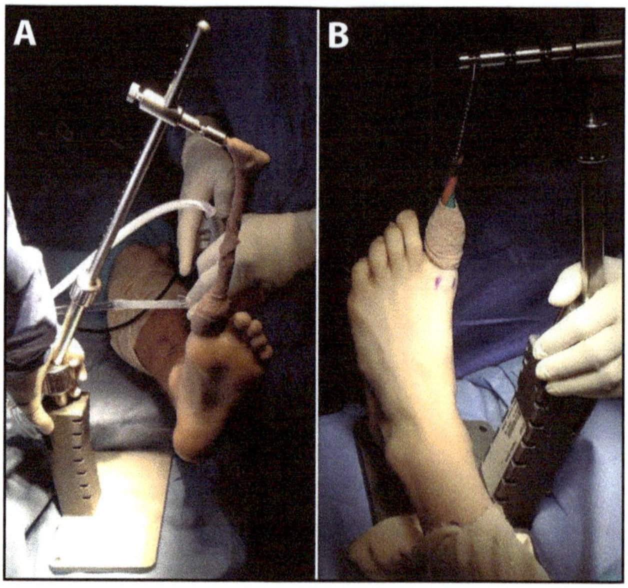

Figure 22-3. Surgical positioning demonstrated on (A) plantar and (B) dorsal views.

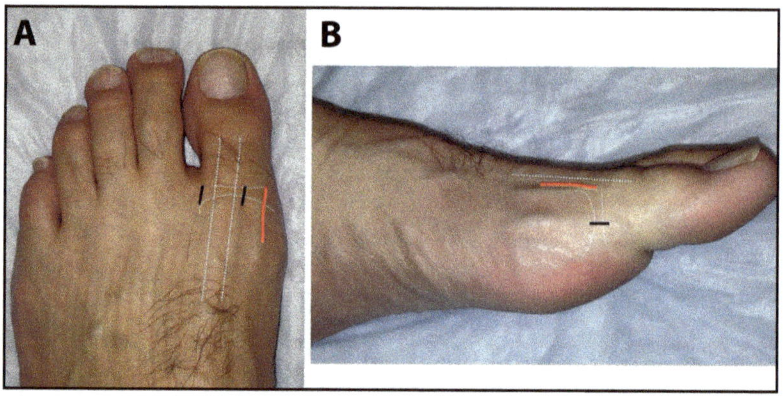

Figure 22-4. Marking anatomic landmarks and location of arthroscopic portals. (A) White longitudinal lines represent the EHL tendon; white tranverse lines represent the joint space; black lines represent portal locations (dorsomedial and dorsolateral); and the red line shows the location of the nerve. (B) Medial portal location shown (black line).

The authors prefer a tourniquet applied on the proximal thigh because an ankle or calf tourniquet may interfere with excursion of the EHL or flexor hallucis longus tendon.

- Marking anatomic landmarks and location of arthroscopic portals (Figure 22-4)
  - Marking of surface anatomy and portals sites is required prior to skin incision.
  - The lateral and medial edges of the EHL tendon, proximal edge of the first proximal phalangeal bone, and distal edge of the first metatarsal bone should be identified and marked out with a surgical pen (see Figure 22-4).
  - Marking of the dorsal cutaneous nerves on the medial and lateral aspects of the hallux should be carried out (see Figure 22-4).
    - The dorsomedial cutaneous nerve can often be palpated approximately 10 mm medial to the dorsomedial portal site. It is important to palpate and perform a Tinel's test before any incision is made to establish if there is any pre-existing nerve compression.[4]
  - Six portal sites for the first MTP joint arthroscopy are described. The dorsomedial and dorsolateral are the most commonly utilized. Others include medial, medial plantar, toe web, and proximal medial portals. The authors prefer dorsomedial, dorsolateral, and medial portals.

- Dorsomedial, dorsolateral, and medial portals
  - The dorsolateral portal should be marked out prior to establishing the portal. It is positioned at the level of the first MTP joint line, 2.0 mm lateral to the lateral edge EHL tendon.
  - A line is drawn from the bisector line of the first metatarsal bone to the proximal phalanx when the joint is in neutral alignment.
  - The dorsomedial portal should be positioned approximately 2.0 mm medial to the EHL tendon. This will generally avoid the neurovascular structures, which are located approximately 4 mm medial to the EHL tendon.
  - Portals located too close to the EHL tendon may cause interference between the instrument and arthroscope due to the small joint space.
  - The medial portal(s) should be marked at the level of the MTP joint line and 2.0 mm inferior to the bisector line (see Figure 22-4B).
- Plantar medial portal
  - A plantar medial portal has been described to access the metatarsosesamoid compartment, particularly when soft tissue release is required in the hallux valgus.[16]
  - Location of the plantar medial portal is 4.0 mm proximal to the joint line between the abductor hallucis tendon and the medial head of the flexor hallucis brevis.
- Toe web lateral
  - A toe web portal has been described for medial soft tissue release in the hallux valgus and sesamoidectomy.
  - The portal site is on the dorsal surface of the first web approximately 4.0 mm proximal and medial.

Step-by-Step Description of the Procedure

- Step 1: Creating the dorsolateral portal
  - With the great toe placed in traction, the joint line should be identified with palpation.
  - A 22-gauge needle is inserted into the first MTP joint via the dorsolateral portal site marked previously. Penetration of the joint capsule is often noted as a "popping" type of sensation as the needle tip passes through it.
  - Once the joint space is entered, 5.0 mL of saline is then injected into the first MTP joint (Figure 22-5A).
  - A vertical skin incision 3.0 to 5.0 mm in length is made over the dorsolateral joint. Care should be taken to avoid damage to the cartilage by only incising the superficial tissues (Figure 22-5B).
  - Subcutaneous, blunt dissection is then performed using a small hemostat through the skin incision (Figure 22-5C). Again, care should be taken to avoid damage to the cartilage.
- Step 2: Creating the dorsomedial portal and medial portal
  - The arthroscope sleeve with a blunt trocar is introduced via the dorsolateral portal and carefully advanced into the joint space (Figure 22-6A).
  - Once the cartilage is palpated with the trocar, the arthroscope is introduced (Figure 22-6B).
  - With the operating room lighting dimmed or off, the arthroscopic view of the dorsomedial joint may highlight the silhouette of dorsomedial cutaneous nerve through the skin.

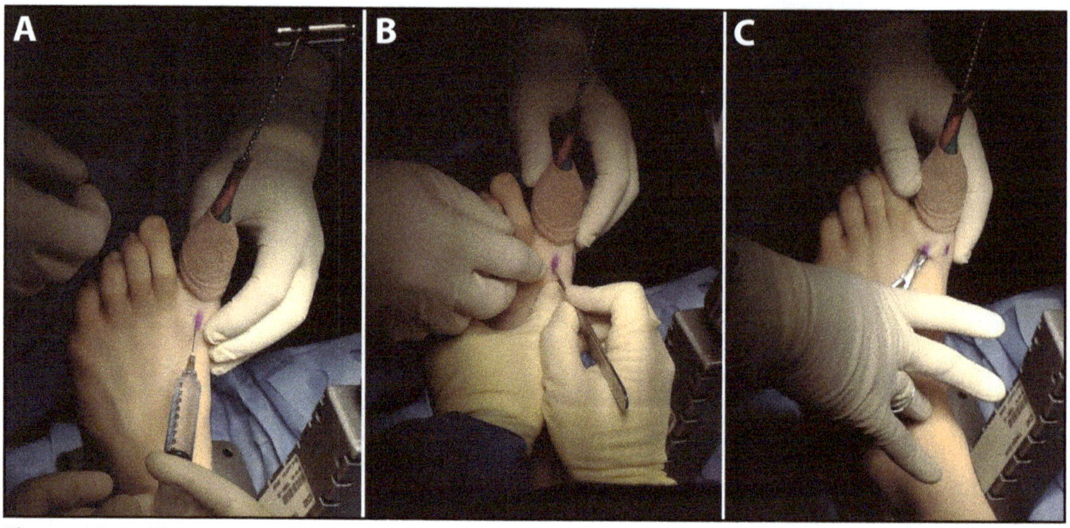

Figure 22-5. (A) Five-mL saline injected into joint space. (B) A vertical skin incision(s) 3.0 to 5.0 mm in length is made over the dorsolateral aspect of the joint. Care should be taken to avoid damage to cartilage by only incising the superficial tissues. (C) Subcutaneous, blunt dissection is then performed using a small hemostat through the skin incision.

Figure 22-6. (A) The arthroscope sleeve with a blunt trocar is introduced via a dorsolateral portal and judiciously advanced into the joint space. (B) Once cartilage can be palpated with the trocar, it is switched out to the arthroscope.

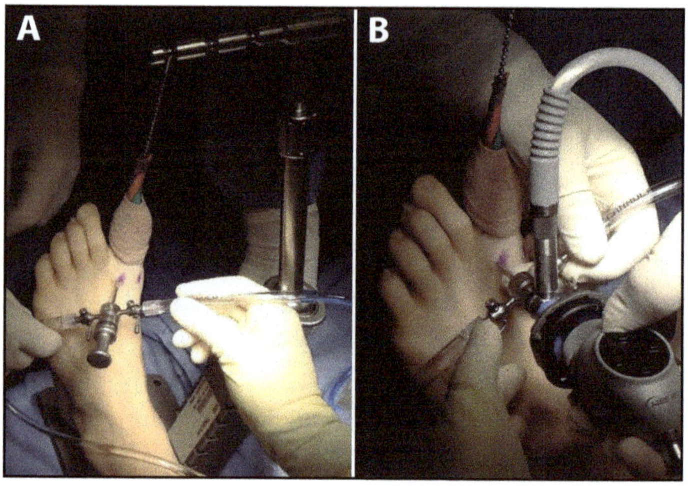

- ▹ If the previously marked dorsomedial portal site avoids the nerve, then a 22-gauge needle may be inserted into the joint at this point under direct visualization (Figure 22-7).
- ▹ After confirming that the tip of the needle is in the joint, the needle is removed and a vertical skin incision 3.0 to 5.0 mm in length is made over the marked portal position.
- ▹ Subcutaneous blunt dissection(s) using a mosquito clamp or hemostat is performed. Care should be taken to avoid damage to the cartilage by this maneuver.
- ▹ As with the dorsolateral portal, a blunt trocar should first be introduced and then removed after confirming a good position arthroscopically.

- ► Step 3: Debridement of soft tissue
  - ▹ Debridement of soft tissue with the shaver via dorsomedial or medial portals is performed. Poor visualization is not an uncommon finding as a result of the soft tissue inflammation and cicatrization (Figure 22-8).

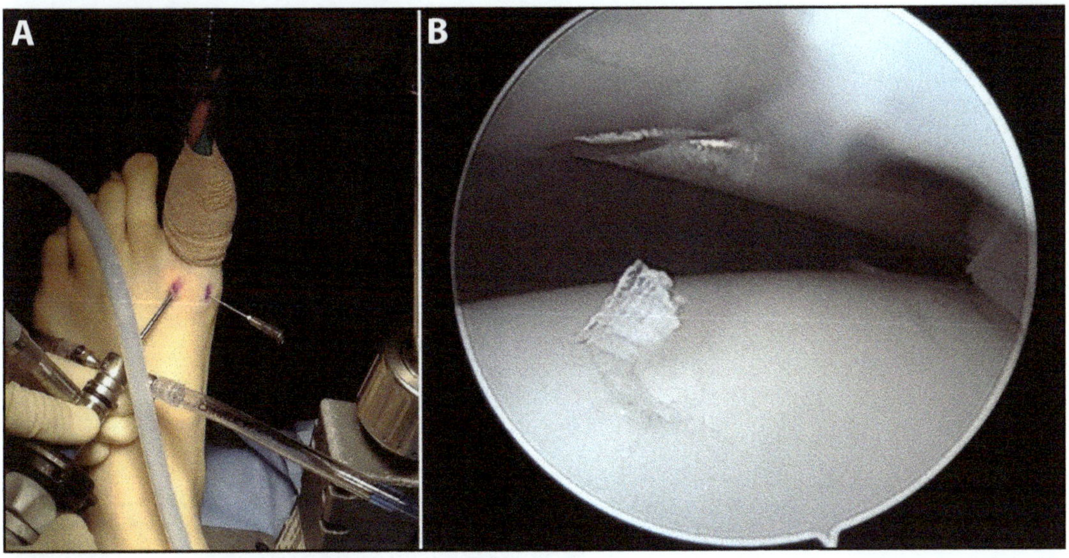

Figure 22-7. (A) With the arthroscope in the lateral portal, (B) a 22-gauge needle can be inserted at this point into the joint space under direct visualization.

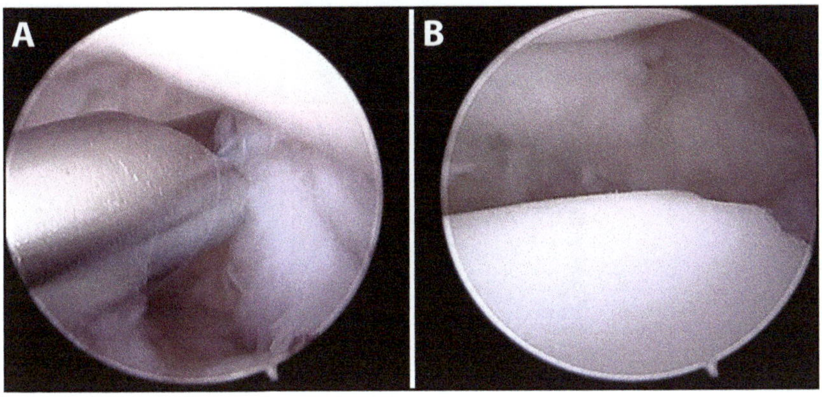

Figure 22-8. (A) Soft tissue inflammation and cicatrization cleared with a 2.5-mm shaver to improve view (B) before any further intra-articular pathology can be addressed.

- ▹ The shaver blade must always be visible to avoid iatrogenic injury to healthy tissue.
- ▹ Portals for the arthroscope and shaver are switched when necessary for optimal access to all pathology and to achieve adequate debridement.
- ▹ Once appropriate debridement of synovitis and scar is achieved, the cartilage of the first MPT joint can be evaluated.

- ▸ Step 4: Evaluation for pathological lesions
  - ▹ A standard probe is utilized under direct visualization to evaluate for any pathological disorder.
  - ▹ The authors prefer a systematic review proposed by Ferkel.[17]
- ▸ Step 5: Treatment of each pathological lesion
  - ▹ Hallux rigidus (grade 1 or 2 in grading of Coughlin and Shurnas)
    - ◆ Osteophytes are debrided using a 2.5-mm aggressive shaver via the dorsal portals. Both portals can be utilized to introduce the shaver as this will facilitate improved visualization and debridement of osteophytes and soft tissue impingement (Figure 22-9).

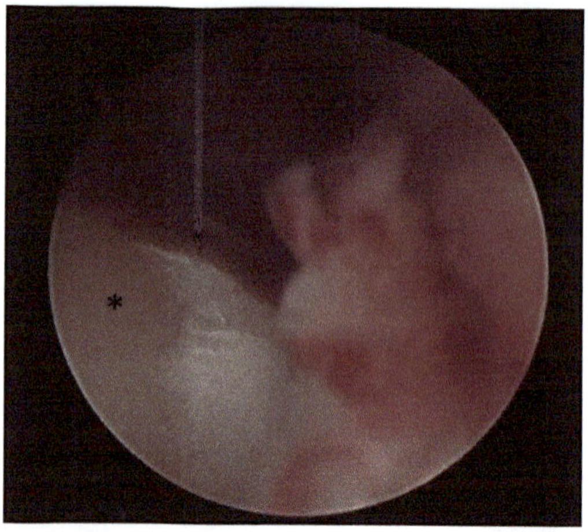

Figure 22-9. Both portals can be utilized to introduce the shaver as this will facilitate improved visualization and debridement of osteophytes and soft tissue impingement. * represents metatarsal head.

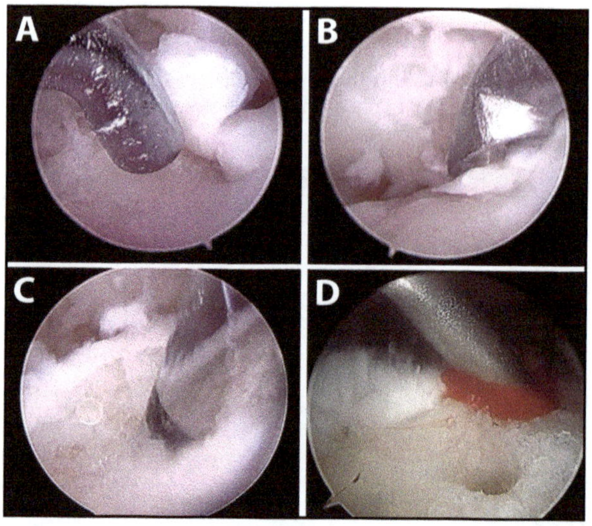

Figure 22-10. Osteochondral lesion (lesion size less than 50 mm^2). (A) Loose cartilage. (B) Spinal curette debridement. (C) Micro-awl with a 1.0 mm diameter is used for BMS. (D) Biologic adjunct injected to subchondral bone.

- Once appropriate debridement of the bony prominence is achieved, traction should be removed and passive range of motion tested under direct or fluoroscopic views. Dorsiflexion and plantarflexion angles achieved under anesthetic should be recorded.

▹ Osteochondral lesion (lesion size less than 50 mm^2; Figure 22-10)

- Dorsomedial, dorsolateral, and medial portals are sufficient for the treatment of osteochondral lesions of the first MTP joint.
- Unstable cartilage is debrided using a small curette and a 2.5-mm shaver until exposure of stable cartilage rim is achieved (see Figure 22-10).
- Once appropriate debridement for bony prominence is achieved, the lesion size is measured under the arthroscopic view.
- BMS is performed when the lesion is less than 50 mm^2. The authors utilize a 1.0-mm microfracture pick to make 3.0-mm deep perforations at 3-mm intervals in order to prevent destruction of underlying subchondral bone.
- Bleeding of subchondral bone following BMS can be confirmed by reducing the tourniquet pressure momentarily and stopping water flow. This bleeding signifies adequate BMS to allow migration of mesenchymal stem cells, growth factors, and formation of fibrin clot at the site of injury.

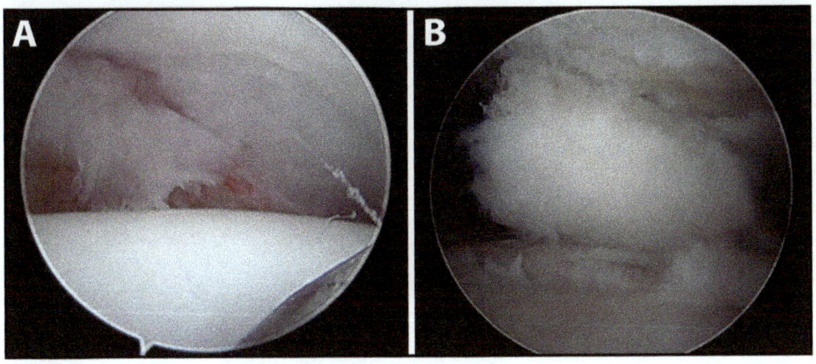

Figure 22-11. (A) Debridement of cicatrization tissue and area of synovitis is achieved using a 2.5-mm shaver. (B) Loose bodies, once identified, should be removed.

- [Optional] Biologic enhancement with PRP or bone marrow concentrate (BMC) can be performed at the BMS site.

▹ Synovitis and soft tissue impingement

- Dorsomedial, dorsolateral, and medial portals are sufficient for the treatment of synovitis and soft tissue impingement.
- Debridement of cicatrization tissue and the area of synovitis is achieved using a 2.5-mm shaver (Figure 22-11A).
- Care should be taken to avoid iatrogenic damage to articular cartilage.

▹ Loose bodies

- Loose bodies should be removed (Figure 22-11B).
- Care should be taken to avoid damage to the cartilage.
- The authors prefer to suction loose bodies whenever possible as the surfaces of loose bodies are often too smooth to be easily grasped using hemostats.
- Some cases will require the use of small hemostats, and this should always be done with full arthroscopic visualization of the tips of the hemostats.

► Step 6: Evaluation following each procedure

▹ Fluoroscopy can be used to assess postoperative alignment and range of motion of the first MTP joint.

► Step 7: [Optional]

▹ PRP and BMC can be injected into the first MTP joint (Figure 22-12).

► Step 8: Skin closure

▹ Nylon is used to suture skin incisions.

► Step 9: Immobilization

▹ Compressive bandage immobilization is applied.

Postoperative Protocol

First MTP arthroscopy is typically performed as an outpatient procedure with patients returning home the same day. Patients are instructed to keep the operative limb elevated with ice applied to reduce pain and swelling. Nonsteroidal anti-inflammatory medications may be useful in the acute phase. Suture removal can be done at postoperative week 2. Physiotherapy can be initiated soon after surgery. Range of motion exercise and full weightbearing as tolerated are advised soon after surgery. Returning to sports activity can be permitted after complete skin healing.

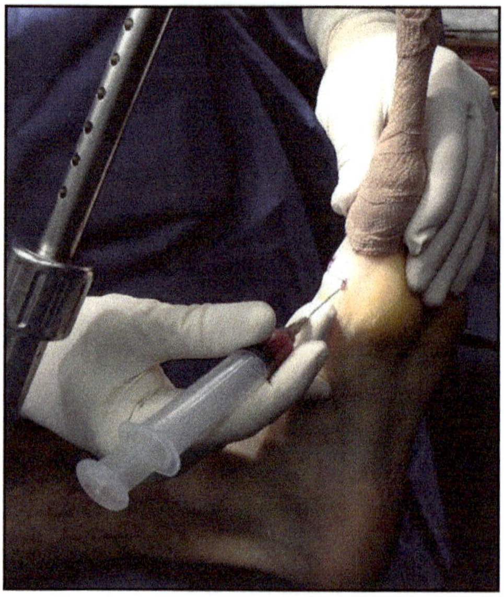

Figure 22-12. PRP and BMC can be injected into the first MTP joint at the end of the procedure where there is concern for cartilage loss or wear.

Potential Complications

The potential complications of hallux metatarsal joint arthroscopic procedures include wound complication, nerve injury, scar formation, persistent pain, and iatrogenic cartilage lesions.

Debnath and colleagues showed that 2 of 20 patients treated with this procedure had neurapraxia, while one patient with a large central chondral defect of the metatarsal head remained symptomatic despite synovectomy, debridement of the defect, and BMS.[2] In a study of 59 patients, Ahn and colleagues had one case (1.69%) with superficial wound infection and one case (1.69%) with transient neurapraxia of the dorsomedial aspect of first MTP joint.[3]

In the current literature, the number of iatrogenic cartilage lesions at the time of the first MTP joint arthroscopy has not been reported. However, these procedures are inherently associated with a relatively high risk of iatrogenic cartilage injury due to the limited working space of the joint and the high technical difficulty associated with this procedure.

Top Technical Pearls for the Procedure

1. Indications for hallux metatarsal joint arthroscopy include hallux rigidus (grade 1 or 2 in Coughlin and Shurnas grading), osteochondral lesion (lesion size less than 50 mm^2), synovitis, soft tissue impingement, and loose bodies.
2. The dorsal portals must be located far enough from the EHL tendon to allow good visualization while still avoiding the cutaneous nerves in the area.
3. The use of a third portal can improve the arthroscopic view and facilitate operative procedures and should be used if required.[4]
4. The shaver blade must always be used under a direct arthroscopic view because of the high risk of iatrogenic damage to the articular cartilage.
5. Biologic adjuncts may improve the biology of MTP joint and may reduce scar tissue and inflammation.

References

1. Siclari A, Piras M. Hallux metatarsophalangeal arthroscopy: indications and techniques. *Foot Ankle Clin.* 2015;20(1):109-122.
2. Debnath UK, Hemmady MV, Hariharan K. Indications for and technique of first metatarsophalangeal joint arthroscopy. *Foot Ankle Int.* 2006;27(12):1049-1054.
3. Ahn JH, Choy WS, Lee KW. Arthroscopy of the first metatarsophalangeal joint in 59 consecutive cases. *J Foot Ankle Surg.* 2012;51(2):161-167.
4. Vaseenon T, Phisitkul P. Arthroscopic debridement for first metatarsophalangeal joint arthrodesis with a 2- versus 3-portal technique: a cadaveric study. *Arthroscopy.* 2010;26(10):1363-1367.
5. Carreira DS. Arthroscopy of the hallux. *Foot Ankle Clin.* 2009;14(1):105-114.
6. van Dijk CN, Veenstra KM, Nuesch BC. Arthroscopic surgery of the metatarsophalangeal first joint. *Arthroscopy.* 1998;14(8):851-855.
7. Davies MS, Saxby TS. Arthroscopy of the first metatarsophalangeal joint. *J Bone Joint Surg Br.* 1999;81(2):203-206.
8. Hunt KJ. Hallux metatarsophalangeal (MTP) joint arthroscopy for hallux rigidus. *Foot Ankle Int.* 2015;36(1):113-119.
9. Kim YS, Park EH, Lee HJ, Koh YG, Lee JW. Clinical comparison of the osteochondral autograft transfer system and subchondral drilling in osteochondral defects of the first metatarsal head. *Am J Sports Med.* 2012;40(8):1824-1833.
10. Coughlin MJ, Shurnas PS. Hallux rigidus. Grading and long-term results of operative treatment. *J Bone Joint Surg Am.* 2003;85-A(11):2072-2088.
11. Lui TH, Chan KB, Chow HT, Ma CM, Chan PK, Ngai WK. Arthroscopy-assisted correction of hallux valgus deformity. *Arthroscopy.* 2008;24(8):875-880.
12. Lui TH. First metatarsophalangeal joint arthroscopy in patients with hallux valgus. *Arthroscopy.* 2008;24(10):1122-1129.
13. Siclari A, Decantis V. Arthroscopic lateral release and percutaneous distal osteotomy for hallux valgus: a preliminary report. *Foot Ankle Int.* 2009;30(7):675-679.
14. Wang CC, Lien SB, Huang GS, et al. Arthroscopic elimination of monosodium urate deposition of the first metatarsophalangeal joint reduces the recurrence of gout. *Arthroscopy.* 2009;25(2):153-158.
15. Stroud CC. Arthroscopic arthrodesis of the ankle, subtalar, and first metatarsophalangeal joint. *Foot Ankle Clin.* 2002;7(1):135-146.
16. Lui TH, Ng S, Chan KB. Endoscopic distal soft tissue procedure in hallux valgus surgery. *Arthroscopy.* 2005;21(11):1403.
17. Ferkel RD. *Surgery of the Foot and Ankle.* 8th ed. Philadelphia, PA: Mosby Elsevier; 2007.

Please visit www.routledge.com/9781617119989 to access additional material.

SECTION VI

Fractures

23

Arthroscopic Ankle Fracture Reductions Including Syndesmosis

Alastair Younger, MB, ChB, ChM, MSc, FRCSC

Introduction

Arthroscopic treatment of ankle fractures is beneficial in assisting in reduction and assessing associated injuries.[1] However, the fixation method should complement the minimally invasive nature of ankle arthroscopy if the benefit of minimally invasive treatment is to be achieved. Many patients have vascular compromised skin and bone fragments. An arthroscopic approach assists in maintaining blood supply to these structures while still allowing the surgical goals to be achieved. Arthroscopy allows the assessment of associated chondral injuries.[2]

Indications

- A reduction should be achievable based on the surgeon's assessment of the fracture and his or her abilities. The indications for arthroscopic open reduction and internal fixation include a fracture that can be reduced with minimally invasive techniques such as isolated or combined malleolar fractures and syndesmosis injuries that can be treated by percutaneous fixation.
- Arthroscopic open reduction internal fixation is of value in patients at risk of wound complications such as those patients with diabetes.[3]

Contraindications

Patient factors are rarely a contraindication to arthroscopic reduction. However, the following are relative contraindications:

- Chronic or delayed diagnosis of fracture. Ideally, the patient should be taken to the operating room within 1 week after fracture because the contracture of the soft tissue envelope will compromise reduction. After 2 to 3 weeks, fracture healing may prevent reduction, and while both are not complete contraindications, the reduction will be much harder to achieve later and the percutaneous approach does not allow dissection of fracture callus and soft tissue release that an open approach affords.

Stone JW, Kennedy JG, Glazebrook M, eds. *The Foot and Ankle: AANA Advanced Arthroscopic Surgical Techniques* (pp 223-231).

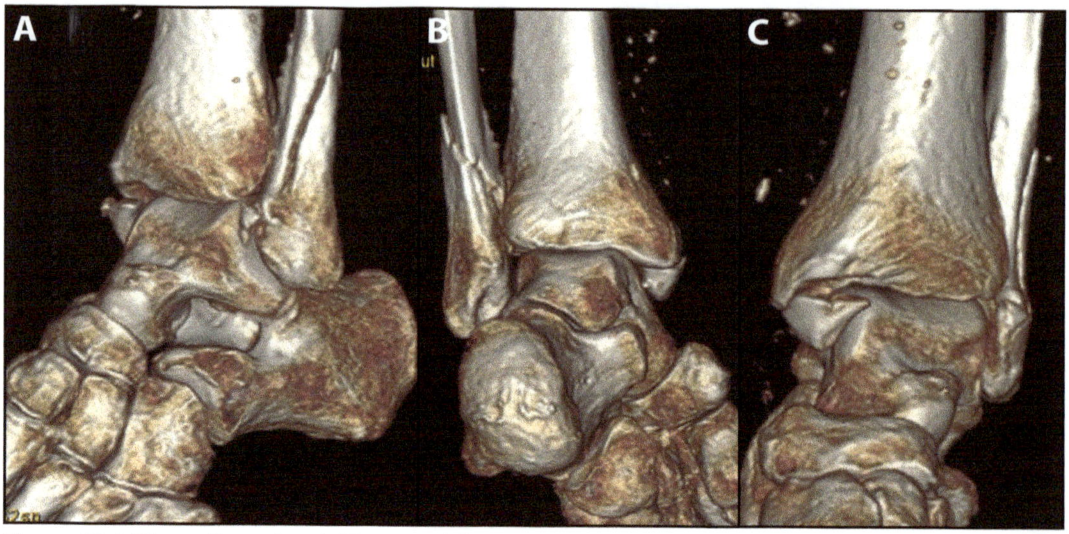

Figure 23-1. Three-dimensional CT views of the injured ankle showing the shape of the medial malleolar fracture and the displacement of the lateral malleolar fracture. If a posterior malleolar fracture or a distal tibial fracture is suspected on plain x-ray, a CT is essential. For arthroscopic reduction, a better knowledge of the 3-dimensional anatomy of the fracture is really helpful.

Pertinent Physical Findings

- The skin should be examined for compound wounds and fracture blisters.
- A neurovascular assessment is required.
- Patients with fractures higher in the tibia or fibula need to be examined to rule out compartment syndrome.
- An isolated injury to the syndesmosis may be hard to identify. A tape test can be performed.[4] For some syndesmosis injuries, the diagnosis is made at the time of ankle arthroscopy.[5]

Pertinent Imaging

- Plain radiographs after the ankle has been reduced and splinted are required.
- If there is any question with regard to the fracture pattern, a computed tomography (CT) scan is required.
- Three-dimensional reconstructions can be helpful in assessing how to perform the reduction and fixation (Figure 23-1).
- Magnetic resonance imaging can be of benefit if the injury is an isolated injury to the syndesmosis.

Equipment

- Standard ankle arthroscopy equipment will be required.
- A screw fixation system will be required for medial and posterior malleolar fractures. This may include headless, headed, or cannulated screw systems. The author prefers full thread screws as they allow better rotational control of fracture fragments.

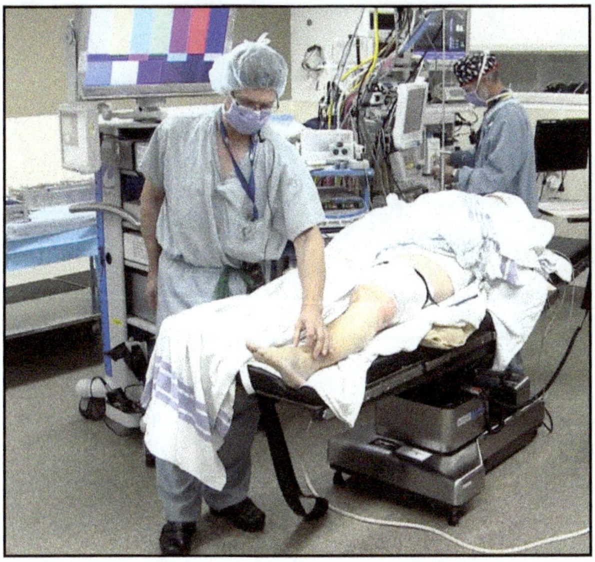

Figure 23-2. The positioning of the patient on the table. The hip is internally rotated and the leg brought to the end of the bed. The arthroscopy tower is placed to the top end of the bed on the opposite side. The C-arm is brought in from the same side of the bed to the surgeon's left for a left-side procedure. The scrub table is placed to the surgeon's right.

- Intraoperative imaging is essential. A mini C-arm unit is more maneuverable than the large C-arm.
- Reduction forceps are also essential. However, standard small fragment set reduction forceps are hard to use within the confines of the soft tissue envelope. Instead, large fragment forceps have a larger radius of curvature and will allow the reduction and immobilization of the bone fragments through the soft tissue envelope.
- If the lateral malleolus is to be reduced and percutaneous fixation used with the fracture being at or above the lateral malleolus, a fibular nail is a useful adjunct to care.

Positioning and Portals

The patient is positioned toward the bottom of the bed. The hip is elevated on the operative side so that the lateral side of the ankle is accessible. The arthroscopy tower is placed on the opposite side of the bed to the operative limb. A thigh tourniquet is used because a calf tourniquet may interfere with the operative field (Figure 23-2).

Step-by-Step Description of the Procedure

After induction of anesthesia, the patient is positioned. The operative hip is elevated to allow access to the lateral side of the ankle. A time-out is performed to confirm the patient identity, procedure, and consent and correct side. Antibiotic prophylaxis is given.

Arthroscopy is performed using anteromedial and anterolateral portals. The joint will require irrigation to remove the blood within the joint to allow visualization. After irrigation, the fracture fragments can be assessed and loose fragments removed (Figure 23-3). Cartilage damage is recorded and the syndesmosis inspected. The nature of ligamentous injury is defined.

On occasion, accessory portals may be required. A medial portal next to the posterior tibial tendon can allow assessment of the syndesmosis viewed from the posterior side with the ankle in dorsiflexion. The posterior malleolar reduction can also be viewed through this portal. A posterior lateral portal can also be used to assess the back of the ankle.

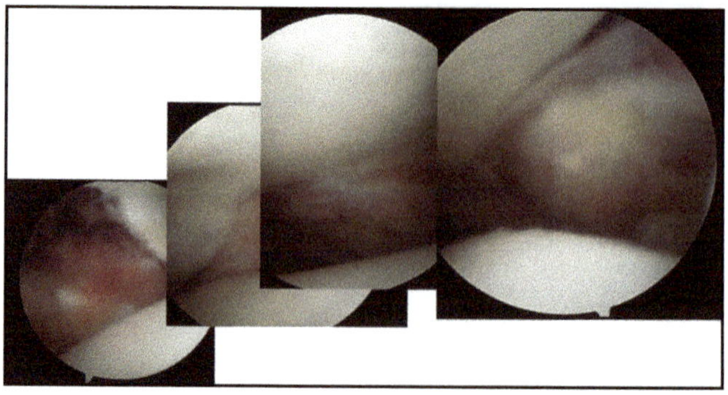

Figure 23-3. Intraoperative arthroscopic view showing the medial malleolar fracture, the posterior ankle with a posterior tibiofibular ligament injury, and a widened syndesmosis. A view looking from the anterior lateral corner back (not illustrated) shows disruption of the anterior tibiofibular ligament. There is no cartilage damage to the talus in this patient's fracture.

An accessory lateral portal can be used in the lateral gutter to assess the lateral reduction after syndesmosis fixation or to debride the lateral gutter to assist in visualization.

Isolated Syndesmosis Injury

For an isolated syndesmosis injury, the syndesmosis is inspected and the instability confirmed. The anterior and posterior tibiofibular ligaments are often disrupted. There may also be an associated cartilage injury.[6] In some cases, ankle arthroscopy is the method of diagnosis.[5]

Reduction is performed with the ankle in dorsiflexion. Plantarflexion will result in tension of the anterior talofibular ligament. Plantarflexion will therefore bring the fibula anterior and into internal rotation.

To correctly reduce the syndesmosis, the fibula must be reduced into the synchondrosis. With an intact fibula, the syndesmosis may be malreduced by the fibula being too anterior, too posterior, too lateral, too internally rotated, and too externally rotated.

The reduction is therefore best performed with a percutaneous clamp onto the fibula. The clamp can then be used to internally and externally rotate the fibula on the dorsiflexed talus to define the neutral position. Typically, the fibula can rotate about 10 degrees in this position. Once rotation is correctly assessed, the fibula is pushed posteriorly and pinned into the tibia transversely with a 2-mm Kirschner wire (K-wire). A pelvic reduction clamp is placed between the fibula and tibia in approximately 20 to 30 degrees of external rotation in the transmalleolar axis.

Once placed, the reduction is checked on the C-arm and with the arthroscope placed into the lateral gutter to make sure that the fibula is correctly orientated on the tibia. The fibula should rest just behind the origin of the talofibular ligament, and the ligament ends may also line up.

After confirmation of the reduction, fixation can be achieved using either percutaneous screws or a suture anchor system. The author prefers lagged, cortical, large fragment screws.

Lateral Malleolar Fractures

Lateral malleolar fractures at or above the level of the syndesmosis can be reduced using a fibular nail.[7] Isolated lateral malleolar ankle fractures are associated with medial osteochondral defects.[8]

After the arthroscopy, the leg is moved to the side of the operating room table and positioned over the C-arm. The fracture is reduced under the C-arm control using percutaneous reduction forceps to distract the distal fibula, while a second reduction forceps is placed percutaneously to hold the fracture reduced (Figure 23-4). The reduction is confirmed on the C-arm views. At this point, it may be helpful to hold the reduction if anatomic with an anterior and posterior K-wire between the anterior and posterior fibula into the distal tibia.

After reduction, the guide wire for the fibular rod is placed centrally in the distal fibula. The wire can be left in while a second wire is placed using the first wire as a guide to reposition into

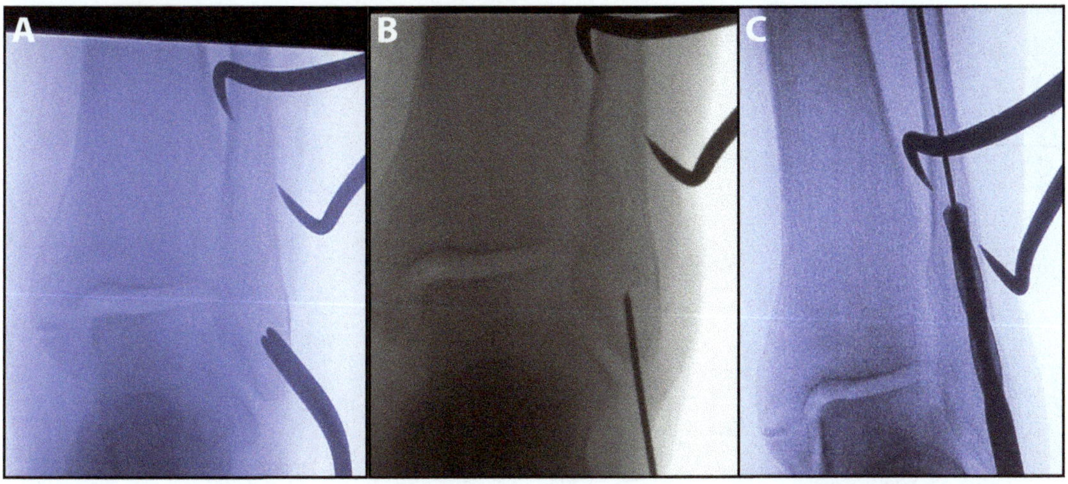

Figure 23-4. (A) Initial reduction using 2 reduction forceps percutaneously, (B) followed by wire positioning in the distal fibula followed by distal reaming (not illustrated), then (C) hand reaming.

the correct orientation. The drill hole is 6 mm in diameter and needs to start slightly lateral to a vertical point dropped down from the shaft of the fibula in an anteroposterior and lateral plane. The nail has a bow in it of 10 degrees, and this accommodates the bowed position.

The fibula is then reamed to an appropriate depth, and the reamers should be sunk to the end of the drill portion. This will allow enough space for the distal segment of the nail. If the reamer is not completely sunk, then the nail may become hung up in the isthmus of the fibula.

A hand reamer is used to broach up the proximal fibula. The proximal nail has 2 diameters, so the smaller reamer is used first and the larger second if the canal will accommodate it. The author prefers to use the largest nail available as this best controls flexion and extension, varus and valgus at the fracture site, and also helps to control translation at the fracture site.

The nail is mounted on the jig and inserted. The nail should be left 1 to 2 mm proud on the distal end as this will assist in fixation in the cortex and subcortical bone of the distal fibula.

The nail is best inserted in 20 to 25 degrees of external rotation and pointing across the transmalleolar axis. This will result in the anteroposterior locking screws starting lateral in the fibula and ending medial to the path of the peroneal tendons. This also affords better bone for the fixation. Two anteroposterior screws of sufficient length are placed to capture the anterior and posterior fibular cortices.

Once the distal locking screws are placed and their position on the C-arm is confirmed, the final fracture and syndesmosis reduction needs to be performed. The fracture at this point may be shortened and internally or externally rotated. The syndesmosis may also be open, and the fibula at the level of the syndesmosis may be translated or rotated even with an anatomic fracture reduction.

The reduction can be achieved on both levels if still malreduced by traction on the jig with the ankle held in dorsiflexion. In this position, only a small amount of rotation of the fibula on the lateral side of the talus is possible in this position as the talus is held locked in the ankle mortise in dorsiflexion. A neutral position is chosen, traction is maintained, the fibula is pushed slightly posterior, and K-wire or drill fixation is achieved between the tibia and fibula. C-arm views are obtained and the arthroscope is reinserted to confirm the reduction. If the locking screw has been placed, the foot can be plantarflexed to confirm reduction.

The 2 proximal locking screws are then placed using the appropriate holes in the jig. The screws are of sufficient length to immobilize the fibula and transfix the fibula to the tibia.

Final images are obtained of the locking screws to confirm the correct placement and of the fracture and syndesmosis to confirm reduction.

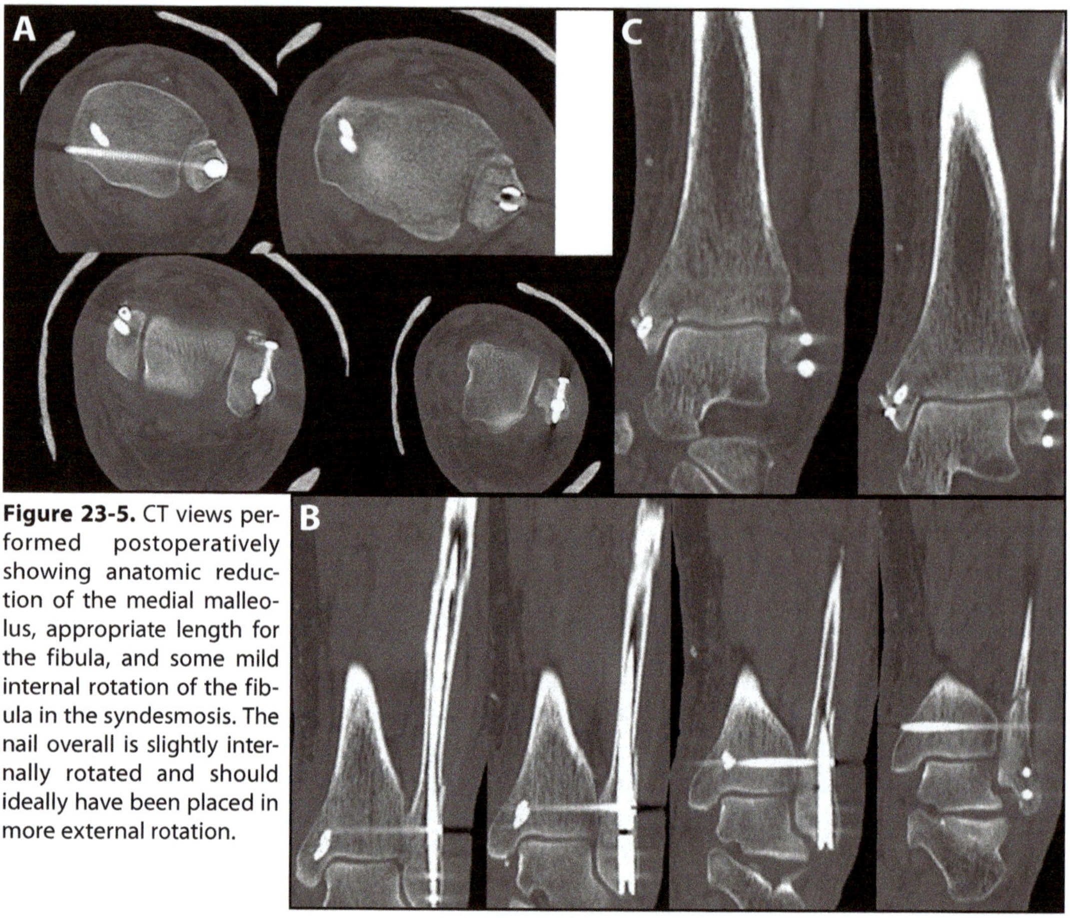

Figure 23-5. CT views performed postoperatively showing anatomic reduction of the medial malleolus, appropriate length for the fibula, and some mild internal rotation of the fibula in the syndesmosis. The nail overall is slightly internally rotated and should ideally have been placed in more external rotation.

Medial Malleolar Reduction and Fixation

The medial malleolus can be reduced and the reduction confirmed using arthroscopy and the C-arm. Alternatively, a small medial incision can be made, dependent on the comfort level of the surgeon. However, the arthroscopic reduction may be more accurate.[9] Medial malleolar fractures treated with arthroscopic reduction did better than patients with open reduction.[10]

The medial malleolus can be reduced using a percutaneous clamp into the malleolus, and then distraction and rotation can be performed. Because the deltoid ligament can be tensioned with the ankle plantarflexed, it is best to reduce the medial malleolus with the ankle dorsiflexed. K-wires can be placed to hold the reduction and C-arm views are obtained, as well as arthroscopic visualization of the reduction. If the reduction is incomplete, then a repeat reduction can be performed.

Fixation is achieved using 2 or 3 headed or headless screws. If required, lag fixation can be achieved by overdrilling the medial malleolar segment. Fully threaded screws are preferable after one lag screw is placed as they will better control rotation and bending movements through the fracture site (Figure 23-5).

Posterior Malleolar Fractures

Posterior malleolar fractures can be reduced arthroscopically and fixated percutaneously. The author prefers to reduce and transfix all posterior malleolar fractures of a size large enough to fixate going from posterior to anterior. The reduction of the joint surface is important to maintain joint congruity and possibly to prevent arthritic pain. The anatomic reduction of the insertion of the posterior tibiofibular ligament is also important in maintaining the correct reduction of the fibula and syndesmosis. A malreduced posterior malleolar fragment may hold the syndesmosis malreduced.

The arthroscope is used first to visualize the fragments. The fibula is best reduced first as this will assist in the reduction of the posterior malleolus through the posterior tibia to fibula ligament.

The posterior malleolus is best then reduced further by removing the arthroscope, dorsiflexing the ankle, and immobilizing the fracture using pelvic reduction forceps placed into the central aspect of the fragment from posterior with one tine through a stab wound just lateral to the Achilles tendon at the level of the ankle, and a second stab wound for the anterior tine just lateral to the medial malleolus. The fracture reduction is confirmed using the arthroscope and the C-arm. Once confirmed, K-wires can be placed posterior to anterior in the distal tibia. As the posterior malleolar piece can be fairly small, the fixation may be best achieved using cannulated full-threaded headed screws with washers. For larger fragments, headless full-thread screws can be placed.

The final reduction is confirmed using the arthroscope and C-arm views. The correct positioning of the hardware is also confirmed.

Cartilage and Capsule Injuries

During the fracture, damage can occur to the cartilage surface. The cartilage should be inspected for osteochondral injuries outside the area of fracture. It is common, particularly with a Weber C fracture, to have an injury to the talar dome.[11] The cartilage fragment may require removal. Cartilage injuries exist in approximately 70% of acute ankle fractures.[12] The osteochondral defect may benefit from microfracture or debridement and can be located on the medial side of the talus, lateral side of the talus, or distal tibia.[13] Cartilage injuries are more likely in Weber C compared with Weber B fractures.[14]

Capsule and ligament injuries may also impinge within the joint. Debridement may therefore be beneficial in preventing ongoing pain.[15]

At the end of the procedure, the incisions are sutured with 3-0 nylon.

Postoperative Protocol

The limb is best placed in a well-padded back slab at the end of the procedure. The patient is kept nonweightbearing and reviewed back in the clinic 2 weeks postoperatively. The limb is kept elevated above the level of the heart to prevent bleeding, swelling, and pain.

At 2 weeks, the cast and sutures are removed. Physiotherapy is initiated. Weightbearing can be initiated at this point if the fracture construct is stable enough to allow it. Regardless, range of motion should be initiated and compression stockings used to prevent swelling. If needed, a plain x-ray is obtained at this point. A walker boot is used from this visit through 10 weeks. The walker boot can be worn at night to maintain dorsiflexion ankle joint range.

At 6 weeks, the patient is re-examined. X-rays are obtained and the fracture construct reviewed. Weightbearing is progressed at that point to partial or full. Physiotherapy and range of motion exercises are continued to the 16-week mark.

At 3 months, a final x-ray is obtained. Patients are encouraged to resume normal activities other than those involving impact.

Hardware removal can be performed after 1 year. The author does not routinely remove syndesmosis screws, but instead informs the patients of the potential of screw removal and discusses the risks and benefits of screw removal and screw retention.

Potential Complications

Complications are less frequent than with open surgery, which is why arthroscopic surgery is preferable. Infection risk and wound breakdown are much less prevalent, and postoperative pain, stiffness, and swelling are much less prevalent than in the open procedure.

Technical challenges from the arthroscopic procedure may result in incomplete reduction, malposition of the hardware, or inadequate fracture fixation. If this is recognized intraoperatively, it can be managed by repositioning the hardware or conversion to an open procedure. Postoperatively recognized, this may compromise the final result or require revision surgery.

Superficial nerve injuries may also occur. On the author's review, superficial nerve injuries are more prevalent in combined open and arthroscopic procedures compared to isolated arthroscopic procedures. Damage to the superficial branch of the peroneal nerve is the most common complication after ankle arthroscopy.

Top Technical Pearls for the Procedure

1. Position the patient correctly with the foot at the bottom of the bed and bumped appropriately to ensure access to the lateral ankle. A bean bag can be deflated to allow access to the medial side of the ankle after lateral fixation.
2. Transfix the lateral malleolus first, the medial malleolus second, and the posterior malleolus third unless the medial malleolus has a vertical shear component. In this case, the medial malleolus should be reduced and transfixed first so that the lateral malleolus can be correctly reduced.
3. Ensure that you have a clear plan for fracture fixation and the correct equipment and reduction tools available before surgery. A bailout plan B should be considered should the arthroscopic surgery not be achievable.
4. Most of the reduction should be done with the ankle in dorsiflexion. In this position, the length and rotation of the fibula can be confirmed against the lateral side of the talus. The anterior talofibular ligament is detensioned in this position, and the posterior malleolus is more likely to reduce.
5. The surgery should be done within 1 week of injury because the ability to mobilize the soft tissue envelope is less during arthroscopic surgery. However, the contraindication to early surgery, namely the risk of wound breakdown secondary to swelling, is much less of a risk.

References

1. Atesok K, Doral MN, Whipple T, et al. Arthroscopy-assisted fracture fixation. *Knee Surg Sports Traumatol Arthrosc.* 2011;19(2):320-329.
2. Yoshimura I, Naito M, Kanazawa K, Takeyama A, Ida T. Arthroscopic findings in Maisonneuve fractures. *J Orthop Sci.* 2008;13(1):3-6.
3. Thevendran G, Younger A. Arthroscopic reduction and fibula nailing in high-risk diabetic ankle fractures: case reviews and technical tip. *Foot Ankle Spec.* 2012;5(2):124-127.
4. Hunt KJ, Phisitkul P, Pirolo J, Amendola A. High ankle sprains and syndesmotic injuries in athletes. *J Am Acad Orthop Surg.* 2015;23(11):661-673.

5. Takao M, Ochi M, Naito K, et al. Arthroscopic diagnosis of tibiofibular syndesmosis disruption. *Arthroscopy.* 2001;17(8):836-843.
6. Sri-Ram K, Robinson AH. Arthroscopic assessment of the syndesmosis following ankle fracture. *Injury.* 2005;36(5):675-678.
7. Kong C, Kolla L, Wing K, Younger AS. Arthroscopy-assisted closed reduction and percutaneous nail fixation of unstable ankle fractures: description of a minimally invasive procedure. *Arthrosc Tech.* 2014;3(1):e181-e184.
8. Thordarson DB, Bains R, Shepherd LE. The role of ankle arthroscopy on the surgical management of ankle fractures. *Foot Ankle Int.* 2001;22(2):123-125.
9. Swart EF, Vosseller JT. Arthroscopic assessment of medial malleolar reduction. *Arch Orthop Trauma Surg.* 2014;134(9):1287-1292.
10. Turhan E, Doral MN, Demirel M, et al. Arthroscopy-assisted reduction versus open reduction in the fixation of medial malleolar fractures. *Eur J Orthop Surgery Traumatol.* 2013;23(8):953-959.
11. Ono A, Nishikawa S, Nagao A, Irie T, Sasaki M, Kouno T. Arthroscopically assisted treatment of ankle fractures: arthroscopic findings and surgical outcomes. *Arthroscopy.* 2004;20(6):627-631.
12. Takao M, Ochi M, Uchio Y, Naito K, Kono T, Oae K. Osteochondral lesions of the talar dome associated with trauma. *Arthroscopy.* 2003;19(10):1061-1067.
13. Loren GJ, Ferkel RD. Arthroscopic assessment of occult intra-articular injury in acute ankle fractures. *Arthroscopy.* 2002;18(4):412-421.
14. Hintermann B, Regazzoni P, Lampert C, Stutz G, Gachter A. Arthroscopic findings in acute fractures of the ankle. *J Bone Joint Surg Br.* 2000;82(3):345-351.
15. Ogilvie-Harris DJ, Reed SC. Disruption of the ankle syndesmosis: diagnosis and treatment by arthroscopic surgery. *Arthroscopy.* 1994;10(5):561-568.

Please visit www.routledge.com/9781617119989 to access additional material.

24

Arthroscopic-Assisted Calcaneal Fracture Reduction

Alastair Younger, MB, ChB, ChM, MSc, FRCSC

Introduction

When performing posterior subtalar arthroscopy, the fixation method should complement the minimally invasive nature if the benefit of minimally invasive treatment is to be achieved. Many patients have compromised vasculature of skin and bone fragments. An arthroscopic approach assists in maintaining blood supply to these structures while still allowing the surgical goals to be achieved. Arthroscopy allows assessment of associated chondral injuries. If care is taken, appropriate reductions can be achieved,[1] and outcome reviews show that wound complications can usually be avoided.[2] A computed tomography (CT) scan is often required prior to treatment to determine whether the fracture is amenable to arthroscopic treatment and percutaneous fixation. A reduction should be achievable based on the surgeon's assessment of the fracture and his or her surgical abilities, and a plan for fixation needs to be in place prior to surgery. Fixation may include cannulated headless or headed screws or solid screws. A sinus tarsi plate may be a way of complementing the reduction without an extensile lateral exposure when the reduction cannot be performed percutaneously. Usually, plate fixation negates the benefit of arthroscopy. The tuberosity fragment can be transfixed to the anterior and sustentacular segments of the calcaneus once held together.

Indications

The indications for arthroscopic open reduction and internal fixation of calcaneal fractures need to be carefully considered. Not all fractures can be reduced in a minimally invasive fashion. It is therefore important to assess the following factors:

- Timing: The fracture should be relatively recent as scarring of the medial soft tissues will restrict distraction and prevent reduction of the tuberosity and fracture fragments. Early callus formation may also restrict mobilization of the fragments.
- Fracture pattern: Highly comminuted fractures or those with small residual sustentacular segments are not amenable to arthroscopic treatment.[3]

Stone JW, Kennedy JG, Glazebrook M, eds. *The Foot and Ankle: AANA Advanced Arthroscopic Surgical Techniques* (pp 233-242).

- It is particularly useful in tongue-type fractures with minimal fracture line widening and minimal anterior comminution.
- Patients at high risk of wound or other surgical or anesthetic complications. If arthroscopic reduction can be achieved, the operation may be shorter, wound complications fewer, and a similar radiographic reduction achieved.[4,5]

Contraindications

- Anterior or plantar comminution
- Fractures > 7 to 10 days old represent a relative contraindication.
- Noncompliant patient
- Patient factors are rarely a contraindication to arthroscopic reduction.
  - Patient factors may necessitate the need for a percutaneous reduction if an extensive lateral incision is considered too risky for those at risk of wound healing complications.[6]

Pertinent Physical Findings

- The diagnosis of a calcaneal fracture should be reasonably clear.
- The skin must be examined for compound wounds and fracture blisters.
- The degree of swelling and soft tissue injury is important in the timing of surgery.
- A neurovascular assessment is always required.
- Examine for compartment syndrome as there is a risk of foot compartment syndrome.
  - In this instance, an urgent compartment release may be required.
  - The role for foot compartment release is debated, but if left untreated, it may compromise the late function of the foot secondary to clawing of the brevis and intrinsic muscles in the foot.

Pertinent Imaging

- Plain radiographs after the foot has been splinted
  - Anteroposterior and lateral views of the foot and ankle and a calcaneal axial view are beneficial (Figure 24-1).
- A preoperative CT scan is always required because the 3-dimensional (3D) anatomy of the calcaneal fracture is quite complicated. 3D reconstructions can be very helpful in assessing how to perform the reduction and fixation (Figure 24-2).

Equipment

- A plating system with sinus tarsi plates may be required should the surgeon choose to use a sinus tarsi plate with the arthroscopic assessment. Ideally, the incision required to place this plate should be avoided.
- A screw fixation system will be required. The choices include headless, headed, or cannulated screw systems. Fully threaded screws are often used as they allow better rotational control of

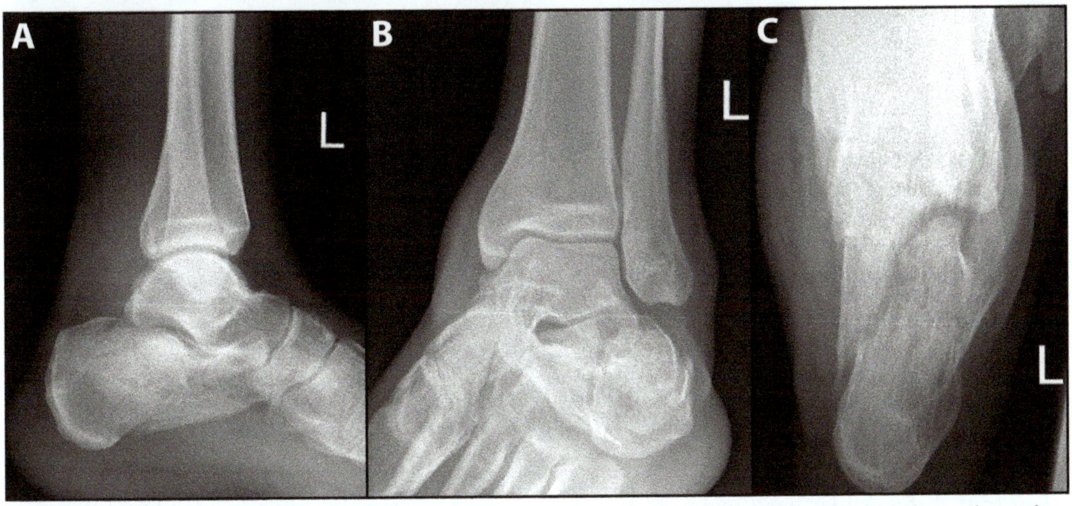

Figure 24-1. A posterior facet fracture with depression. The medial wall is displaced on the calcaneal axial view. The fracture is 3 weeks old and therefore not ideal for percutaneous management. (A) Anteroposterior view. (B) Mortise view. (C) Calcaneal axial view.

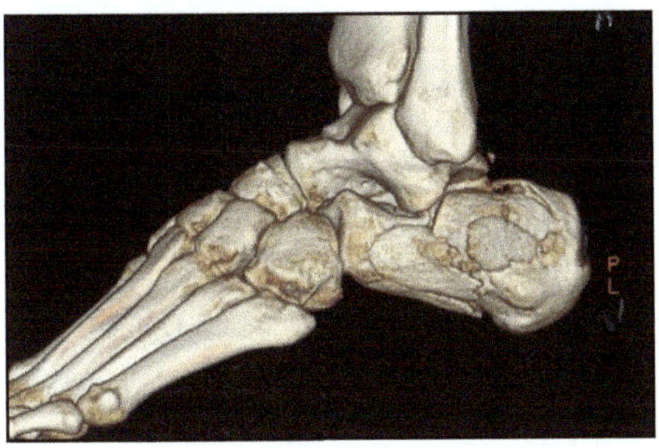

Figure 24-2. A 3D reconstruction of the CT scan demonstrating the depression of the lateral portion of the posterior facet; the lateral wall blow out; the shortened medial wall; and the lateralized, shortened, and varus position of the tuberosity fragment.

fracture fragments. Therefore, a set with screws up to 70-mm long with small heads to reduce the subcutaneous irritation of the screw heads is required.

- Intraoperative imaging (fluoroscopy) is essential. A mini C-arm unit is more maneuverable than the large C-arm and is therefore favorable.
- Reduction forceps are also essential; however, standard small fragment set reduction forceps are hard to use within the confines of the soft tissue envelope. Instead, large fragment forceps have a larger radius of curvature and will allow the reduction and immobilization of the bone fragments through the soft tissue envelope.
- 2.4- or 2.9-mm, 30-degree arthroscope
- Small oscillating shaver is required
- Standard arthroscopy equipment

Positioning and Portals

The patient is positioned toward the bottom of a fully radiolucent operating table. The patient is placed in the full lateral position (Figure 24-3). Padding is used on the lower limb and care is

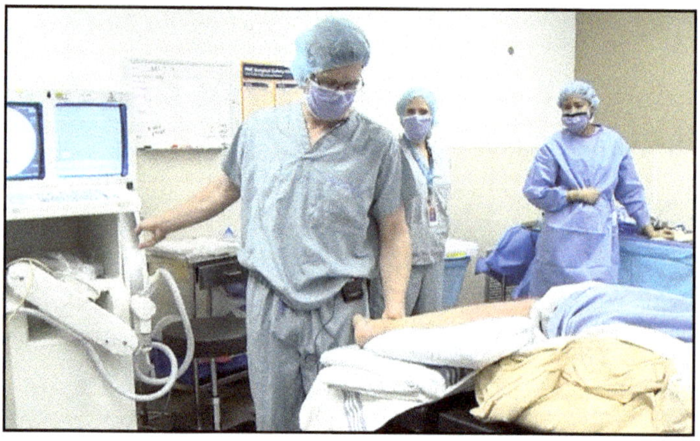

Figure 24-3. Positioning of the patient on the table. The lateral position is used, with the lower limb padded. The surgeon sits at the foot of the bed toward the injured side (in this case, the left side) with the arthroscopy tower to the right side at the head of the bed.

taken to pad the fibular head region to prevent peroneal nerve palsy. Pillows are placed between the limbs. The shoulders and arms are also appropriately padded and protected. A full lateral position allows the limb to be placed in traction to achieve reduction. The C-arm is placed behind the surgeon and brought in as necessary. The scrub table is positioned on the opposite side of the table to the operative limb.

The arthroscopy tower is placed on the opposite side of the bed to the operative limb. A thigh tourniquet is used because a calf tourniquet may interfere with the operative field and tighten the calf muscles, preventing reduction.

Step-by-Step Description of the Procedure

Preoperative Considerations

After induction of anesthesia, the patient is positioned. A time-out is performed to confirm the patient identity, procedure, and consent and correct side. Intravenous antibiotic prophylaxis is administered preoperatively and a thigh tourniquet is applied to the upper thigh and inflated to 250 mm Hg.

Access and Portal Placement

Arthroscopy can be performed using sinus tarsi, direct lateral, and Achilles tendon portals (Figure 24-4). The subtalar joint will require irrigation to remove the hematoma within the joint, and then 5 to 10 mL of normal saline (NaCl 0.9%) injected into the joint will help allow visualization. After irrigation, the fracture fragments can be assessed and loose fragments removed. Cartilage damage is recorded intraoperatively (Figure 24-5). A 2.4- or 2.9-mm, 30-degree arthroscope can be used and a power shaver is required for debridement of the fracture site and for soft tissue clearance if there is an obstructing view. Additionally, the shaver can be used to clear any unstable osteochondral fragments. Use of a 2.9-mm arthroscope, while having a larger cannula, can be more effective for fluid flow, although the larger size means a resultant tighter fit within the confines of the joint, leading to less working space. The subtalar joint facet is harder to see once the fracture is reduced and usually needs to be visualized from behind with the arthroscope outside of the joint. The posterior facet can be seen on an arthroscopic view, as can the edge of the floor of the sinus tarsi. The medial facet, however, cannot be visualized using this technique.

On occasion, accessory portals may be required. A portal lower or higher than the Achilles portal can assist in the reduction and visualization. An accessory sinus tarsi portal can also be used.

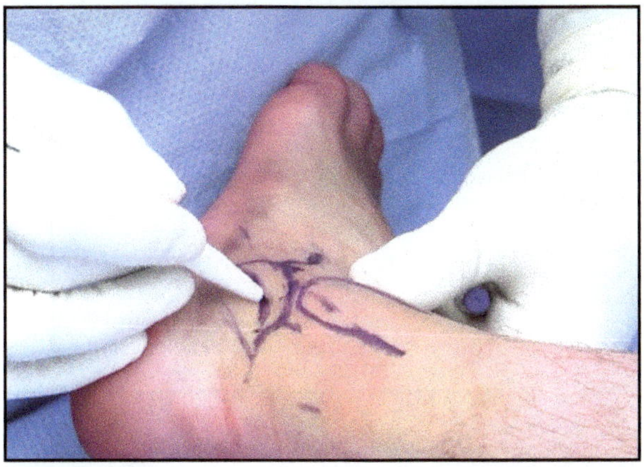

Figure 24-4. Portals are placed in the edge of the sinus tarsi, at the tip of the fibula, and at the edge of the Achilles tendon.

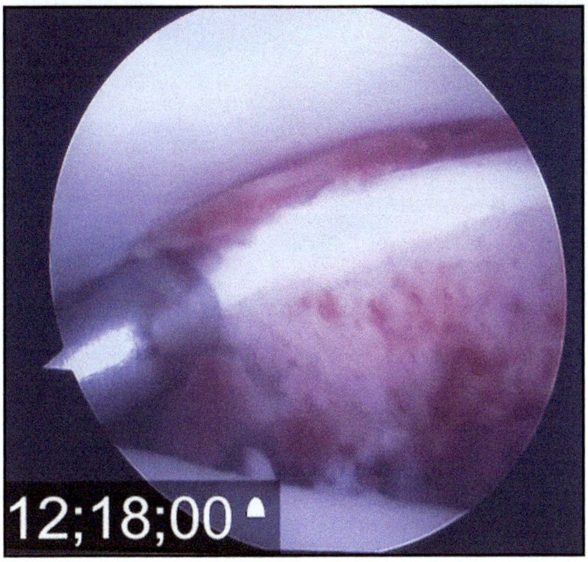

Figure 24-5. A view of the subtalar joint after removal of the fracture clot. Cartilage damage was demonstrated both on the talar and calcaneal surfaces of the joint.

Reduction of Fracture

Closed Reduction of the Tuberosity

After initial arthroscopy of the posterior facet, the tuberosity is reduced. A large Kirschner wire (K-wire; 4-mm diameter) or Steinmann pin is placed in the tuberosity fragment as posterior as possible. The wire should just penetrate the medial cortex. If necessary, the fracture lines can be mobilized using a small elevator through the arthroscopy portals or through a separate stab incision. The fractures should be mobile before a reduction is attempted. It is important to note that fractures treated within the first 7 days are usually easier to treat as the medial soft tissues have not yet formed contractures.

The reduction can often require up to 3 attempts. An assistant is placed on the opposite side of the operating table to provide countertraction to the knee. The surgeon can then pull to mobilize the tuberosity fragment. If needed, an elevator can be passed back through a portal and fracture line to be used to leverage the medial wall.

The reduction is performed by bringing the tuberosity out to length, medializing the tuberosity with respect to the sinus tarsi, and then derotating the tuberosity by bringing it back out of varus.

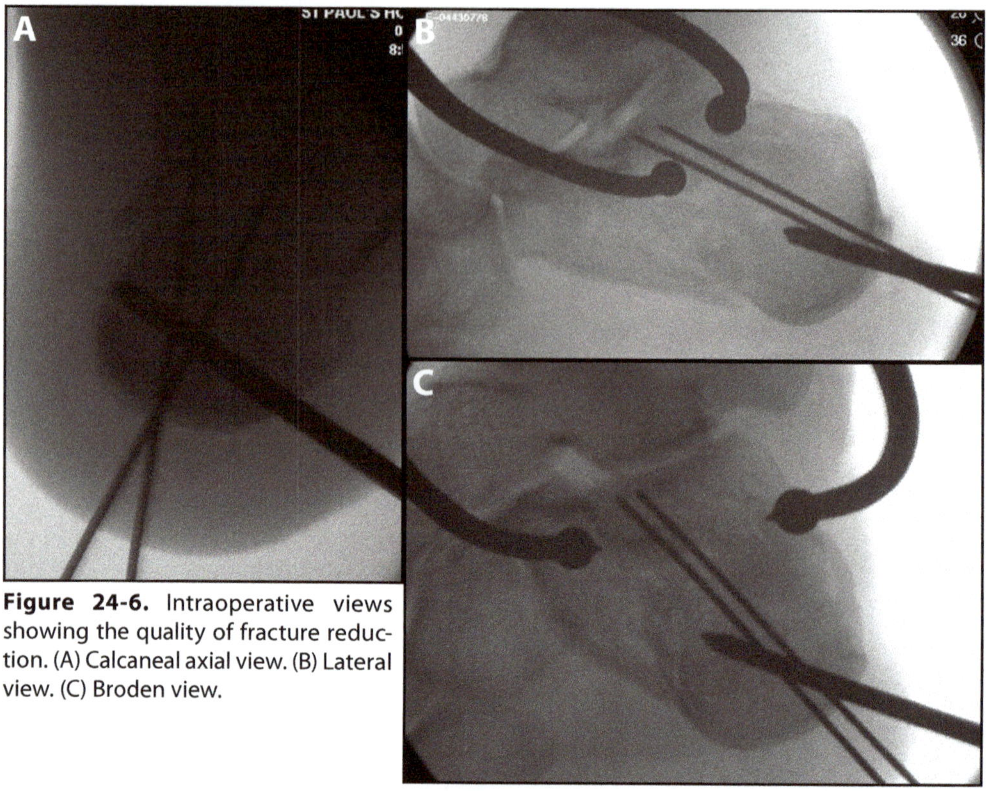

Figure 24-6. Intraoperative views showing the quality of fracture reduction. (A) Calcaneal axial view. (B) Lateral view. (C) Broden view.

The second assistant then drives a 2-mm K-wire up from the tuberosity, along the medial wall of the calcaneus and into the sustentaculum tali. A calcaneal axial view is obtained to assess the quality of reduction (Figure 24-6). A lateral view of the foot allows visualization of Bohler's angle and aids in the confirmation of appropriate reduction.

If the calcaneal axial view indicates that the tuberosity of the calcaneus is shortened, laterally translated, or still in varus (the most common concern), then the reduction needs to be repeated. This is the most critical step of the procedure as the tuberosity must be made anatomic if the reduction of the posterior facet is to be achieved.

Once the tuberosity is reduced, 2 to 3 K-wires are fixed in place to maintain reduction.

Subtalar Joint Reduction

Once the tuberosity is reduced and held, the sinus tarsi and posterior facet can be reduced. Large fragment or pelvic reduction forceps may be required to assist in reduction, as well as in elevation of the lateral part of the posterior facet using an accessory portal and elevator.

The lateral segment of the posterior facet is pushed back using the elevator so that it is medialized and derotated. Initial fixation can be achieved using K-wires going from lateral to medial into the sustentaculum tali. The wire may need to be angled in approximately 10 to 20 degrees of external rotation and aimed slightly inferiorly on the medial side.

The reduction forceps can be used to medialize the fragment with one tine on the posterior lateral fragment and the second tine on the prominence of the sustentaculum tali.

The scope is then reinserted and the calcaneus distracted to allow visualization (Figure 24-7). It is important to note that after reduction, it is often hard to reinsert the scope because the subtalar joint can be much tighter following the reduction of the fragments, and working room can be significantly reduced.

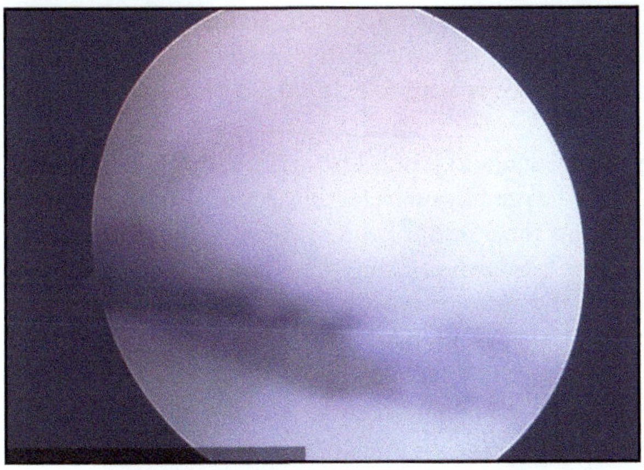

Figure 24-7. Assessment of fracture reduction via the arthroscope posterior to the joint.

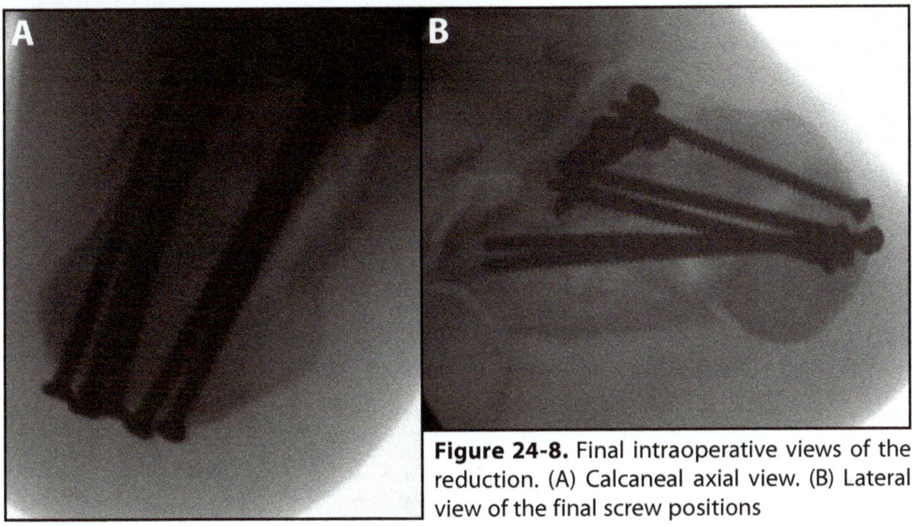

Figure 24-8. Final intraoperative views of the reduction. (A) Calcaneal axial view. (B) Lateral view of the final screw positions

Intraoperative fluoroscopy, ideally with the use of a mini C-arm, is also used to assess reduction and confirm that it is congruent and anatomical. The lateral side of the floor of the sinus tarsi should be anatomic. The posterior facet fragment often falls under the sinus tarsi floor. A lateral view, anteroposterior view, and internal rotation and mild plantarflexion view of the posterior facet will allow the posterior facet to be visualized and ensure that the reduction is complete.

If necessary, the lateral wall can now be reduced. This is important to allow the peroneal tendons to reduce back into the fibular groove. The lateral wall is reduced by using reduction forceps or an appropriately placed elevator through a lateral stab incision.

Endoscopy can then be used to visualize the peroneal tendons within the peroneal sheath as well as the posterior aspect of the fibula. This is done to ensure that the tendons are reduced.

Placement of Hardware

Once the calcaneal reduction is anatomic, hardware is placed to maintain fracture position and stability. A lag screw is first placed from the lateral posterior facet fragment into the sinus tarsi. A compression headless screw approximately 3 mm in diameter or a 3.5-mm small fragment screw can be used. The drill needs to be angled to follow the subchondral course of the posterior facet and will end up in the most medial aspect of the sustentaculum tali. The 3.5-mm lag drill should penetrate only to the medial side of the lateral facet fragment. Fluoroscopy should be used for guidance (Figure 24-8).

A screw and washer are then placed. This screw, if correctly placed, should be from 36 to 40 mm long. A second screw is placed parallel to the first screw, and this can be done using either a lagged or nonlagged technique. A third screw, if space is available, is placed anterior or inferior to the first 2 screws.

If needed, a reduction is performed of the calcaneocuboid joint. The arthroscope can be placed in the calcaneocuboid joint using 2 lateral portals. Large fragment forceps can be used to assist in the reduction placed from dorsal to plantar holding the anterior process down. Two stab wounds are required. A medial-to-lateral reduction can be performed using a lag screw. Reduction forceps cannot easily be placed on the medial side of the anterior process of the calcaneus; therefore, K-wires can be used for this initial reduction. Screws can be placed in the anterior process in a lateral-to-medial and superior-to-inferior orientation, and a lagged technique can be employed if necessary. An additional screw may need to be placed in the posterior-to-anterior direction in the floor of the sinus tarsi to maintain adequate reduction. A headless screw is useful for this purpose.

Once the anterior aspect of the calcaneus is reduced, fixation is achieved from the tuberosity to the reconstructed anterior half of the calcaneus. Two or 3 axial screws should be placed along the medial wall of the calcaneus and into the sustentacular fragment using the K-wire tracts. Screw fixation can also be placed from the tuberosity to the anterior process of the calcaneus. Fluoroscopy views are obtained to ensure that the fragments are correctly transfixed and that the tips of the screws are extra-articular. A final view of the joint surface can be obtained at this juncture. Sutures are placed to close the portals and Steri-Strips (3M) are added if required. Dressings are applied and the patient's limb is then placed in a well-padded back slab at the end of the procedure.

Postoperative Protocol

The patient is kept nonweightbearing and reviewed back in the clinic at 2 weeks postoperatively. During this time, the limb should be kept elevated above the level of the heart to prevent bleeding, swelling, and pain. At 2 weeks, the cast is removed, wound checked, and sutures removed as well. Physiotherapy is initiated. Range of motion exercises should be initiated at 2 weeks and compression stockings used to prevent swelling. A plain x-ray film is obtained at this point (Figure 24-9). The wounds at 6 weeks after surgery are shown in Figure 24-10. A walker boot is used from this visit until 10 weeks postoperatively and should be worn at night to maintain dorsiflexion of the ankle joint.

At 6 weeks, the patient is re-examined and anteroposterior and lateral views of the foot, ankle, and calcaneal axial view x-rays are obtained so the fracture structure can be reviewed. If there is any concern about the quality of reduction, a CT scan can be obtained. A CT is also useful to review the placement of hardware and quality of reduction, especially for surgeons who are newer to this technique.

Weightbearing is progressed at the 6-week review to partial or full. Physiotherapy and range of motion exercises are continued until week 16 postoperatively.

At 3 months, a final x-ray is obtained. Patients are encouraged to partake in normal activities, except for those involving high impact. Hardware removal can be performed after 1 year.

Potential Complications

Complications during arthroscopic procedures are rarer than open surgery, which is why arthroscopic surgery is preferable if possible. Infection risk and wound breakdown are much less prevalent, and postoperative pain, stiffness, and swelling are much less prevalent than in open procedures.[7]

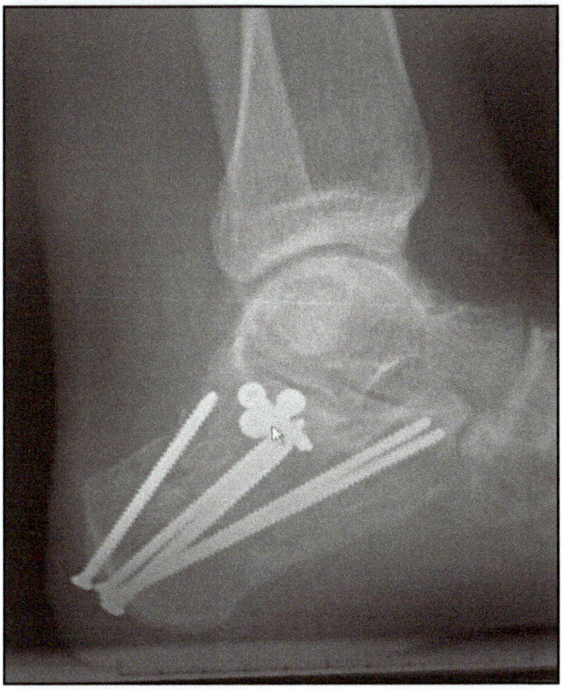

Figure 24-9. Postoperative view at 6 weeks after reduction.

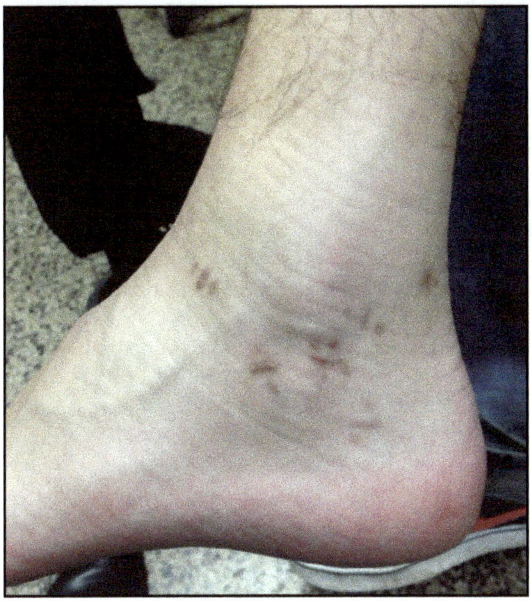

Figure 24-10. Picture of the foot at 6 weeks.

Technical challenges from the arthroscopic procedure may result in incomplete reduction, malposition of the hardware, or inadequate fracture fixation. If this is recognized intraoperatively, it can be managed through repositioning of the hardware or conversion to an open procedure. Postoperatively recognized, this may compromise the final result or require revision surgery.

Superficial nerve injuries may also occur. Sural nerve palsy is the most likely to occur during this procedure. It is rarely possible to change the outcome of a nerve injury after the procedure, so care should be taken to ensure that the nerves are not damaged during the development of portals or the placement of screws.[7]

Top Technical Pearls for the Procedure

1. Position the patient correctly with the foot to the bottom of the bed and in the lateral position. Incorrect positioning will compromise the ability to arthroscope the joint, reduce the tuberosity, and obtain the correct angles of the screws.
2. Reduce the tuberosity anatomically. A number of attempts may be required. Without a correct reduction of the tuberosity fragment assessed on the calcaneal axial view, the rest of the calcaneus cannot be reduced appropriately.
3. The arthroscope is used to assess the size, position, and reduction of the articular fracture fragments. The joint can be hard to visualize once the posterior facet is reduced.
4. The lateral wall needs to be reduced to allow relocation of the peroneal tendons. Peroneal tendoscopy can be performed to ensure that they are reduced.
5. The surgery should be done within 1 week of injury as the ability to mobilize the soft tissue envelope is less during arthroscopic surgery. However, the contraindication to early surgery, namely the risk of wound breakdown secondary to swelling, is much less of a risk.

References

1. Sivakumar BS, Wong P, Dick CG, Steer RA, Tetsworth K. Arthroscopic reduction and percutaneous fixation of selected calcaneus fractures: surgical technique and early results. *J Orthop Trauma.* 2014;28(10):569-576.
2. Hammond AW, Crist BD. Percutaneous treatment of high-risk patients with intra-articular calcaneus fractures: a case series. *Injury.* 2013;44(11):1483-1485.
3. Woon CY, Chong KW, Yeo W, Eng-Meng Yeo N, Wong MK. Subtalar arthroscopy and flurosocopy in percutaneous fixation of intra-articular calcaneal fractures: the best of both worlds. *J Trauma.* 2011;71(4):917-925.
4. Weber M, Lehmann O, Sagesser D, Krause F. Limited open reduction and internal fixation of displaced intra-articular fractures of the calcaneum. *J Bone Joint Surg Br.* 2008;90(12):1608-1616.
5. Rammelt S, Amlang M, Barthel S, Gavlik JM, Zwipp H. Percutaneous treatment of less severe intraarticular calcaneal fractures. *Clin Orthop Relat Res.* 2010;468(4):983-990.
6. Rammelt S, Zwipp H. Calcaneus fractures: facts, controversies and recent developments. *Injury.* 2004;35(5):443-461.
7. Epstein N, Chadran S, Chou L. Current concepts review: intra-articular fractures of the calcaneus. *Foot Ankle Int.* 2012;33(1):79-86.

Please visit www.routledge.com/9781617119989 to access additional material.

Financial Disclosures

Dr. Jorge I. Acevedo is a consultant for and receives royalties from Arthrex.

Dr. Francesco Allegra has no financial or proprietary interest in the materials presented herein.

Dr. Annunziato Amendola has no financial or proprietary interest in the materials presented herein.

Dr. William Bugbee is a consultant for and has received research support from Joint Restoration Foundation, a not-for-profit tissue bank.

Dr. James D. F. Calder receives institutional funding from Arthrex, Smith & Nephew, and DGO Global.

Dr. Woojin Choi has no financial or proprietary interest in the materials presented herein.

Dr. Mark E. Easley has no financial or proprietary interest in the materials presented herein.

Dr. Richard D. Ferkel is a consultant for Smith & Nephew and Geistlich. He receives royalties from Lippincott Williams & Wilkins and institutional support from Smith & Nephew, DJO, and Depuy Mitek.

Dr. Ethan J. Fraser has no financial or proprietary interest in the materials presented herein.

Dr. Richard Freeman has no financial or proprietary interest in the materials presented herein.

Arianna L. Gianakos has no financial or proprietary interest in the materials presented herein.

Dr. Mark Glazebrook receives research/institutional support from and is a consultant for Smith & Nephew, Ferring Inc, and Cartiva Inc. He is also a consultant for Wright and Stryker. He is a journal reviewer for *F&A International*, *JBJS*, and *CORR*. Dr. Glazebrook is also a Board or Committee member for COFAS, COA, and AOFAS.

Dr. Alberto Gobbi is a scientific consultant for Anika USA.

Dr. Christopher E. Gross has no financial or proprietary interest in the materials presented herein.

Dr. Stephane Guillo has no financial or proprietary interest in the materials presented herein.

Dr. Beat Hintermann has no financial or proprietary interest in the materials presented herein.

Dr. Georgios Karnatzikos has no financial or proprietary interest in the materials presented herein.

Dr. John G. Kennedy is a consultant for Arteriocyte, Inc and receives research support from Ohnell Family Foundation, Mr. & Mrs. Michael J. Levitt, and Arteriocyte, Inc. He is also a board member of European Society of Sports Traumatology, Knee Surgery, and Arthroscopy (ESSKA); International Society for Cartilage Repair of the Ankle (ISCRA); American Orthopaedic Foot and Ankle Society (AOFAS) Awards and Scholarships Committee; and International Cartilage Repair Society (ICRS) finance board.

Dr. Dnyanesh Lad has no financial or proprietary interest in the materials presented herein.

Dr. Peter Mangone receives royalties and is a paid consultant for Arthrex, Inc. He is also a paid consultant for Amniox, Inc.

Dr. Alberto Marangon has no financial or proprietary interest in the materials presented herein.

Dr. Adam F. Meisel has no financial or proprietary interest in the materials presented herein.

Dr. Gokhan Meric has no financial or proprietary interest in the materials presented herein.

Dr. Xavier Martin Oliva is an AO fundation Member and AO faculty. He participates like faculty in some courses for Smith & Nephew and Arthrex.

Dr. Jason A. Patterson has no financial or proprietary interest in the materials presented herein.

Dr. Phinit Phisitkul has no financial or proprietary interest in the materials presented herein.

Dr. Steven M. Raikin receives research support from Zimmer (unrelated to current chapter).

Andrew W. Ross has no financial or proprietary interest in the materials presented herein.

Dr. Chamnanni Rungprai has no financial or proprietary interest in the materials presented herein.

Dr. James W. Stone is on the board of directors, for Arthroscopy Association of North America (AANA) and is a paid speaker for Smith & Nephew.

Dr. Masato Takao has no financial or proprietary interest in the materials presented herein.

Dr. C. Niek van Dijk is a consultant for Smith & Nephew.

Dr. Jin Woo Lee has no financial or proprietary interest in the materials presented herein.

Dr. Youichi Yasui has no financial or proprietary interest in the materials presented herein.

Dr. Alastair Younger receives personal fees from Acumed, Cartiva, and Wright Medical. He also receives grants from COA - Hip Hip Hooray, University of British Columbia, St. Paul's Hospital Foundation, American Orthopaedic Foot and Ankle Society, Canadian Orthopaedic Research Legacy Fund, Bioset, Orthopaedic Research Excellence Fund, Integra Life Sciences Corporation, Cartiva, Acumed, Smith & Nephew, Synthes, DePuy, Bioventus, Amniox Medical, and Zimmer. In addition, Dr. Younger has a patent for a fastening device for total ankle arthroplasty.

Dr. Ruben Zwiers has no financial or proprietary interest in the materials presented herein.

Index

For Product Safety Concerns and Information please contact our EU
representative GPSR@taylorandfrancis.com
Taylor & Francis Verlag GmbH, Kaufingerstraße 24, 80331 München, Germany

www.ingramcontent.com/pod-product-compliance
Ingram Content Group UK Ltd.
Pitfield, Milton Keynes, MK11 3LW, UK
UKHW052216190926
475702UK00006B/1039
* 9 7 8 1 6 1 7 1 1 9 9 8 9 *